AF667468

Management of Extended Parotid Tumors

Victor-Vlad Costan
Editor

Management of Extended Parotid Tumors

Springer

Editor
Victor-Vlad Costan
University of Medicine and Pharmacy
Iasi
Romania

ISBN 978-3-319-26543-8 ISBN 978-3-319-26545-2 (eBook)
DOI 10.1007/978-3-319-26545-2

Library of Congress Control Number: 2016931902

Springer Cham Heidelberg New York Dordrecht London
© Springer International Publishing Switzerland 2016
This work is subject to copyright. All rights are reserved by the Publisher, whether the whole or part of the material is concerned, specifically the rights of translation, reprinting, reuse of illustrations, recitation, broadcasting, reproduction on microfilms or in any other physical way, and transmission or information storage and retrieval, electronic adaptation, computer software, or by similar or dissimilar methodology now known or hereafter developed.
The use of general descriptive names, registered names, trademarks, service marks, etc. in this publication does not imply, even in the absence of a specific statement, that such names are exempt from the relevant protective laws and regulations and therefore free for general use.
The publisher, the authors and the editors are safe to assume that the advice and information in this book are believed to be true and accurate at the date of publication. Neither the publisher nor the authors or the editors give a warranty, express or implied, with respect to the material contained herein or for any errors or omissions that may have been made.

Printed on acid-free paper

Springer International Publishing AG Switzerland is part of Springer Science+Business Media (www.springer.com)

Preface

The surgery of the parotid gland is apparently simple, but in reality numerous pitfalls must be overcome in order to arrive to the desired results. When tumors invade the glandular tissue as well as the adjacent structures, achieving superior functional and aesthetic results becomes even more challenging. On the one hand this is due to the structures involved by the tumor and on the other hand to the existing comorbidities that usually favor the development of such extensive tumor invasion in the patients necessitating extended parotidectomy.

When the limits between the tumor, the parotid tissue, and the structures surrounding the gland become unclear, the entire management of the case becomes more complex, and this is why this book will cover issues regarding the diagnosis, treatment, and reconstructive options with the main purpose of assisting clinicians in the overall structuring and following of the case in multidisciplinary teams for best outcomes. The personal experience of the authors regarding extended parotid gland tumors is shared by images of clinical cases in order to enhance the understanding and facilitate decision making in these complicated cases.

This book aims to achieve an overview of the potential patterns of tumor evolution toward and from the glandular tissue and a review of the possibilities for reconstructing the postoperative tissue loss, by the use of various surgical techniques chosen to suit both the defect and the general condition of the patient, that significantly limits the reconstructive options in certain cases. General anesthesia and special postoperative care must be ensured and are dictated by the tumor invasion and the coexisting general disorders influencing the general state of the patient. Important details related to the practical aspects of the surgery of extended parotid gland tumors are outlined according to the experience of the authors in this regard.

Since extended parotidectomy is usually performed for malignancy, there was an evident need to address a few pages of this book to the radiotherapy and chemotherapy treatment with either curative or palliative purpose.

Iasi, Romania — Victor-Vlad Costan, MD, DMD, PhD

Contents

Contributors

Julio Acero, MD, DMD, PhD Department of Maxillofacial Surgery, Ramón y Cajal University Hospital, University of Alcala, Madrid, Spain

Otilia Boisteanu, MD, PhD Department of Anesthesiology, "Grigore T. Popa" University of Medicine and Pharmacy, Faculty of Dental Medicine, Iasi, Romania

Hartmut Peter Burmeister, MD, Priv.-Doz. Dr. med. habil. Institute of Diagnostic and Interventional Radiology, Neuroradiology, and Nuclear Medicine, Klinikum Bremerhaven Reinkenheide, Bremerhaven, Bremen, Germany

Constantin-Cătălin Ciocan-Pendefunda, MD, DMD, PhD Department of Oral and Maxillofacial Surgery, Fachklinik Hornheide Münster, Münster, Germany

Victor-Vlad Costan, MD, DMD, PhD Department of Oral and Maxillo-Facial Surgery, Faculty of Dental Medicine, "Grigore T. Popa" University of Medicine and Pharmacy, "St. Spiridon" University Hospital, Iasi, Romania

Marius Dabija, MD, PhD Department of Neurosurgery, Faculty of General Medicine, "Grigore T. Popa" University of Medicine and Pharmacy, Iasi, Romania

Mihai Danciu, MD, PhD Pathology Department, "Grigore T. Popa" University of Medicine and Pharmacy, Iasi, Romania

Cristian Ilie Drochioi, DMD, MD Department of Oral and Maxillofacial Surgery, "Sfântul Spiridon" Emergency Hospital, Iasi, Romania

Dan Ferariu, MD, PhD Department of Pathology, Regional Institute of Oncology, Iasi, Romania

Belen Guerra, MD, DMD Department of Oral and Maxillofacial Surgery, Quiron Madrid University Hospital, European University Madrid, Madrid, Spain

Department of Maxillofacial Surgery, Quiron Madrid University Hospital, Madrid, Spain

Orlando Guntinas-Lichius, MD Department of Otorhinolaryngology, University Hospital Jena, Jena, Germany

Dragos Iancu, MD, PhD Department of Radio-oncology, "Grigore T. Popa" University of Medicine and Pharmacy, Regional Institute of Oncology, Iasi, Romania

Bogdan F. Iliescu, MD, PhD Department of Neurosurgery, "Prof. Dr. Nicolae Oblu" Clinical Emergency Hospital, Iasi, Romania

Felix P. Koch, MD, DMD, MBA, PhD Department of Oral, Cranio-Maxillofacial and Facial Plastic Surgery, University Hospital Frankfurt, Frankfurt, Germany

Mihai V. Marinca, MD, PhD Medical Oncology, Faculty of Medicine, "Grigore T. Popa" University of Medicine and Pharmacy, Iasi Regional Institute of Oncology, Iasi, Romania

Christian N. Mihaila, MD Department of Radio-oncology, Hôpital du Valais, Sion, Valais, Switzerland

Lucian Miron, MD, PhD Medical Oncology, Faculty of Medicine, "Grigore T. Popa" University of Medicine and Pharmacy, Iasi Regional Institute of Oncology, Iasi, Romania

Ion Poeata, MD, PhD Department of Neurosurgery, "Grigore T. Popa" University of Medicine and Pharmacy, Iasi, Romania

Dragoş Cristian Popescu, MD, PhD Department of Morpho-Functional Sciences (Anatomy Discipline), Faculty of Medicine, "Grigore T. Popa" University of Medicine and Pharmacy, Iasi, Romania

Eugenia I. Popescu, DMD, PhD Department of Surgery (Dentoalveolar Surgery, Oral and Maxillofacial Surgery), Faculty of Dental Medicine, "Grigore T. Popa" University of Medicine and Pharmacy, Iasi, Romania

Robert A. Sader, MD, DDS, PhD Department of Oral, Cranio-Maxillofacial and Facial Plastic Surgery, University Hospital Frankfurt, Frankfurt, Germany

Tatiana V. Taranu, MD, PhD Department of Dermatology, "Grigore T. Popa" University of Medicine and Pharmacy, University Clinical Railways Hospital, Iasi, Romania

Mihaela Paula P. Toader, MD, PhD Department of Dermatology, "Grigore T. Popa" University of Medicine and Pharmacy, University Clinical Railways Hospital, Iasi, Romania

Daniela A. Trandafir, MD, PhD Department of Surgery (Dentoalveolar Surgery, Oral and Maxillofacial Surgery), Faculty of Dental Medicine, "Grigore T. Popa" University of Medicine and Pharmacy, Iasi, Romania

1 Anatomical Landmarks in the Surgery of Extended Parotid Gland Tumors

Dragoş Cristian Popescu

Abstract

The anatomy of the parotid region is complex and its content diverse and rich in important neurovascular structures both inside and around the parotid gland. Due to its location at the convergence point between the head and neck and irregular shape, the parotid gland will come in close contact with various adjacent structures that can become involved by malignant tumors developing here. The unique characteristics of the parotid gland are the presence of a very important functional structure, the facial nerve, crossing the gland, as well as the presence of lymph nodes inside the glandular tissue. The surgical anatomy of the parotid region is comprised of several layers, each one influencing the pattern of tumor spread, layers that will be traversed by the surgeon upon performing the tumor removal, and the same layers will have to be reconstructed at the end of the surgery in terms of volume but also function for best postoperative results.

1.1 Introduction

Detailed knowledge of the anatomy of the parotid gland and surrounding structures is imperative, especially in the surgery of extended tumors when local anatomy is distorted by the presence of the parotid mass obstructing direct vision of crucial structures by its volume, while also modifying the position of local tissues, including important nerves and vessels. Common anatomical landmarks used for orientation in the surgical field might be displaced or even infiltrated by the tumor and impossible to access. Familiarity with the anatomy of the region and ability to identify numerous anatomical landmarks will provide the surgeon with increased security and ability to modify the surgical access to suit the removal of tumors exhibiting very different patterns of spread in surrounding structures.

Extended parotidectomy usually results in complex defects involving several tissue layers

D.C. Popescu, MD, PhD
Department of Morpho-Functional Sciences (Anatomy Discipline), Faculty of Medicine, "Grigore T. Popa" University of Medicine and Pharmacy, Iasi, Romania
e-mail: dragospopescu1975@yahoo.com

© Springer International Publishing Switzerland 2016

V.-V. Costan (ed.), *Management of Extended Parotid Tumors*, DOI 10.1007/978-3-319-26545-2_1

that will require versatile reconstructive techniques for good aesthetical results. Attention to detail and understanding of the surface anatomy will help in choosing the best reconstructive method for each individual case.

1.2 Situation and Boundaries

The parotid region marks the transition area between the face, the neck, and the cranial vault. Superiorly, the parotid gland is bounded by the zygomatic arch, but also the temporomandibular joint and the external auditory meatus [1]. Recent imagistic studies have shown that the glandular tissue can sometimes extend above the zygoma and external auditory canal [2]. The inferior part of the gland overflows the posterior belly of the digastric muscle and comes in contact with the sternocleidomastoid muscle toward its insertion on the mastoid tip. The tail of the parotid gland can extend for variable distances on the anteromedial margin of the sternocleidomastoid muscle. Anteriorly, the superficial portion of the parotid gland runs across the ascending mandibular ramus and overlying masseter muscle, extending toward the anterior border of the masseter for variable distances [3]. An accessory parotid gland may be found sometimes anteriorly, in close association to the Stensen's duct, lying on the masseter muscle, but apart from the main parotid gland [4]. Medially, the deep portion of the parotid gland lies in the prestyloid compartment of the parapharyngeal space. The styloid process and its attached muscles separate the parotid gland from the neurovascular structures of the poststyloid compartment, mainly from the internal carotid artery and internal jugular vein [1]. Extensions from the deep part of the gland are often found toward the pharynx or the medial pterygoid muscle [5].

1.3 Anatomical Layers of the Parotid Region

To facilitate the understanding of tumor growth as well as the reverse pathway that will be performed during surgery for tumor removal, the anatomy of the parotid region can be described in layers from superficial to deep. Marking the contents of the layers and the relation between them provides the surgeon with a useful map to arrive to the correct dissection plane and find and protect key structures.

The concentric soft tissue layers clothe the bony surfaces and at the same time provide volume and contour to the area. This particular aspect will be important in the reconstruction of the postoperative defect.

The skeletal frame is created by the mandibular ascending ramus anteriorly, the temporomandibular joint and the external acoustic meatus posterosuperiorly, the styloid process situated medially, and the mastoid process posteriorly.

The masseter, the medial pterygoid, and the temporal muscles attached to these bony elements form a different frame of the region, delineating and supporting the soft tissue layers [5].

Covering the bony and muscle background are the soft tissue layers of the region. From superficial to deep, we encounter the skin, the subcutaneous layer, the SMAS, and the parotid fascia, followed by the parotid gland. Inside the gland, neurovascular structures can also be grouped in planes according to the depth and spatial relations between them [5]. In this aspect we initially find the nerve plane represented by the facial nerve and its branches coursing through the parotid gland. Underneath the nervous layer we usually encounter the venous plane – the retromandibular vein and its branches, and deep to the venous layer there is the arterial plane consisting of the external carotid artery. Deep to the parotid bed, we find the masseter muscle and periosteum of the ascending branch of the mandible in its anterior superficial part. Deep to the retromandibular part of the gland, there is the parapharyngeal space with its complex neurovascular anatomy. The proximity of the TMJ, external auditory canal, and skull base will also influence tumor spread and subsequent removal.

The characteristics of each layer will be detailed in the following subchapters.

1.4 Surface Anatomy, Skin, and Subcutaneous Tissue

The parotid region is a transition region between the cheek, the neck, the external ear, temporal region, and scalp, situated at the convergence point of the face, the neck, and the cranial vault. Therefore the skin of this area will vary in thickness, color, and texture at different levels of the region. In this particular area, the skin must be extremely mobile on the underlying tissues, to allow the mandibular movements. The extensibility of the skin in this region allows for easy elevation by tumors developing underneath. Another important thing to consider is that this is a hair-bearing area in the male patient (Fig. 1.1).

The subcutaneous tissue provides volume to the region and mobility of the overlying skin in relation to the deeper structures (Fig. 1.2). This particular characteristic is ensured by the fibrous retinacular cutis that provides a connection between the dermis and the underlying SMAS. Both elements vary in amount, proportion, and arrangement across the different areas of the face.

The volume of the region is provided by the underlying soft tissues supported by the bony framework. It is shaped in contours and depressions that should be observed and restored. The contour of the region is mainly provided by the mandibular angle, ramus, and the parotid gland. The contour and position of the tragus and the ear lobule should also be preserved during surgery as well as the small pretragal depression.

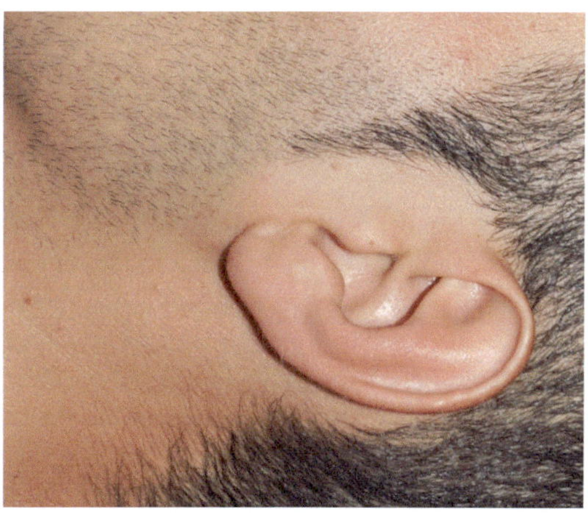

Fig. 1.1 In men the presence of hair at the level of the parotid region makes it difficult to place the incision lines so that the symmetry of the skin can be preserved. (Courtensy of Victor-Vlad Costan)

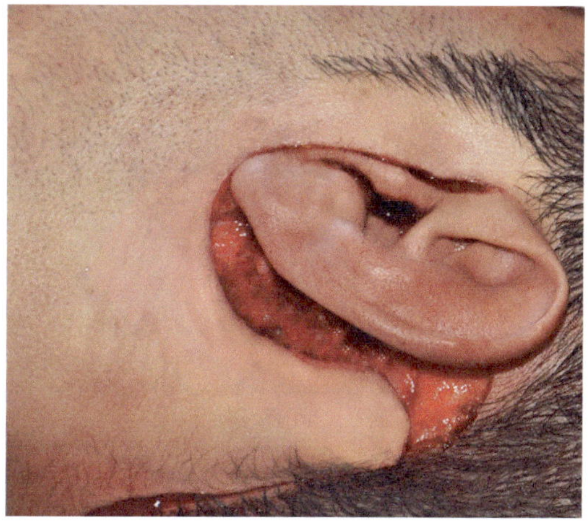

Fig. 1.2 The fibrous retinacular cutis allows the easy dissection of the skin from the SMAS and the sternocleidomastoid muscle. (Courtensy of Victor-Vlad Costan)

1.5 Enveloping Structures: The Parotid Fascia and SMAS

Following the skin and subcutaneous tissue, there is the superficial musculoaponeurotic system (SMAS), a fanlike structure continuous with the superficial temporal fascia above the zygomatic arch and with the platysma muscle inferiorly (Fig. 1.3). It is firmly attached to the periosteum of the zygomatic arch superiorly and to the cartilaginous external auditory canal and mastoid posteriorly. At its anterior limit, the SMAS inserts on the modiolus, zygomaticus major muscle, and depressor anguli oris muscle. By its fixed points provided by the zygomatic arch and external auditory meatus, and its insertions on the facial muscles, the SMAS provides a suspensory sheet that helps distribute the forces of facial expression.

The SMAS is thicker in the parotid region and becomes thinner while progressing anteriorly. It can be undermined as far as the nasolabial fold. Dissection on the deep surface is safe in the area of the parotid gland where the branches of the

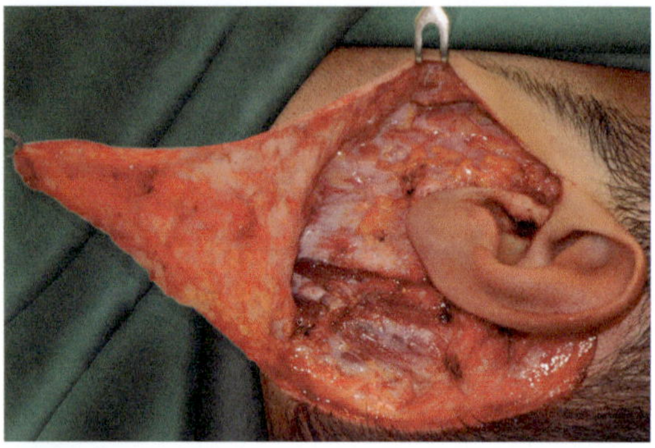

Fig. 1.3 After the dissection of the skin, the SMAS is revealed anteriorly and the sternocleidomastoid muscle posteriorly. (Courtensy of Victor-Vlad Costan)

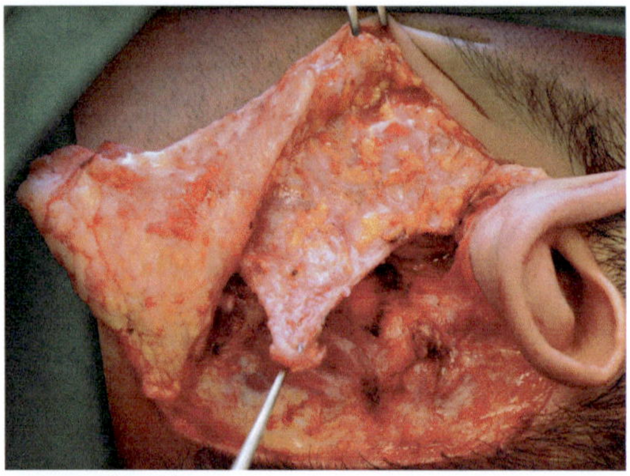

Fig. 1.4 The SMAS layer dissected from the parotid bed and mobilized. (Courtensy of Victor-Vlad Costan)

facial nerve are protected by the parotid tissue and fascia (Fig. 1.4).

The parotid gland fascia varies in thickness and fixation to surrounding structures. The presence of the fascia directs and partially contains tumor growth and extension to neighboring spaces, behaving as an anatomical barrier [6].

The lateral surface of the parotid gland is covered by a thick and inelastic fascia. Superiorly the fascia is attached firmly to the zygomatic arch and posteriorly to the sternocleidomastoid muscle [7]. This dense fascia of the lateral surface progressively thins out into loose areolar tissue toward the cheek to meet the fascia covering the masseter muscle [7]. The anterior limit of the parotid tissue in this area is difficult to define. Between the posterior aspect of the parotid gland and in front of the tragal and conchal cartilage, the fascia is quite thin and can be separated easily by digital pressure, developing a potential fascial space. Inside this easily divided space, the facial nerve can be found in the precartilaginous and pre-sternocleidomastoid plane, announced by the presence of the stylomastoid artery [8].

In the area of the mastoid process, the fascia becomes thicker and firmly attaches the gland to the mastoid. It then thins out over the surface of the sternocleidomastoid muscle. Toward the tail of the parotid gland, the fascia becomes thick again to form a membrane that separates the parotid gland from the posterior surface of the submandibular gland [6].

The medial extension of the parotid fascia is thin and sometimes incomplete making it difficult to define the borders of the parotid tissue [7]. The fascial layers adjacent to the styloid process form the stylomandibular membrane that expands to the posterior border of the ascending mandibular ramus. Toward the inferior part, the fascial elements converge to form the stylomandibular ligament, a crucial structure in the surgical exposure of deep lobe parotid tumors or other parapharyngeal space tumors [3, 6].

1.6 The Surgical Anatomy of the Parotid Gland/ Architecture of the Parotid Gland

The parotid gland fills the irregular space between the ascending mandibular ramus, external auditory canal, mastoid process, and sternocleidomastoid muscle (Fig. 1.5). It has been described as having a superficial lobe situated lateral to the nerve, a deep lobe medially to the nerve, and an isthmus between the two main divisions of the facial nerve, plastically compared to a “nerve sandwich” [9]. Due to the absence of clear anatomical delineation, it is now considered that the parotid gland is a unilobular structure subdivided by the presence of the facial nerve into a large superficial part and a smaller deep part, for the sole purpose of surgical simplicity [2] (Fig. 1.6). The anterior surface of the parotid gland is grooved by the ascending mandibular

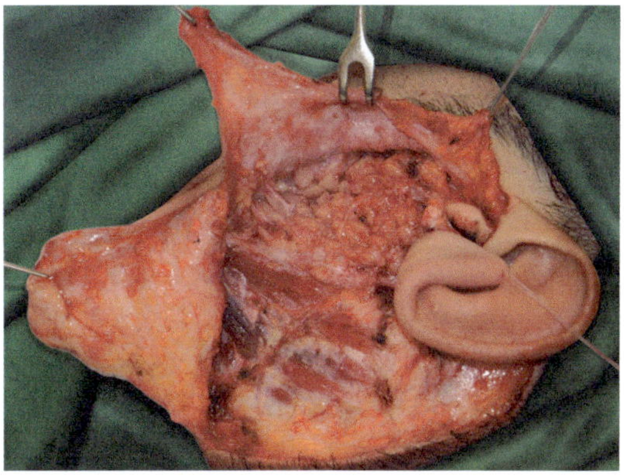

Fig. 1.5 Parotid tissue pertaining to the superficial lobe revealed under the SMAS. (Courtensy of Victor-Vlad Costan)

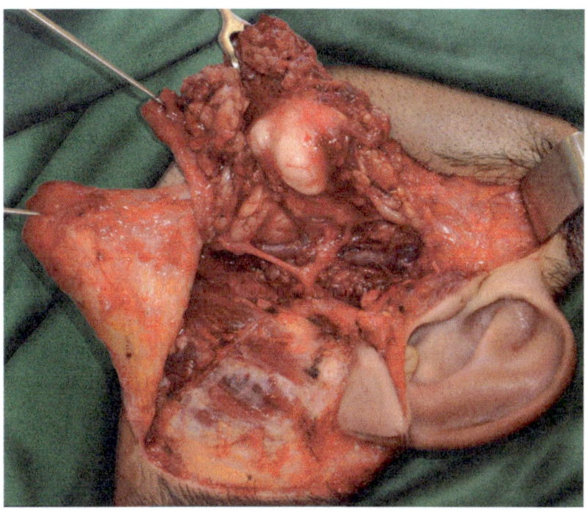

Fig. 1.6 The superficial parotid lobe containing a tumor mass is lifted off the facial nerve, revealing the main divisions of the nerve, the underlying retromandibular vein and the glandular tissue of the so-called deep parotid lobe. (Courtensy of Victor-Vlad Costan)

ramus, wrapping around it to follow the anterior aspect of the masseter muscle [7].

Although often described as having a roughly pyramidal shape with a superior base and inferior apex, this is just an approximation of the morphology of the main body of the parotid gland. The actual shape of the gland has been proven to be quite irregular, showing increased individual variations [2]. The parotid tissue extends to form multiple processes of variable shapes and sizes that fill the space between the different anatomical structures in the area. We can identify a mastoid process, a temporomandibular process, temporal process, inferior process, duct process, pterygomandibular process, and parapharyngeal process [10]. The number of processes and their size and volume will provide an irregular, complex shape of the parotid and increased difficulty in the removal of the entire glandular tissue during surgery. Their presence explains the unusual location of some parotid gland tumors and different patterns of tumor extension. The greatest surgical surgically, the greatest significance is attributed to the medial extensions of parotid tissue because of their deep location, in relation to important anatomical structures in the parapharyngeal space and difficult surgical access. Parotid gland tissue may extend for variable distances deep to the temporomandibular joint and lateral pterygoid muscle and on the pharyngeal wall.

Cadaveric dissections have demonstrated the presence of an accessory parotid gland, lying on the masseter muscle, in close relation to the Stensen's duct, but completely separated from the main parotid gland in 21–61 % of individuals [4].

The parotid duct emerges from the anterior extension of the parotid gland, running along the anterior surface of the masseter, and then turns medially at the anterior border of the muscle, pierces the buccinators, and opens into the oral cavity on the buccal mucosa close to the second upper molar. The length of the duct is approximately 5 cm. It travels along an imaginary line from the tragus to the middle of the upper lip, parallel to the zygoma, approximately 1 cm below it [3]. The buccal branch of the facial nerve runs with the Stensen's duct.

1.7 Nervous Structures

1.7.1 The Facial Nerve

The nervous structure most famously associated with the parotid gland is the facial nerve, whose branches are protected inside the parotid tissue for a variable distance in order to finally arrive to the facial muscles. The course of the facial nerve in its relation with the parotid tissue can be divided into retroglandular, intraglandular, and preglandular segments.

The initial extraparotid portion of the seventh nerve is approximately 1.3 cm long, allowing extension due to mandibular or glandular protraction [8]. It exits the skull base through the stylomastoid foramen. Initially it gives off motor branches to the auricular muscles, stylohyoid muscle, posterior belly of the digastric muscle, and the occipital end of the occipitofrontal muscle [8]. It also provides sensory (vagal) fibers to parts of the external auditory canal and external ear, including the ear lobule [11].

The stylomastoid artery, a branch of the posterior auricular artery or occipital artery, usually announces the proximity of the facial nerve, found just a few millimeters inferior and medially to the artery [12]. A cartilaginous landmark is represented by the external auditory meatus that forms a "pointer" indicating the direction of the nerve trunk, approximately 1.0–1.5 cm deep and slightly anterior and inferior to its inferior border [13]. The single most constant landmark is the stylomastoid foramen that can be traced following adjacent anatomical structures. The posterior belly of the digastric muscle can be followed to its insertion on the mastoid process situated immediately below the stylomastoid foramen. The facial nerve can be found approximately 1 cm deep to this medial attachment of the muscle [13]. A more reliable bony landmark is represented by the tympanomastoid suture line. The nerve trunk can be encountered 6–8 mm deep to it [13], forming the bisector of the angle between the mastoid and the osseous auditory canal [8]. It lies on the posterolateral aspect of the styloid process near its base, traveling obliquely across it. In the case of large tumors obstructing view or local recurrences, the facial nerve trunk can also be identified by performing a mastoidectomy and then following its course toward the exit [13].

After leaving the foramen, the trunk of the nerve turns to become more superficial as it enters the substance of the parotid gland where it divides into a superior temporofacial division and an inferior cervicofacial division (Fig. 1.7). The splitting point is plastically called pes anserinus, the Latin name for a goose's foot. The temporofacial division is usually larger and can be easily identified and traced during surgery. Inside the parotid tissue the facial nerve branches are commonly situated above the vascular plane represented by the posterior facial vein and external carotid artery. The further branching pattern of the facial nerve into temporal, zygomatic, buccal, marginal mandibular, and cervical branches is highly variable, with the first three usually arising from the superior division and the last two from the inferior one [11]. The buccal branch can arise from either one of the main two divisions, but it can also arise separately from the main trunk of the nerve as a third division [8].

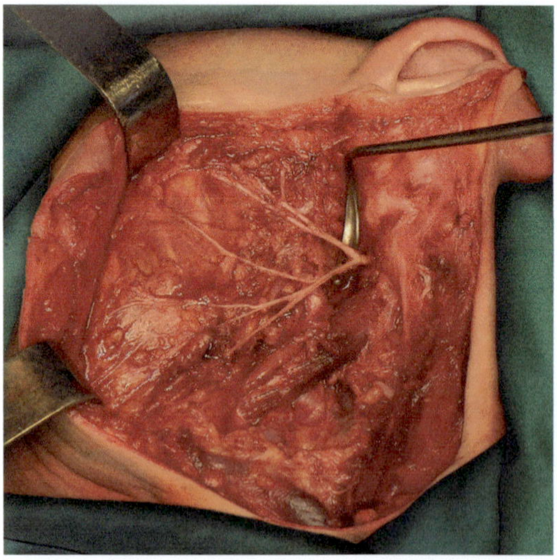

Fig. 1.7 The branches of the facial nerve emerge from the main trunk as soon as it enters the parotid gland. These branches that form anastomoses between each other form a network that separates the deep lobe from the superficial lobe. (Courtensy of Victor-Vlad Costan)

The five terminal branches spread resembling the fingers of a hand, and they become thinner and more superficial in their anterior course, developing multiple anastomoses [8]. They eventually leave the gland traveling superficially to reach the mimetic muscles where they form a veritable nervous plexus. After exiting the parotid tissue at the anterior border of the gland, the facial branches are most prone to injury during surgery.

The cervical branch supplies the platysma muscle and is of little surgical importance since its division does not lead to important functional disturbances. The marginal mandibular branch can be identified traveling along the inferior border of the parotid gland, in a plane beneath the platysma muscle and superior to the retromandibular vein and facial vein, to eventually reach the lower lip and chin muscles [3]. The buccal branch runs parallel with the parotid duct, either superior or inferior to it to supply the upper lip, the nostril muscles, and the buccinator muscle [3, 14]. The zygomatic branches reach the zygomatic, orbital, and infraorbital muscles traveling over the periosteum of the zygomatic arch. They can be found 2.5 cm anterior to the tragus on a line between the intertragic notch and the external canthus [15] and should be protected during surgery because of their important functional role. The temporal branch can be identified traveling parallel to the superficial temporal vessels across the zygoma toward the frontal belly of the occipitofrontalis muscle, the anterior and superior auricular muscles, the orbicularis oculi, and corrugator supercilii [3]. It can be found in the area of Pitanguy's line, defined by an imaginary line from a point 0.5 cm inferior to the tragus to a point 1.5 cm superior and lateral to the eyebrow [14].

1.7.2 The Great Auricular Nerve

It travels parallel to the external jugular vein on the lateral aspect of the sternocleidomastoid muscle, toward the tail of the parotid gland. At this point it splits to form its two branches. The anterior one provides sensory innervation to the skin overlying the parotid area, while the posterior branch supplies the inferior portion of the ear, the posterior surface of the ear, and lobule [3, 6] (Fig. 1.8).

1.7.3 The Auriculotemporal Nerve

The auriculotemporal nerve departs from the mandibular division of the trigeminal nerve, passing posteriorly around the neck of the mandibular condyle, close to the deep portion of the parotid gland, and then travels parallel to the superficial temporal vessels to eventually supply the skin of the anterior upper ear, the external acoustic meatus, the temporomandibular joint, and the temporal region to the top of the scalp [6]. It also carries the parasympathetic secretory fibers from the otic ganglion to the parotid gland, fibers involved in the development of Frey syndrome [6].

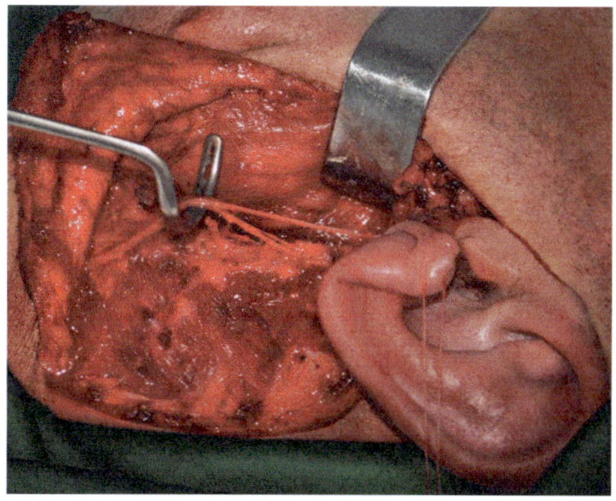

Fig. 1.8 The great auricular nerve is practically intercepted every time during dissection for parotidectomy. (Courtensy of Victor-Vlad Costan)

1.8 Surrounding Muscles

The muscles in the parotid area contribute to the volume of the region, filling the space delineated by the skeletal frame. At the posterior and inferior part of the gland, there is the sternocleidomastoid muscle, while the parotid bed in the anterior part is formed by the masseter muscle. On the medial side, the multiple extensions of the gland come in close contact with the medial pterygoid muscle, the posterior belly of the digastric muscle, the stylohyoid, and the parapharyngeal muscles. The parotid tissue insinuates between the muscular structures, while the muscles create grooves on the surface of the gland, contouring its shape. The pressure provided by the muscular contractions might contribute to the physiologic emptying of the gland [6]. They also form partial anatomical barriers opposing and directing the extension of tumors developing in the parotid area.

1.9 Neighboring Bony Structures and Cartilages

Bony structures in the regions surrounding the parotid gland define the frame of this complex space and are mainly represented by the components of

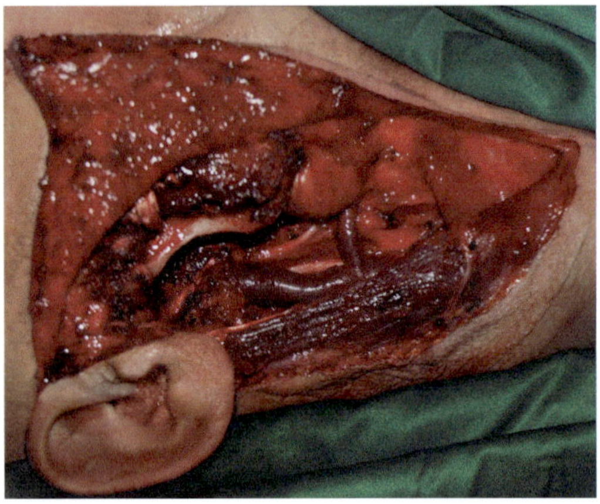

Fig. 1.9 After the removal of the parotid gland, of the masseter muscle partially, of the posterior belly of the digastric muscle, but also the removal of the superior cervical lymph nodes, the mandibular ascending ramus is revealed as well as the proximity of the great vessels. (Courtensy of Victor-Vlad Costan)

the temporal bone, the mandibular ascending ramus, zygomatic arch, and pterygoid plates (Fig. 1.9).

The parotid gland is grooved and shaped by the various adjacent bony structures. The bones in this region represent fixed landmarks that are reliable for orientation during surgery. Palpating the styloid process alerts the surgeon to the close proximity of the internal carotid artery and internal jugular vein situated medially to it. The mastoid process, the tympanomastoid suture, and styloid process are useful landmarks in the identification of the facial nerve. The deep extension of the tragal cartilage, named the tragal pointer, is one of the most commonly used landmarks in the identification of the main facial nerve trunk. The external auditory canal communicates directly with the parotid gland through certain specific sites that facilitate tumor spread from one compartment to the other, the fissures of Santorini and the foramen of Huschke. Two horizontal fissures have been demonstrated in the cartilaginous external ear canal, named the fissures of Santorini. Their purpose is to allow more flexibility of the canal, but they also provide a gateway for tumor passage in case of a developing malignancy. Another direct communication is achieved through a gap of the anteroinferior portion of the canal, termed the foramen of Huschke [6].

1.10 Important Vascular Structures

The main vascular structures associated with the parotid region are the external carotid artery and the retromandibular vein, running through the substance of the parotid gland under the facial nerve branches.

The parotid gland itself is not highly vascularized, and dissection of the parotid tissue can be achieved with only minor bleeding if it is carefully performed above a fasciovenous plane described by Patey, lying just deep to the facial nerve branches [7].

The external carotid artery, traveling deep to the posterior belly of the digastric muscle, enters the parotid space giving rise to the posterior auricular artery. This vessel provides the origin for the stylomastoid artery that lies superficially and in close proximity to the main trunk of the seventh nerve. The external carotid artery enters the parotid tissue on the medial side of the gland, and within the gland, it will rest in a plane deep to the facial nerve and retromandibular vein. Reaching the neck of the mandibular condyle, it gives its terminal branches, the internal maxillary artery and superficial temporal artery. The transverse facial artery originates in the proximal part of the superficial temporal artery and travels just superior to the parotid duct. The internal maxillary artery turns medially around the mandibular condyle to enter the infratemporal fossa [5].

Venous drainage generally parallels the arterial supply. The superficial temporal vein and maxillary vein unite to form the retromandibular vein, also named the posterior facial vein. It travels inside the parotid tissue under the nervous plane and above the arterial layer, ending at the tail of the gland by giving off anterior and posterior branches (Fig. 1.10).

The posterior branch and the posterior auricular artery form the external jugular vein, while the anterior branch unites with the anterior facial vein, forming the common facial vein that eventually empties in the internal jugular vein.

The internal carotid artery and internal jugular vein lie in the poststyloid compartment

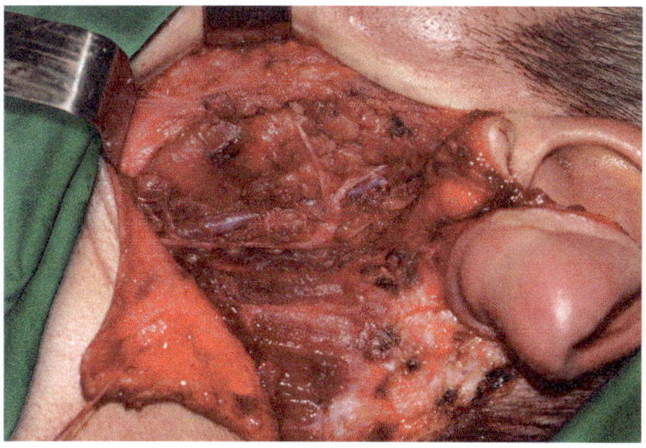

Fig. 1.10 Generally, the facial nerve crosses the retromandibular vein found underneath. (Courtensy of Victor-Vlad Costan)

of the parapharyngeal space, protected by the styloid process and attached muscles and ligaments.

1.11 The Parapharyngeal Space

The prestyloid compartment is located anterior to a line from the styloid process to the medial portion of the medial pterygoid plate, and it contains the deep lobe of the parotid gland, minor salivary glands, the internal maxillary artery, the ascending pharyngeal artery, the inferior alveolar nerve, the lingual nerve, and the auriculotemporal nerve. The poststyloid compartment lies posterior to the line described, and it contains vital structures like the internal jugular vein, internal carotid artery and vagus nerve, glossopharyngeal nerve, accessory nerve, hypoglossal nerve, and the cervical sympathetic chain [3]. Maybe the most important fact to remember during surgery in this area is to not confuse the external carotid artery situated in the prestyloid compartment with the internal carotid artery located deeper in the poststyloid compartment. The internal and external carotid arteries are separated by the styloid process, the stylohyoid ligament, the stylopharyngeus muscle, and glossopharyngeal nerve. To help in the differentiation, it is important to always search for emerging branches from the artery since it is a known fact that the internal carotid artery does not have any branches in the neck [5].

1.12 Lymph Nodes

The lymphatic system is organized in rich networks of vessels and approximately 20–30 lymph nodes located inside and around the parotid tissue [13]. The lymph nodes in the parotid region are uniquely organized in groups located inside the gland and adjacent to it, in a superior, inferior, or posterior position, but not anterior to the gland [7]. According to the depth of the lymph nodes, they are divided in superficial suprafascial nodes, subfascial nodes, and deep intraglandular nodes. The majority of the parotid nodes (90 %) are located between the glandular tissue and the capsule of the gland [3].

The superficial, suprafascial preauricular group is found in front of the tragus or above it, along the course of the superficial temporal vessels under the skin, within the subcutaneous tissue of the area. Next are the subfascial lymph nodes situated outside the parotid tissue and divided in two groups, a superior one, located in front of the ear, and an inferior one under the ear, in close proximity to the external jugular vein. The superficial nodes and the superior subfascial group drain the lymph from the frontal region, the root of the nose, the upper eyelid and the external half of the lower eyelid, the external ear and external auditory canal, upper lip, cheek, and Eustachian tube.

The inferior subfascial group collects the lymphatic fluid from the parotid gland, the nose, the upper eyelid, the mucosa of the cheek, and gingival mucosa corresponding to the molars and retromolar triangle [16]. In rare cases, the inferior paraglandular nodes together with a perimeter of parotid tissue can be included in the process of a neck dissection if there is extensive metastasis of the high region of the neck to ensure free margins, but if involvement of the parotid nodes is suspected, a parotidectomy should be performed [6].

The deep intraglandular nodes are usually located lateral to the facial nerve and external jugular vein. They drain the lymph from the parotid gland, the skin in the frontal and parietal areas, lacrimal gland, middle ear, posterior nasopharynx, and soft palate [3, 16]. A few lymph nodes can also be found in the deep lobe of the gland, medial to the facial nerve. This is an important fact considering the surgical treatment that aims the removal of all the lymph nodes possibly involved by metastasis [17].

The paraparotid and intraparotid nodes are interconnected [6]. They drain mainly into the superficial and deep cervical lymph systems. The lymph fluid from the superficial and deep parotid nodes is transported to the superior part of the internal jugular lymph group. They are closely related to the accessory nodes, explaining the frequent nodal metastasis from parotid tumors to this area. Additionally, the posterior part of the gland is sometimes drained in the accessory chain. In rare cases, a lymph collector starting from the anterior inferior part of the parotid gland, following the masseter muscle, transports the lymph fluid to the submandibular chain [18].

References

1. Ellis H. Clinical anatomy. A revision and applied anatomy for clinical students. London: Blackwell Publishing; 2006.
2. Medbery R, Yousem DM, Needham MF, Kligerman MM. Variation in parotid gland size, configuration, and anatomic relations. Radiother Oncol. 2000;54(1):87–9.
3. Myers EN, Ferris RL. Salivary gland disorders. Berlin: Springer; 2007.
4. Ramachar SM, Huliyappa HA. Accessory parotid gland tumors. Ann Maxillofac Surg. 2012;2:90–3. PMCID: PMC3591091.
5. Fischer JE, Bland KI, Callery MP. Mastery of surgery, vol. 1. Philadelphia: Lippincott Williams & Wilkins; 2006.
6. Conley J. Salivary glands and the facial nerve. Stuttgart: George Thieme Publishers; 1975. p. 313–25.
7. Attie JN, Sciubba JJ. Tumors of major and minor salivary glands: clinical and pathologic features. Chicago: Year Book Medical Publisher; 1981.
8. Gola R, Chossegros C, Carreau P. Anatomie chirurgicale de la région parotidienne. Rev Stomatol Chir Maxillofac. 1994;95(6):395–410.
9. Hamilton B. Surgical anatomy of the parotid gland. Br Med J. 1948;2(4569):245–8. PMCID: PMC2091022.
10. Xu Yongzhao, Li Nan. The anatomic study of the morphology of parotid gland and its duct in Chinese. J Cap Med Univ. 1994;15(3):165–71.
11. Rodrigues DCA, Andreo JC, Menezes DFL, Chinellato PT, Rosa-Júnior GM. Anatomy of the facial nerve and its implication in the surgical procedures. Int J Morphol. 2009;27(1):183–6.
12. Upile T, Jerjes W, Nouraei SA, Singh SU, Kafas P, Sandison A, Sudhoff H, Hopper C. The stylomastoid artery as an anatomical landmark to the facial nerve during parotid surgery: a clinicoanatomic study. World J Surg Oncol. 2009;7:71. doi:10.1186/1477-7819-7-71.
13. Cernea CR, Dias FL, Fliss D, Lima RA, Myers EN, Wei WI, editors. Pearls and pitfalls in head and neck surgery. Basel: Karger; 2008. p. 106–7.
14. Davies JC, Agur AMR, Fattah AY. Anatomic landmarks for localization of the branches of the facial nerve. OA Anat. 2013;1(4):33.
15. Chatellier A, Labbé D, Salamé E, Bénateau H. Skin reference point for the zygomatic branch of the facial nerve innervating the orbicularis oculi muscle (anatomical study). Surg Radiol Anat. 2013;35(3):259–62.
16. Ricbourg B. Système lymphatique de la tête et du cou. Encyclopédie Médico-Chirurgicale, 22-001-B-40.
17. Pisani P, Ramponi A, Pia F. The deep parotid lymph nodes: an anatomical and oncological study. J Laryngol Otol. 1996;110(2):148–50.
18. Werner JA, Davis RK. Metastases in head and neck cancer. New York: Springer Science & Business Media; 2004.

Part I

Characterization of Extended Parotid Tumors

2 Extended Parotid Tumors with Origin in the Parotid Tissue

Eugenia I. Popescu and Victor-Vlad Costan

Abstract

Primary tumors of the parotid gland arise either in the superficial lobe, deep lobe, isthmus, accessory lobe, or Stensen's duct, which will result in different behaviors concerning local spread and different clinical presentations. The various topographic and histologic possibilities, especially in the presence of extended tumors, will lead to a difficult differential diagnosis. Primary tumors must be differentiated from involvement of the parotid gland by direct invasion from tumors in neighboring areas and from metastatic disease to the parotid gland. Clinical suspicion is extremely important in order to properly address unusual individual cases and avoid the trap of approaching all parotid masses in the same manner that could eventually lead to either unnecessary or incomplete treatment. The suspicion is raised first by clinical examination and will be strengthened by further imaging studies, and eventually the final diagnosis will be confirmed by pathology. A great variety of histological types have been described in primary as well as secondary tumors to this area. Although statistical data suggests a great prevalence of certain malignant parotid tumors over others, the surgeon must not underestimate the possibility of rare tumors arising in this area that may require a different therapeutic approach. It is a challenge for the surgeon to manage certain complex tumors encountered in the parotid area. The aim of establishing the origin of the extended parotid gland tumor is to tailor the treatment according to the known behavior of tumors originating in the parotid tissue and to avoid the danger of under- or overtreatment.

E.I. Popescu, DMD, PhD
Department of Surgery (Dentoalveolar Surgery, Oral and Maxillofacial Surgery), Faculty of Dental Medicine, "Grigore T. Popa" University of Medicine and Pharmacy, Iasi, Romania

V.-V. Costan, MD, DMD, PhD (✉)
Department of Oral and Maxillo-Facial Surgery, Faculty of Dental Medicine, "Grigore T. Popa" University of Medicine and Pharmacy, "St. Spiridon" University Hospital Iasi, Iasi, Romania
e-mail: victorcostan@gmail.com

© Springer International Publishing Switzerland 2016

V.-V. Costan (ed.), *Management of Extended Parotid Tumors*, DOI 10.1007/978-3-319-26545-2_2

2.1 Introduction

In the presence of an advanced parotid tumor extended to neighboring structures, determining the origin of the malignancy can prove to be quite challenging, and it can imply true detective work. Therefore, a good understanding of the anatomy and tumor behavior is needed, together with a thorough history of the patient, careful clinical examination, and adequate imaging. Summing up the different clues provided by each step of the investigation will help distinguish intrinsic from extrinsic lesions with positive outcomes on the overall management of the case.

2.2 Epidemiology

Salivary gland malignancies account for approximately 12 % of oral and pharyngeal cancers, 3–6 % of head and neck cancers, and 0.3 % of all malignancies. Studies have shown some geographic variation in the frequency of tumor types, possibly related to higher ultraviolet radiation in certain areas. Seventy-five percent of salivary gland malignancies occur in the parotid gland. On average, only 20 % of tumors originating in the parotid gland are malignant [1]. Approximately 90 % of parotid gland tumors arise in the superficial lobe, while the other 10 % represent tumors of the deep lobe.

The accessory parotid gland is present in 21 % of individuals. Tumors arising here account for 1–7.7 % of parotid gland tumors, and they are associated with a higher rate of malignant tumors than the main parotid gland – one-quarter to half of the tumors originating here are primary malignant [2–4].

Incidence of malignancy has been proved to be slightly higher in men, and two-thirds of the tumors are generally diagnosed in patients over 55 years old [1].

2.3 Diagnosis

The clinical and imaging diagnoses of extended parotid gland tumors are detailed in Chaps. 10 and 11.

The diagnosis of an extended parotid gland tumor with origin in the parotid tissue is made after ruling out contiguous spread to the parotid from adjacent structures and metastatic disease by lymphatic or hematogenous dissemination.

Careful history and clinical examination of the entire head and neck area, including an intraoral exam of the lateral pharyngeal wall in particular, summed with adequate imaging, will guide the surgeon toward a probability preoperative diagnosis. FNAC can sometimes help the diagnosis in uncertain cases but it is not always reliable. Biopsy is possible in tumors ulcerated to the skin. The final diagnosis will be provided by histology, but in certain cases, tumor origin is still difficult to establish due to the wide variety of malignant tumors that can involve the parotid gland as well as other structures, leading to an extremely challenging differential diagnosis.

2.3.1 Extended Parotid Gland Tumors Arising in the Superficial Lobe

Tumors arising in the superficial lobe are more easily detectable, since they cause deforming of the region and facial asymmetry. The tumor growth is more noticeable and patients may present in earlier stages. Malignant tumors tend to involve the branches of the facial nerve and then extend to the deep portion of the gland, progressively even to the masseter muscle and mandibular bone and become fixated to the deep structures. The dense parotid fascia on the lateral side initially contains the tumor spread, providing a safe surgical resection above it. Eventually, in more advanced stages, the tumor will erode through the parotid fascia, SMAS layer, and overlying skin, becoming fixated to the superficial structures, and might even erode through the skin to form an ulcerated tumor and increase difficulty in establishing the starting point of the tumor (Fig. 2.1a, b). The main differential diagnosis is of a skin malignancy invading the parotid gland.

But in the case of an ulcerated skin tumor continuous with underlying structures, including the

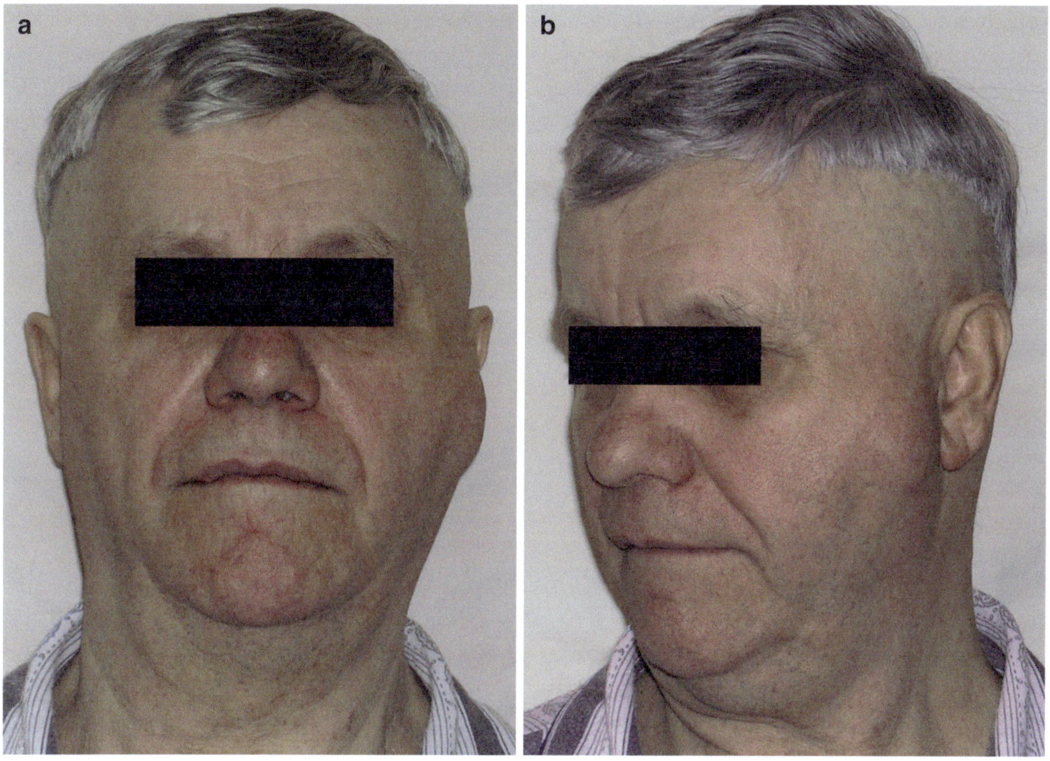

Fig. 2.1 (**a**, **b**) Adenoid cystic carcinoma of the left parotid gland extended to the skin. The clinical exam shows signs of invasion of the superior branch of the facial nerve

parotid gland, performing a biopsy is relatively easy and safe and will help determine the histology and, of course, the treatment plan.

2.3.2 Extended Parotid Gland Tumors Arising in the "Tail" of the Gland

The inferior portion of the parotid gland, the "tail" of the gland, is not well defined and can extend for variable distances in the cervical region, in front of the sternocleidomastoid muscle and toward the mastoid. Tumors arising in this part of the gland can lead to confusions in diagnosis, presenting like cervical masses, and they can extend to involve the skin, the marginal mandibular branch of the facial nerve, mandibular basilar border, the sternocleidomastoid muscle, and even vascular and nervous structures found deep to the muscle. In the presence of a cervical mass located in the upper third or even upper two-thirds of the SCM, a tumor of the tail of the parotid gland must be suspected and approached accordingly, since they can perfectly mimic metastatic cervical lymph nodes that are more frequently encountered in this region.

Toward the inferior part, the parotid fascia becomes thicker to form the stylomandibular ligament, which separates the parotid gland from the submandibular gland, and also represents a barrier in the pathway of a tumor developing in proximity, delaying spread toward the submandibular space [5].

2.3.3 Extended Parotid Gland Tumors Arising in the Accessory Parotid Gland

Even more difficult to diagnose are tumors arising from the accessory lobe of the parotid gland, usually found on the central one-third of the line running from the middle of the tragus to a point between the ala of the nose and vermillion border of the upper lip, along the line of the Stensen's duct. Awareness of their possible occurrence together with good knowledge and understanding of the regional anatomy will raise the surgeon's suspicion in the presence of a midcheek mass that can also sometimes protrude intraorally [3, 4]. Adjacent soft tissue invasion is common due to absence of anatomical barriers to tumor extension [4]. The contents of the buccal space, the overlying skin or mucosa, the zygomatic branches of the facial nerve, and the masseter muscle are all prone to tumor invasion. The buccal fat pad in particular, once penetrated by malignant tissue, is an area where the tumor can slide freely to surrounding spaces, through the extensions of the fat pad. The presence of pain, facial nerve paralysis, and Stensen's duct obstruction and fixation to overlying skin are signs of malignancy [6]. Parotid gland origin of a midcheek mass is not a common finding, but the key to diagnosing it is being aware of its possible occurrence.

2.3.4 Extended Parotid Gland Tumors Arising in the Stensen's Duct

Malignant primary tumors of the Stensen's duct are extremely rare and often misdiagnosed in early stages, although symptomatic, due to frequent presentation as recurrent parotitis associating less obvious midcheek masses, often masked by inflammatory signs that can be missed on presentation if the clinical examination is superficial. In the presence of obstructive parotitis without salivary calculus and associating a palpable mass, a Stensen's duct tumor should be included in the differential diagnosis [7]. Invasion of adjacent structures is a common finding upon late presentation. In such cases it is a challenge to establish the exact origin of the tumor. When the oral mucosa around the opening of the duct is infiltrated, it can be argued whether the tumor was primary in the duct or it is growing into the duct from the surrounding mucosa. Imaging techniques, such as MR sialography and sialendoscopy, can be very helpful in determining the intraluminal and adjacent tumor growth. The final diagnosis of true Stensen's duct carcinoma will eventually be decided on the basis of clinical presentation, specific radiological findings, and histology.

2.3.5 Extended Parotid Gland Tumors Arising in the Deep Lobe of the Parotid Gland

The deep part of the parotid fascia is thin and often incomplete, making it difficult to define the extension and borders of the medial part of the gland and providing a gateway toward tumor spread [8]. The parapharyngeal space contains the deep lobe of the parotid gland and provides a vertical highway for the extension of malignant processes developing here [9]. Considering the rich neurovascular contents of this space, it is natural to assume a complex differential diagnosis of tumors arising in this area. The poststyloid compartment shelters the great vessels and the important neural structures and must be protected during tumor removal. Invasion of the internal carotid artery or the internal jugular vein close to the base of skull is often an indicator of nonresectability.

Due to the presence of fascial planes directing tumor growth [10], deep lobe tumors growing through the stylomandibular tunnel present as dumbbell shaped due to constriction in between the mandible and the stylomandibular ligament [8].

Tumors extending parapharyngeally can produce the medial displacement of the tonsils and palatal arches. They can displace the superficial parotid lobe laterally with or without invasion, further infiltrating the masticatory space and mandibular ramus. Trismus due to invasion of the medial pterygoid muscle is highly suggestive in this aspect. Compression and involvement of the muscles of the Eustachian tube will cause a feeling of pressure and fullness in the ear. Advanced tumors can also invade the external auditory canal, the skin of the outer ear, temporal bone, zygomatic arch, and temporomandibular joint, leading to difficulty in the diagnosis of the initial tumor location. Extension by directly transgressing fascial planes will lead to advanced tumors filling the infratemporal fossa and then entering the orbit through the inferior orbital fissure, the middle cranial fossa through the foramen ovale and spinosum, and the pterygopalatine fossa through the pterygomaxillary fissure [11]. The presence of an advanced parapharyngeal mass will cause important dysphagia, inanition, obstructive respiratory distress, and possible bleeding that will lead to death [10].

The hidden location of these tumors may lead to late presentation and difficult diagnosis. Extended deep lobe parotid tumors must be differentiated from other tumors arising in the parapharyngeal space and from tumors of the tonsil or other oropharyngeal cancers that can extend to involve the parotid through the parapharyngeal space and present with similar clinical signs.

2.3.6 Extension to Specific Areas and Consecutive Differential Diagnosis Issues

Extension of parotid gland malignancies to the *external auditory canal* is mainly achieved through specific gateways where the two structures communicate directly, the fissures of Santorini and the foramen of Huschke [8, 10]. In the cartilaginous portion of the external canal, two horizontal fissures have been described, termed the fissures of Santorini, which are meant to render more flexibility to the canal, but they also provide a gateway for tumor passage in either direction between the two neighboring structures, the parotid gland and external auditory canal. Failure to complete ossification in the anteroinferior canal in the first 3 or 4 years of life will result in a bony gap, termed the foramen of Huschke, another direct communication site between the EAC and the parotid gland. Clinical signs of EAC invasion may mimic chronic otitis media, presenting with hearing loss, purulence, pain, or presence of a canal mass. This could lead to delayed diagnosis if proper clinical exam and imaging are not performed.

Primary parotid tumors that extend to the *temporal bone* will cause clinical signs like bleeding from the ear, purulent drainage, hearing loss, facial nerve weakness, or paralysis. They can also be confused with inflammatory conditions. Malignant parotid tumors invading the temporal bone must also be differentiated from primary temporal bone tumors invading the parotid gland, tumors arising in the EAC, middle ear, or the skin of the outer ear with consecutive temporal bone and parotid gland involvement. History, imaging, and histology might help the diagnosis, but sometimes it can be very challenging if not impossible to demonstrate the exact starting point. Another significant issue to address is the matter of perineural invasion. There are sometimes cases when concomitant temporal bone and parotid tissue tumors are discovered, and it is extremely challenging to assess tumor origin. This presentation is possible by perineural spread via the facial nerve, through a retrograde fashion, a trait exhibited mainly by certain histological types of malignancy. Preoperative fine-needle biopsy evaluation is imperative for the determination of the type of malignancy and treatment planning. When biopsy shows the presence of an adenoid cystic carcinoma, salivary duct carcinoma, or squamous cell carcinoma in a tumor involving the temporal bone, intracranial extension through the facial nerve must be suspected and investigated appropriately [6]. Another perineural pathway of invasion that has been described is via the auriculotemporal branch of the trigeminal nerve. Tumors follow the nerve course around the posterior border of the mandibular ascending ramus, through the masticator space, and upward, toward foramen ovale and the skull base [6].

Facial nerve status must be properly assessed preoperatively, especially in extended parotid gland tumors. Facial nerve palsy on presentation is a sign of malignancy, but in the absence of clinical signs, facial nerve invasion should be carefully assessed during surgery, since the absence of functional impairment does not rule out malignant involvement, and, although imaging can provide important information concerning relation between the tumor and nerve, it cannot visualize nerve structure and cannot rule out invasion

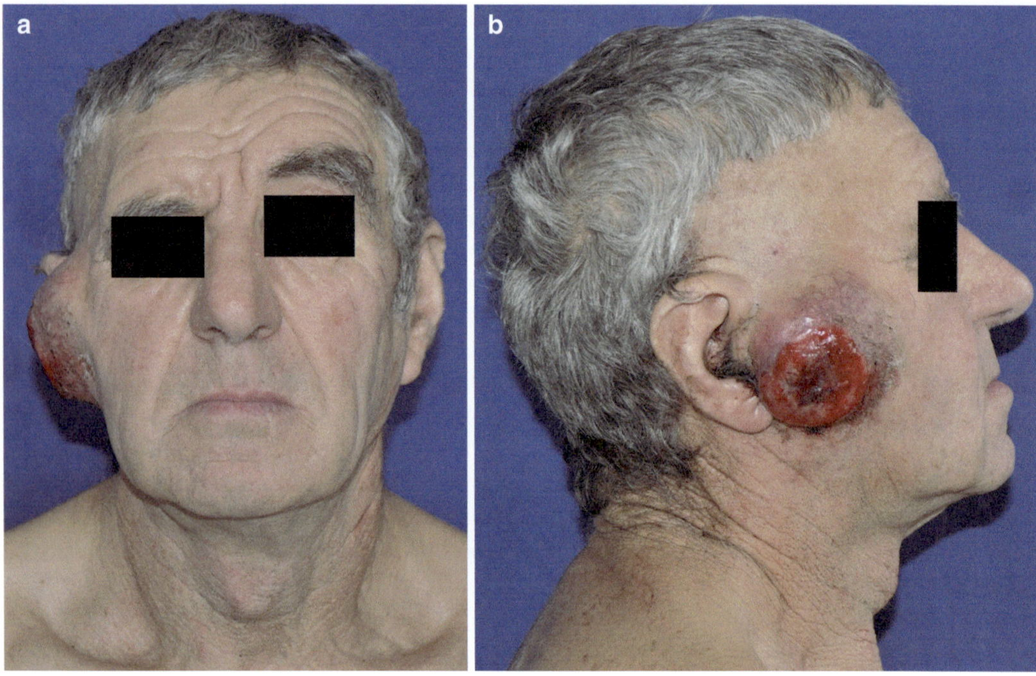

Fig. 2.2 (**a**, **b**) Adenoid cystic carcinoma of the right parotid gland extended to the zygomatic bone. The clinical exam does not show evidence of facial nerve paralysis

(Fig. 2.2a, b). Some studies have correlated facial nerve invasion with tumor size and poor prognosis following treatment [12]. Deep lobe invasion, tumors larger than 4 cm, salivary duct carcinoma [13], and adenoid cystic carcinoma [6] were significantly associated with intraoperative finding of facial nerve involvement.

TMJ involvement is another possibility that must be considered. Malignant tumors of the deep lobe of the parotid gland extended to the TMJ may present as a temporomandibular disorder in the absence of any other clinical sign [14]. Accurate diagnosis is difficult and onset of adequate treatment will be delayed if this rare possibility is not considered.

The anterior surface of the parotid gland is grooved by the ascending mandibular ramus. Malignant tumors can erode through the periosteum and invade the *mandibular bone* and even the *masticatory muscles*, causing trismus. Patients occasionally present with this complaint because of inability to feed properly. Sometimes confusions can be made with odontogenic infections associating trismus, but with careful history and clinical examination, absence of acute inflammatory signs will raise the suspicion of malignancy and avoid unnecessary draining incisions and tumor dissemination.

Advanced deep lobe parotid tumors projected intraorally can sometimes be confused with *tonsil* malignancies due to similar clinical presentation with displacement and sometimes involvement of the tonsils, palatal arches, and lateral pharyngeal wall [15]. It is important to differentiate the two conditions due to different treatment strategies. Radiotherapy alone is usually preferred and proves to be just as successful as surgery in the treatment of usual tonsil cancers [16], whereas most parotid malignancies require combined treatment.

2.4 Imaging and Differential Diagnosis Issues

Differentiating intrinsic from extrinsic parotid masses is not only a clinical but also a radiological challenge and proves to be especially difficult in the presence of large tumors occupying the parapharyngeal space.

There are several imaging techniques available, each showing strengths and weaknesses in the evaluation of salivary gland tumors, and most often need to be combined for a better assessment of tumor origin and spread. MRI is usually preferred in the evaluation of salivary gland tumors, but CT is more available, is quicker to perform, and avoids the contraindications of MRI. CT displays the anatomy of the region with great accuracy so it can be of real help for the surgical planning. MRI seems to be more reliable in assessing tumor margins and perineural spread [6]. MR sialography and sialendoscopy are useful in assessing ductal anatomy when obstruction is suspected.

The detailed imaging of extended parotid gland tumors is fully presented in Chap. 11.

2.5 Pathology and Differential Diagnosis Issues

The broad histological spectrum of salivary gland tumors makes them probably one of the most complex among human neoplasias. From the great variety of histological types, the most frequently encountered malignant tumors are the mucoepidermoid carcinoma, the adenoid cystic carcinoma, ex pleomorphic adenoma carcinoma, and acinar cell carcinoma [1]. Some histological types are more aggressive than others and more likely to invade adjacent structures, like high-grade tumors or tumors exhibiting properties of perineural spread like adenoid cystic carcinoma, salivary duct carcinoma, and squamous cell carcinoma.

The pathology of tumors with origin in the parotid gland is extremely diverse and will be discussed in detail in Chap. 9. However, it is important to outline several factors that have to be considered when differentiating tumors originating in the parotid gland from metastatic tumors and from tumors extended from adjacent structures.

It is worth to mention a common type of skin cancer that is frequently a cause for debate concerning the origin of the malignancy, since it is so often encountered on the skin but such a rare encounter when it comes to the parotid gland. Extended tumors will involve both the gland and the overlying skin making it extremely difficult to state the place of initial development [17]. Primary parotid squamous cell carcinoma is extremely rare, accounting for 1.9 % of salivary gland tumors [6], and the final diagnosis should only be made after ruling out extended and metastatic tumors that are encountered more often [17]. History will clarify the debut of the presenting lesion that may have started as a skin ulceration that progressively extended to deeper tissues, translating a carcinoma of the skin extended to the parotid tissue. If the parotid mass developed first and the skin ulceration followed, then the diagnosis of primary parotid tumor extended to the skin is more likely. The patient's history would also warn us of preexisting, surgically removed skin lesions consistent with this histologic diagnostic in the drainage territory of the parotid gland that could be a clue toward a late metastasis to the parotid from a previous SCC of the head and neck. Squamous cell carcinoma of the oropharyngeal mucosa extended to the gland through the parapharyngeal space or metastatic to the parotid gland is another possible occurrence, and it must be ruled out. The same case can be argued for other less frequent histological types of cancer that can arise in the parotid gland, in tissues surrounding the gland, or in distant tissues.

2.6 Treatment Options

The ultimate aim of establishing the true origin in the parotid tissue and not in adjacent or distant tissues is to avoid either insufficient or, in other cases, unnecessary treatment. These situations will be discussed in detail throughout the next chapters.

In the case of extended parotid tumors arising in the parotid gland, the surgical removal of the tumor with free margins should always be performed when possible, followed by appropriate closure of the defect. The surgical treatment for extended parotid tumors and each type of tissue invasion will be covered in great detail in subsequent chapters.

Management of the neck also varies greatly with tumor origin and type. A neck dissection is usually necessary when dealing with extended tumors originating in the parotid tissue, even for clinically negative neck. The neck dissection is generally started before the actual tumor removal, since it helps prepare the field, controls bleeding, and allows the preparation of the neck vessels for microvascular anastomosis when this type of reconstruction is needed.

Extended tumors originating in the parotid gland will benefit from a multimodal treatment that includes postoperative radiotherapy and chemotherapy, discussed in Chaps. 23 and 24.

2.7 Prognosis and Quality of Life

The prognosis depends on several factors including stage, particularly the N stage, the histologic type and tumor grading, the radicality of the surgical resection, and completion of postoperative radiotherapy [18]. Postoperative radiotherapy improves locoregional control for patients with negative prognostic factors [19]. The prognosis of primary parotid gland tumors tends to be overall better than the one of metastatic lesions to the parotid gland, but it varies according to the factors enumerated above.

The sequelae following extended parotidectomy can impact the quality of life of the patients to a certain degree, mainly by the presence of facial nerve paralysis, sensory disturbances, changes in facial appearance, and Frey syndrome. Increased care for avoiding complications and sparing nervous structures uninvolved by tumor can greatly improve quality of life. Some of the sequelae can be addressed at a later time with good results.

References

1. Ho K, Lin H, Ann DK, Chu PG, Yen Y. An overview of the rare parotid gland cancer. Head Neck Oncol. 2011;14(3):40. doi:10.1186/1758-3284-3-40.
2. Afify SE, Maynard JD. Tumours of the accessory lobe of the parotid gland. Postgrad Med J. 1992;68:461–2.
3. Lin DT, Coppit GL, Burkey BB, Netterville JL. Tumors of the accessory lobe of the parotid gland: a 10-year experience. Laryngoscope. 2004;114(9):1652–5.
4. Tamiolakis D, Chimona TS, Georgiou G, Proimos E, Nikolaidou S, Perogamvrakis G, Papadakis CE. Accessory parotid gland carcinoma ex pleomorphic adenoma. Case study diagnosed by fine needle aspiration. Stomatologija Balt Dent Maxillofac J. 2009;11:37–40.
5. Attie J, Sciubba J. Salivary gland neoplasms. Chicago: Year Book Medical Publishers; 1981.
6. Myers EN, Ferris RL. Salivary gland disorders. Berlin: Springer-Verlag; 2007.
7. Tominaga Y, Uchino A, Ishimaru J, Inokuchi A, Sato S, Kudo S. Squamous cell carcinoma arising from Stensen's duct. Radiat Med. 2006;24(9):639–42.
8. Close L, Larson DL, Shah JP. Essentials of head and neck oncology. New York: Thieme; 1998.
9. Harnsberger H, Osborn A. Differential diagnosis of head and neck lesions based on their space of origin. I. The suprahyoid part of the neck. AJR. 1991;157:147–54.
10. Myers EN, Ferris RL. Master techniques in otolaryngology – head and neck surgery, vol. 2. New York: Thieme; 2013.
11. Arya A, D'Cruz A. Infratemporal fossa, masticator space and parapharyngeal space: can the radiologist and surgeon speak the same language? AIJOC. 2012;4(3): 125–35. doi: 10.5005/jp-journals-10003-1098.
12. Wierzbicka M, Kopeć T, Szyfter W, Kereiakes T, Bem G. The presence of facial nerve weakness on diagnosis of a parotid gland malignant process. Eur Arch Otorhinolaryngol. 2012;269(4): 1177–82. doi:10.1007/s00405-011-1882-6, PMCID: PMC3311986. Published online Dec 18, 2011.
13. Preis M, Soudry E, Bachar G, Shufel H, Feinmesser R, Shpitzer T. Predicting facial nerve invasion by parotid gland carcinoma and outcome of facial reanimation. Arch Otorhinolaryngol. 2010;267(1):107–11. doi:10.1007/s00405-009-0968-x.
14. Miyamoto H, Matsuura H, Wilson DF, Goss AN. Malignancy of the parotid gland with primary symptoms of a temporomandibular disorder. J Orofac Pain. 2000;14(2):140–6.
15. Vourexakis Z. Tonsillar asymmetry from a parotid tumor. N Engl J Med. 2014;370:e20. doi:10.1056/NEJMicm1310638.
16. Mendenhall WM, Amdur RJ, Stringer SP, Villaret DB, Cassisi NJ. Radiation therapy for squamous cell carcinoma of the tonsillar region: a preferred alternative to surgery? J Clin Oncol. 2000;18(11): 2219–25.
17. Marks MW, Ryan RF, Litwin MS, Sonntag BV. Squamous cell carcinoma of the parotid gland. Plast Reconstr Surg. 1987;79(4):550–4.
18. Teo PM, Chan AT, Lee WY, Leung SF, Chan ES, Mok CO. Failure patterns and factors affecting prognosis of salivary gland carcinoma: retrospective study. Hong Kong Med J. 2000;6:29–36.
19. Terhaard CHJ, Lubsen H, Van der Tweel I, Hilgers FJM, Eijkenboom WMH, Marres HAM, et al. Salivary gland carcinoma: independent prognostic factors for locoregional control, distant metastases, and overall survival: results of the Dutch Head and Neck Oncology Cooperative Group. Head Neck. 2004;26(8): 681–92; discussion 692–3.

Extended Metastatic Tumours to the Parotid Gland

3

Victor-Vlad Costan, Constantin-Cătălin Ciocan-Pendefunda, and Eugenia I. Popescu

Abstract

The parotid gland's unique characteristic among other glands is the presence of lymph nodes within the glandular tissue. This contributes greatly to the variety of the tumours that can be found here, by either primary malignancy arising in the parotid nodes or by the presence of lymphatic metastasis that exhibits the characteristics of the tissue of origin. The most common type of malignancy that can lead to lymph node metastasis with this location is represented by skin cancer in the territory of drainage, especially high-risk squamous cell carcinoma.

The lymphatic spread can follow the usual anatomical pathways, but it is not unusual for tumours located beneath the clavicle to metastasise into the parotid gland. This can be explained either by obstruction of the normal lymphatic flow or by the presence of haematogenous metastasis.

In the case of extended tumours, whenever there is important invasion of adjacent structures, it can be extremely difficult to find the tissue of origin of the malignancy, set the right diagnosis and therefore decide upon the most suitable treatment.

Starting with the diagnosis and ending with the decision of appropriate treatment, the entire management of the case is much more complex than for

V.-V. Costan, MD, DMD, PhD (✉)
Department of Oral and Maxillo-Facial Surgery, Faculty of Dental Medicine, "Grigore T. Popa" University of Medicine and Pharmacy, "St. Spiridon" University Hospital, Iasi, Romania
e-mail: victorcostan@gmail.com

C.-C. Ciocan-Pendefunda, MD, DMD, PhD
Department of Oral and Maxillofacial Surgery, Fachklinik Hornheide Münster, Nordrhein-Westfalen, Germany

E.I. Popescu, DMD, PhD
Department of Surgery (Dentoalveolar Surgery, Oral and Maxillofacial Surgery), Faculty of Dental Medicine, "Grigore T. Popa" University of Medicine and Pharmacy, Iasi, Romania

© Springer International Publishing Switzerland 2016

V.-V. Costan (ed.), *Management of Extended Parotid Tumors*, DOI 10.1007/978-3-319-26545-2_3

the usual malignancy arising in the parotid gland, addressing both the primary tumour and the metastasis. There are situations when the treatment of the primary is simple, by tumour removal and primary closure, but the metastasis necessitates an extended parotidectomy followed by complex reconstruction procedures for maximal aesthetic and functional results.

3.1 Introduction

Metastasis to the parotid gland is a rare and unexpected finding among the multitude of tumours involving the parotid gland, but not so rare when reviewing certain groups of patients with skin cancer, a prevalent disease with increasing incidence considering the ageing population and increased sun exposure.

Both regional and distant metastasis can involve the gland, either synchronous with the primary tumour or after the removal of the primary. In addition to the usual management of a parotid mass, the treatment must also address the primary tumour. Extension of the tumour to surrounding tissues makes it difficult to establish the exact origin of the malignancy and therefore difficult to decide an accurate treatment. Furthermore, extended tumours lead to extensive postoperative defects and the need to perform complex reconstruction methods.

3.2 Incidence

Metastatic tumours of the parotid gland are a relatively rare occurrence, representing approximately 8 % of parotid tumours [3]. There is however a geographical variation in the incidence of parotid metastasis due to the increased rate of head and neck skin cancer in certain areas of the world, a type of malignancy that frequently metastasises to the parotid nodes. This is why in Australia, the region with the highest incidence of skin cancer in the world, the most common malignant tumour of the parotid gland is metastatic squamous cell carcinoma [1].

3.3 Anatomy Review

The parotid gland has been described as a reservoir for the metastatic tumours of the head due to the presence of lymph nodes on the surface of the gland as well as inside the parotid tissue. This characteristic is unique among the salivary glands and complicates the pathology of the parotid gland that becomes extremely varied, implying a difficult differential diagnosis.

The parotid comprises rich networks of lymphatic vessels and approximately 20–30 lymph nodes located inside and around the glandular tissue [12]. The nodes in the parotid region collect the lymph mainly from the parotid gland itself, the scalp, the nose, eyelids, external ear and external auditory canal, lacrimal gland, middle ear, posterior nasopharynx and soft palate [6]. It is estimated that the parotid nodes filter the lymph from 75 % of head and neck primaries [16].

Lymph nodes can be found on the surface of the parotid gland, above or deep to the fascia covering the gland [9], at different levels, in front or below the ear. They are also found inside the substance of the parotid, at different depths. The intraglandular nodes are mostly distributed in the superficial lobe of the gland, lateral to the facial nerve. A few lymph nodes can also be found in the deep lobe of the gland [8, 10, 11]. The paraparotid and intraparotid nodal layers are interconnected [6], draining mainly into the superficial and deep cervical nodes.

The distribution of the parotid nodes in and around the gland is important from a surgical view point, dictating the level and extent of tissue removal necessary in order to achieve optimal locoregional control of the disease.

The anatomy of the parotid lymphatic system is described in detail in Chap. 1.

3.4 Mechanism of Spread

Metastasis involves either the parotid tissue or the parotid lymph nodes, considering the spreading mechanism, haematogenous or lymphatic. Most parotid metastasis [70 %] is represented by lymph node metastasis from cutaneous squamous cell carcinoma or melanoma of the head and neck. The rest are split between tumours originating in noncutaneous head and neck regions (15 %) and the ones arising in distant sites, below the clavicle, represented mainly by the kidney, lung and breast tumours (15 %) [2]. Additionally, in our experience, parotid gland metastasis from an unknown primary is a relatively frequent encounter.

The parotid lymph nodes can be involved by either primary (Fig. 3.1a, b) or metastatic tumours (Fig. 3.2). A specific feature of the parotid gland is the enclosure of lymph nodes within the parotid tissue, both in the superficial and deep parts of the gland. In addition, lymph nodes can also be found in proximity to the gland, lying on its surface, in the pretragal area and in the area of the retromandibular vein. This is the reason that allows the parotid gland to be involved by both haematogenous and lymphatic metastasis, in contrast to the submandibular gland that is mostly affected by haematogenous metastasis due to the absence of lymphatic nodes within its structure. It is also the reason why primary parotid gland lymphoma can be encountered as a primary tumour arising in the parotid nodes.

Lymphatic spread is the most common mechanism encountered for the metastatic tumours of the parotid gland, and malignancy usually originates from the drained territories of the head and neck, although in rare cases the lymphatic flow

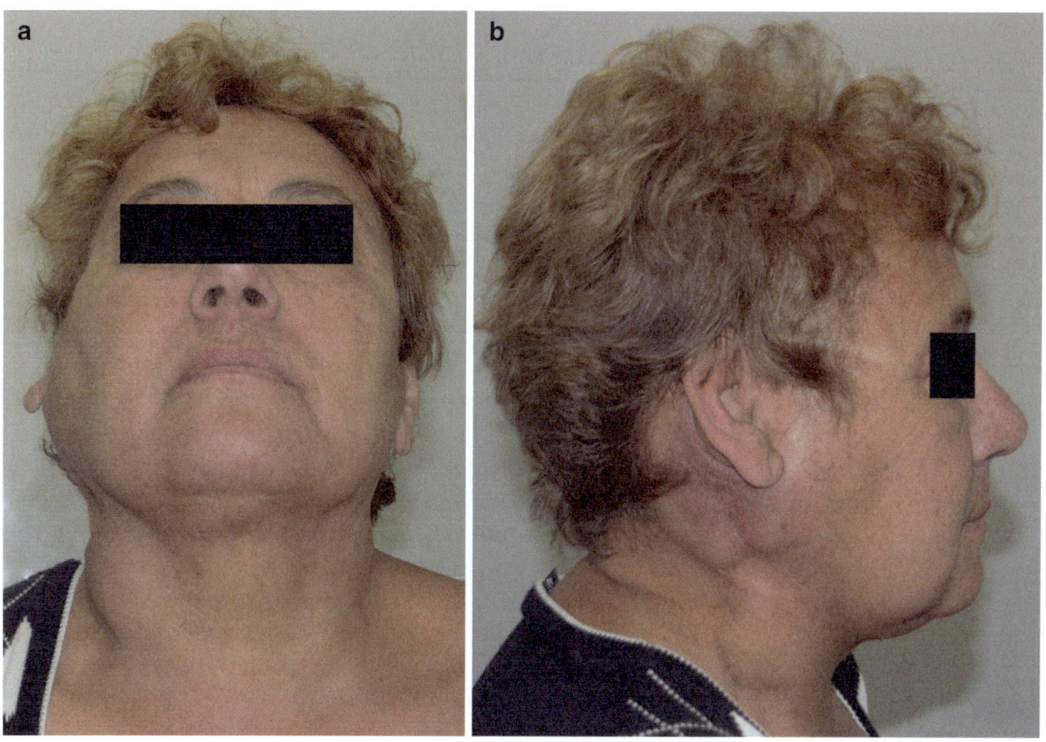

Fig. 3.1 (**a**, **b**) Diffuse non-Hodgkin lymphoma. In this case the treatment will not be a surgical one but eminently chemotherapeutic

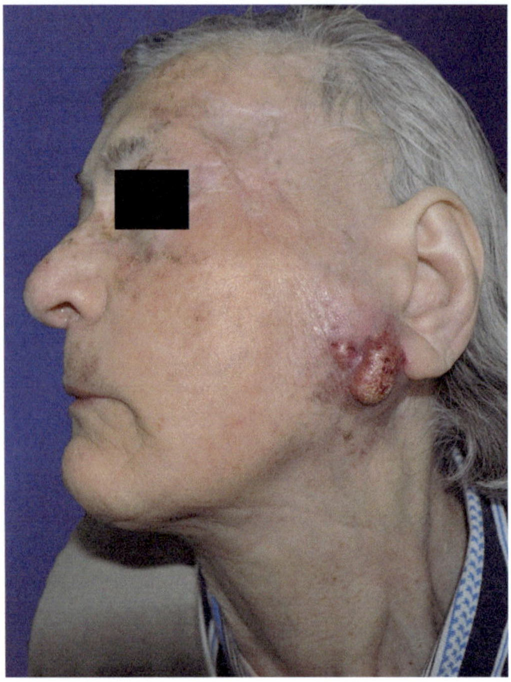

Fig. 3.2 Left intraparotid metastasis from a squamous cell carcinoma located on the left inferior temporal region. The primary lesion had been excised almost 1 year before presentation for the parotid mass

may be disrupted or diverted by important obstructing neck metastasis, presence of inflammation, previous surgery or radiotherapy [7], leading to unusual nodal metastasis involving the parotid gland.

Metastasis to the parotid gland from infraclavicular primaries is most likely the result of haematogenous spread rather than lymphatic dissemination through the thoracic duct. In this aspect a haematogenous route of spread has been described via Batson's venous plexus, a system of valveless paravertebral veins connecting the pelvic and thoracic vessels to the intraspinal veins. It provides a way for the retrograde spread of malignancy, by allowing tumour cells to bypass the pulmonary venous system, resulting in distant metastasis in the absence of secondary lung lesions [5].

Clinical suspicion of metastatic disease to the parotid gland is imperative for adequate management of the case. Furthermore, differentiating lymphatic from haematogenous metastasis is important in regard to the treatment of choice as well as prognosis. Lymphatic metastasis to the parotid gland should raise suspicion to the possible presence of occult nodal disease in the neck, and a neck dissection may be considered in addition to the parotidectomy. If haematogenous metastasis to the parotid gland from a distant site is suspicioned, further neck dissection would not be necessary considering the spreading route.

Knowledge of the main pathways of spread to the parotid gland from local and distant sites allows the surgeon to formulate an initial clinical suspicion and choose an appropriate treatment plan. Unfortunately, due to the rarity of metastatic disease to the parotid gland and the possibility of parotid metastasis occurring years later from the primary or from distant sites, even as a primary manifestation of a distant primary tumour, the diagnosis is sometimes provided only after performing surgery, by the pathology.

Differentiating lymphatic secondary tumours from haematogenous is not always an easy task for the pathologist, since elements of the lymphatic capsule must be identified in order to distinguish the two entities. In the case of extended tumours originating in the parotid nodes, the nodal architecture is usually completely substituted by tumour growth, and the capsule is invaded and efractioned, making it especially difficult to establish the starting point of the tumour.

Haematogenous lesions developing in the parotid gland can grow to engulf adjacent parotid nodes in a tumour block increasing the difficulty in establishing the initial site of development. In addition, there is a great histological variety of primary parotid malignancies that are not always easy to differentiate from metastatic tumours from distant sites, especially in the case of an occult distant primary tumour.

Extension of the tumour to surrounding tissues like skin invasion and ulceration and muscle, bone or even mucosal invasion will lead to large tumour masses and difficulty in establishing the tissue of origin. This in turn makes for a difficult differential diagnosis between a possible extended parotid metastasis and an extended primary tumour.

For all these reasons, in the presence of edifying signs for parotid gland malignancy, metastatic disease should always be considered and ruled out prior to surgery. Furthermore, when the pathology suggests a rare histological type of primary parotid tumour, a metastasis to the parotid gland from a distant site should be considered a possibility and investigated accordingly.

3.5 Diagnosis

History plays a key role in formulating a supposition diagnosis, and it is followed by imaging studies and eventually invasive procedures like FNAC or biopsy. The clinical and imaging diagnosis of extended parotid gland tumours makes the subject of Chaps. 10 and 11.

In the absence of evidence of previous malignancy that could metastasise to the parotid gland, it is the histology of the surgical specimen that raises suspicion of parotid metastasis, and in such a case, a full body investigation must be carried out in search of a primary tumour. The search should not be limited to the territory known to drain into the parotid lymph nodes since it is a known fact that distant metastasis can also be encountered here and both lymphatic and haematogenous pathways are possible.

In the presence of a known previous or synchronous tumour in the head and neck region, clinical suspicion of parotid nodal involvement is formulated based on the knowledge of the preferred pathways of lymphatic drainage in this area. Although these general anatomical backgrounds offer the surgeon important clues, they do not offer accurate basis for adequate surgical management of the case. There are situations when the presence of a cutaneous postoperative scar in close proximity to the malignant parotid mass makes it difficult to establish whether the tumour extension was carried out directly or by means of an intraparotid lymph node metastasis (Fig. 3.3).

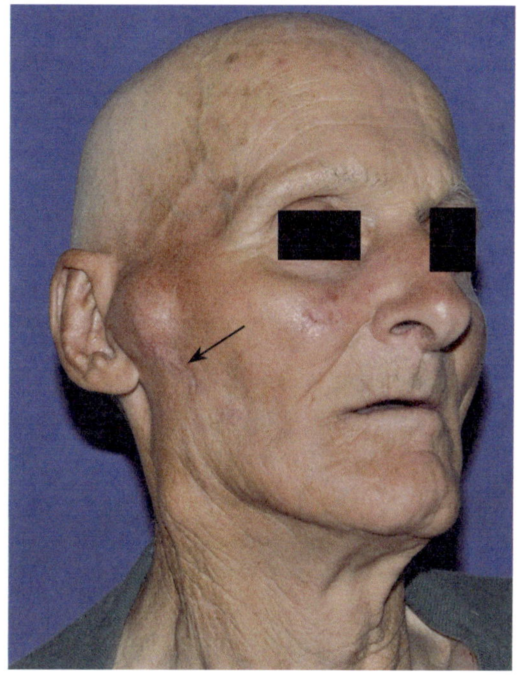

Fig. 3.3 Squamous cell carcinoma of the masseteric region followed by the development 6 months postoperatively of an intraparotid nodular lesion, in contact with the postoperative scar (*arrow*). It is difficult to estimate clinically whether the intraparotid mass represents a lymph node metastasis or the contiguous extension of the masseteric squamous cell carcinoma into the parotid tissue

Location of the primary tumour towards the midline complicates things even further, making it increasingly difficult to predict the nodal stations possibly involved by metastasis or decide upon the surgical treatment of choice.

Lymphoscintigraphy has shown that lymphatic drainage patterns of the head and neck are highly unpredictable clinically, demonstrating drainage in multiple node fields, skip metastasis, contralateral drainage and even upstream metastasis [4, 14]. This is due to individual variation in the lymphatic anatomy but also differences in lymphatic flow that is greatly influenced by the state of the locoregional tissues. Inflammation, blockage due to tumour growth, previous radiotherapy or surgery can modify the direction and rate of the lymph flow leading to unusual sites of metastasis [14]. The presence of locoregional pedicled flaps used for the plasty of the postoperative defect can also alter the direction of lymphatic drainage and provide different pathways for the metastatic cells to reach unusual nodal stations [13].

3.6 Histological Types

The time passed from primary tumour to the development of metastasis, the spreading pattern, clinical behaviour and prognosis depend mainly on the histological type of primary tumour. Although a great variety of tumour types can metastasise to the parotid gland, the most frequent encounter is a secondary tumour from skin cancer, mainly squamous cell carcinoma, followed by melanoma.

3.6.1 Cutaneous Squamous Cell Carcinoma

The head and neck is origin to 95 % of all cutaneous SCC, due to increased sun exposure in this area [18]. Squamous cell carcinoma is the second most common type of skin cancer after BCC. Although less frequent than BCC, the overall incidence of regional metastasis including the parotid nodes is higher because the metastatic potential of SCC is more important than the one for BCC.

The rate of metastasis for cutaneous squamous cell carcinoma in general is considered quite low, in the area of 2–3 % [15]. Certain factors related to the primary tumour, the general condition of the patient and previous treatments can increase the risk of metastasis to regional nodes, including the parotid nodes, above 5 %, up to approximately 20 % [6]. When parotid nodes are involved by lymphatic spread, there is a 25–50 % chance that neck nodes are simultaneously affected, whether clinically evident or occult [6]. Detecting high-risk squamous cell carcinoma is important for the adequate management of the case, with special care in early detection of lymphatic metastases and determining the need for prophylactic or curative treatment, especially since cases presenting with synchronous primary tumour and parotid metastasis are relatively rare (Fig. 3.4a, b). Generally, the onset of metastasis follows after a variable time interval from the removal of the primary (Fig. 3.5a, b).

Immunosuppressed patients are a distinct group known to be at a higher risk in general of developing malignancies and also increased risk of metastasis.

Factors related to the primary tumour that increase the possibility of regional and distant metastasis are represented by tumour size above

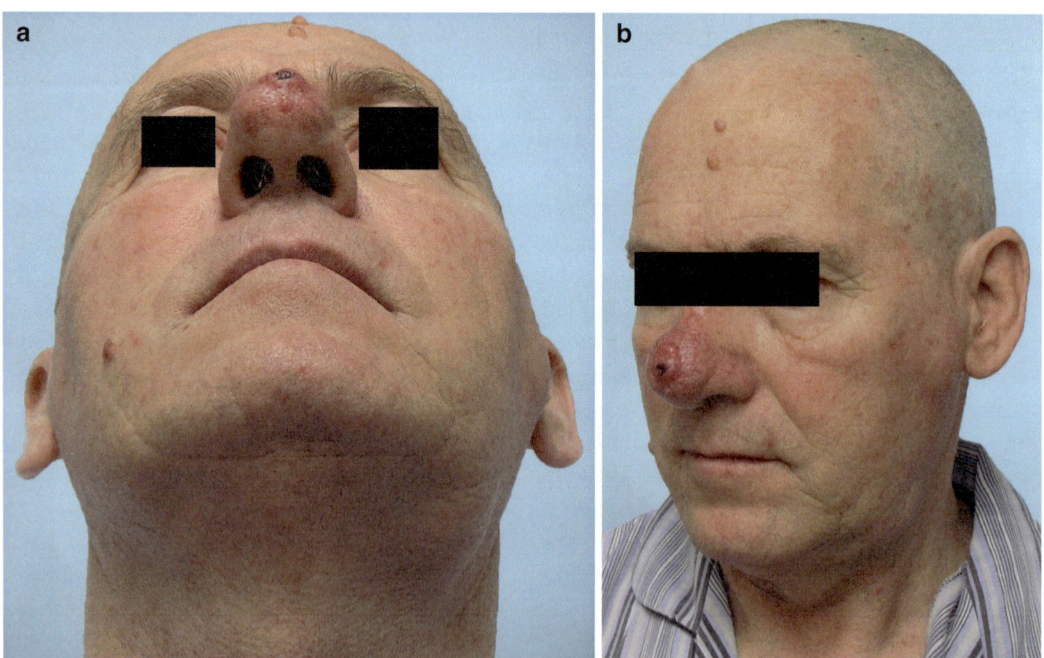

Fig. 3.4 (**a**, **b**) Squamous cell carcinoma of the nose tip and synchronous lymphatic metastasis in the left parotid gland

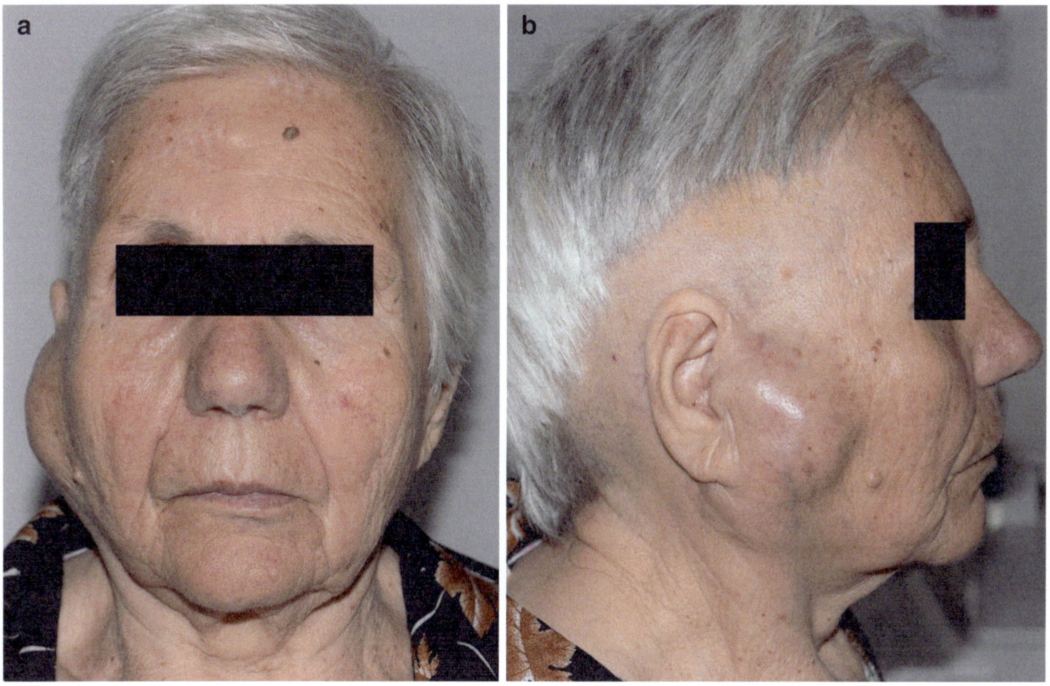

Fig. 3.5 (**a**, **b**) Right parotid lymph node metastasis from a squamous cell carcinoma of the frontal region previously removed and locally healed

2 cm, increased tumour thickness and depth of invasion over 4 mm, positive surgical margins, recurrent tumours, undifferentiated tumours and the presence of perineural and lymphovascular spread [15].

Perineural invasion is an important characteristic of cutaneous SCC, and it is highly associated with larger tumours located on the face, recurrent tumours and poorly differentiated tumours. Some studies have found a higher risk of parotid involvement in the presence of perineural invasion [19]. When extended parotid metastasis occurs, the tumour invasion can follow the facial nerve towards the base of the skull, and this should be anticipated prior to surgery [18].

Another important factor that has been associated with increased risk of lymphatic spread is the location of the primary tumour in the vicinity of the parotid gland [auricular, temporal, frontal and anterior scalp regions] [15]. Furthermore, SCC of the ear and periauricular area demonstrated perineural invasion more often than the ones located in other regions [19].

When high-risk SCC is identified, close follow-up with adequate evaluation of regional lymph nodes must be performed. Prophylactic neck dissection and parotidectomy can be considered since prognosis is influenced by the presence and number of affected nodes.

In the case of extended metastatic SCC of the parotid gland, the diagnosis is not an obvious one, since invasion and ulceration of the overlying skin can lead to confusions about the starting point of the tumour. Multiple SCC lesions can develop in the sun-exposed areas of the face, and secondary lesions can develop years following the primary. Tumours in advanced stages of development with skin ulceration and infiltration of surrounding tissues can be the result of primary cutaneous SCC extended to the parotid tissue, a metastatic tumour extended to the skin or even the rare event of primary SCC of the parotid gland extended to the skin. Proper history can help in establishing the clinical behaviour and most likely tumour origin. The same case can be argued for metastatic tumours originating in the nodes of the deep parotid lobe that can infiltrate the mucosa of the lateral pharyngeal wall.

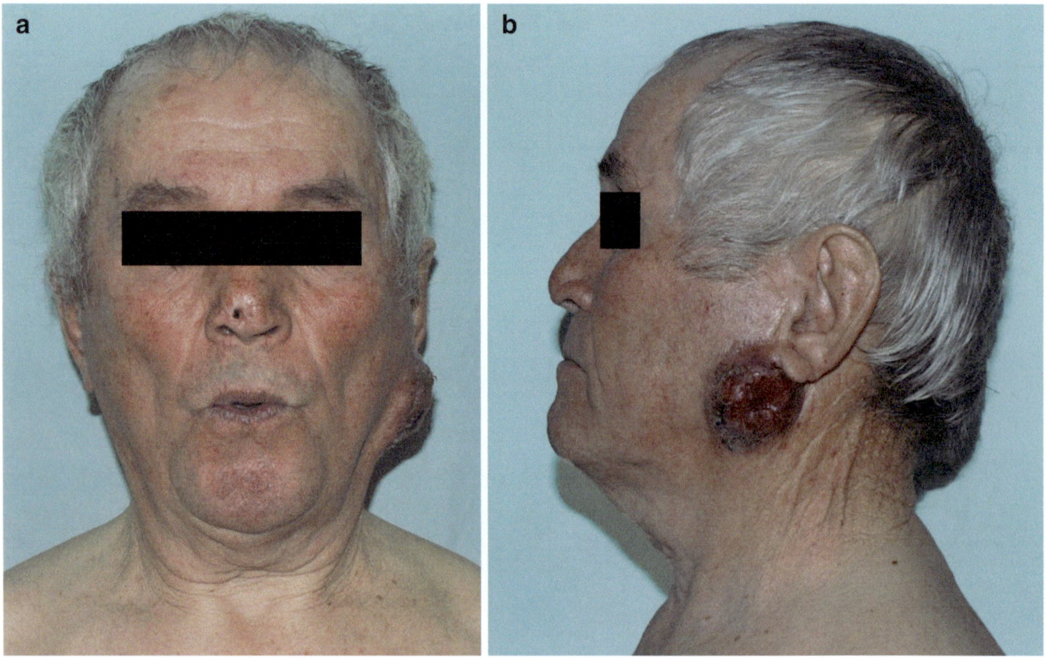

Fig. 3.6 (**a**, **b**) Lymph node metastasis of the left parotid gland starting from a Merkel cell carcinoma of the nose tip that had been previously removed and locally healed

3.6.2 Melanoma

Metastasis from regional malignant melanoma to the parotid gland is the second most common metastatic tumour of the parotid after squamous cell carcinoma [22]. It must be differentiated from primary melanoma of the parotid gland, a rare but possible occurrence, and from invasion of the gland by direct extension of skin melanomas. The presence of parotid metastasis from malignant melanoma is generally an indicator of poor prognosis. The usual treatment for both primary and secondary lesion is wide surgical excision. Additionally to the removal of the extended parotid metastasis, a simultaneous neck dissection on the ipsilateral side is usually performed.

3.6.3 Basal Cell Carcinoma

Although the most frequent type of skin cancer is basal cell carcinoma, this malignancy is known for extremely low metastatic rates, explaining the low incidence among the metastatic tumours of the parotid gland.

The presence of metastasis of BCC carries a very poor prognosis. The gold standard for both primary and secondary tumours is still surgical treatment, since chemotherapy and radiotherapy alone have not been shown to improve prognosis. Association of radiotherapy to parotidectomy in the case of parotid metastasis of BCC has been proven beneficial [17].

3.6.4 Other Histological Types

A great histological variety of tumours have been proved to metastasise to the parotid gland, including the rare Merkel cell carcinoma, thyroid gland cancer, breast cancer, renal cell carcinoma and many others that are discussed in Chap. 9.

The nonspecific appearance of Merkel cell carcinoma (Fig. 3.6a, b) leads to late diagnosis of the primary tumour that can eventually present as a parotid gland metastasis via lymphatic pathways. Although it is a rare encounter, it should not be overlooked upon clinical examination.

Thyroid gland carcinomas can sometimes lead to the developing of intraparotid metastasis,

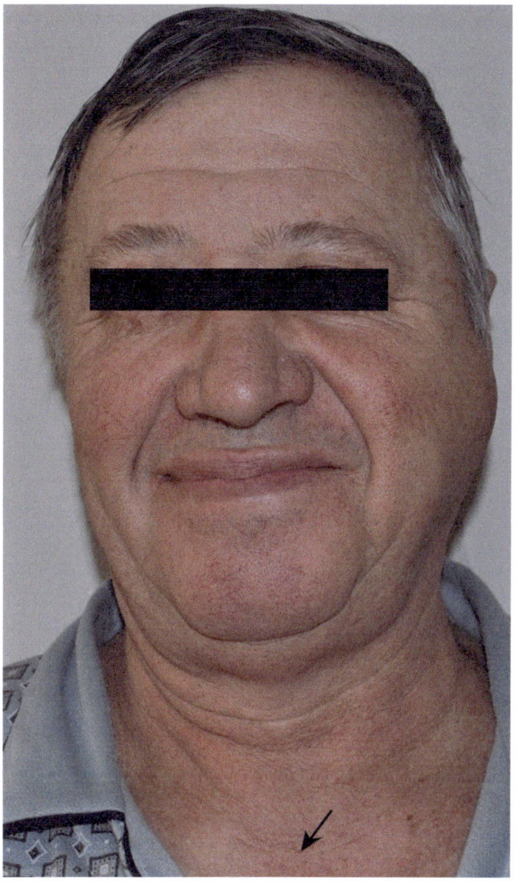

Fig. 3.7 Intraparotid lymph node metastasis from a papillary carcinoma of the thyroid gland operated 2 years previously (*arrow*) by total thyroidectomy followed by radioactive iodine

although infrequently. Considering the location of the thyroid gland above the clavicle, it is not surprising that these metastases are generally produced by lymphatic spread (Fig. 3.7).

A particular case is represented by the finding of a haematogenous metastasis from breast cancer. One particularity in these cases is the difficulty to differentiate the pathology of carcinomas arising in the parotid glandular tissue from metastasis of carcinomas arising in the breast glandular tissue. The purpose is not purely academic but has practical importance since this will set the stage of the disease and will guide the treatment plan.

Renal cell carcinomas have a high rate of haematogenous metastasis that can also involve the parotid gland. Since the primary tumour is not obvious, parotid metastasis can sometimes be the revealing sign of the initial tumour.

3.6.5 Occult Metastasis

The most difficult management is in front of occult parotid gland metastasis. This is an exclusion diagnosis established after the thorough search for a primary tumour at all levels in the body by means of clinical, imagistic, biologic and immunologic investigations, with increased focus on areas of primary concern. It is now known that metastasis can develop in the absence of a primary lesion by site-specific transformation of circulating cells and increased intrinsic metastatic aggressiveness of the malignant cells [21]. The primary tumour can develop and manifest a long time after the diagnosis of occult metastasis. This is why the search for the primary should be continued periodically even after the initial evaluation.

It is not a rare encounter to find that an initially diagnosed occult metastasis eventually proves to be originating in the ORL territory. Parotid metastasis from nasopharyngeal carcinoma should always be investigated whenever the histology suggests a metastasis of lymphoepithelial origin. Lesions in the nasopharynx do not present clinically in early stages and can be easily overlooked upon clinical examination. Fiberscopic view can also miss submucosal tumours developing in the wall of the nasopharynx. For these reasons, MRI should always be performed in order to rule out a possible origin of the metastasis at this level [20]. The diagnosis is especially important since the initial recommended treatment is usually represented by radiotherapy for both the primary and the secondary lesions.

In rare cases the parotid gland metastasis can be the presenting symptom of a distant hidden tumour.

3.7 Treatment

The surgical removal of extended parotid tumours, as well as the plasty of the postoperative defect, is discussed extensively in different chapters according to the type of tumour extension.

In addition to the removal of the extended parotid metastasis, the starting point should also be evaluated and submitted to treatment if this is the case. The overall treatment plan will vary if the parotid metastasis has been diagnosed synchronous with the primary tumour, if it occurred a while after the adequate removal of the primary or if a local relapse of the primary has been proven together with the metastasis.

Considering the type of tumour spread, in the case of a lymphatic metastasis to the parotid gland, it is important to also perform a neck dissection at least on the tumour side, together with the extended parotidectomy. In certain cases of locally advanced tumours, the extensive surgical removal of invaded tissues and additional neck dissection will lead to extensive defects and increased difficulty in preserving or finding suitable ipsilateral vessels for the free flap reconstruction. A neck dissection is not necessary if a haematogenous metastasis to the parotid gland is suspected.

The treatment of intraparotid lymphoma is not a surgical one, but a primarily a medical treatment, conducted by the haematologist. Unfortunately, considering the fact that parotid tumours in particular are operated without having a certain pathological report preoperatively, there are situations where a parotidectomy is performed.

3.8 Prognosis

The prognosis is variable according primarily to the histology of the primary tumour but also the local extension of the metastasis, as well as the sensitivity of the tumours to the complementary radiotherapy and chemotherapy.

References

1. Yeong R, Goh H, Bova R, Fogarty GB. Cutaneous squamous cell carcinoma metastatic to parotid – analysis of prognostic factors and treatment outcome. World J Surg Oncol. 2012;10:117.
2. Barnes L. Metastases to the head and neck: an overview. Head Neck Pathol. 2009;3:217–24. doi:10.1007/s12105-009 0123-4.
3. Gnepp DR. Metastatic disease to the major salivary glands. In: Ellis GL, Auclair PL, Gnepp DR, editors. Surgical pathology of the salivary glands. Philadelphia: WB Saunders; 1991. p. 560–9.
4. Suton P1, Lukšić I, Müller D, Virag M. Lymphatic drainage patterns of head and neck cutaneous melanoma: does primary melanoma site correlate with anatomic distribution of pathologically involved lymph nodes? Int J Oral Maxillofac Surg. 2012;41(4):413–20. doi:10.1016/j.ijom.2011.12.027. Epub 2012 Jan 23.
5. Brook RC, Tung K, Oeppen R. Batson's plexus and retrograde venous spread of malignancy – a pictorial review. Cancer Imaging. 2014;14 Suppl 1:40.
6. Myers EN, Ferris RL. Salivary gland disorders. Berlin: Springer; 2007.
7. Werner JA, Davis RK. Metastases in head and neck cancer. Berlin: Springer; 2004.
8. Marks NJ. The anatomy of the lymph nodes of the parotid gland. Clin Otolaryngol Allied Sci. 1984;9(5):271–5.
9. McKean ME, Lee K, McGregor IA. The distribution of lymph nodes in and around the parotid gland: an anatomical study. Br J Plast Surg. 1985;38(1):1–5.
10. Garatea-Crelgo J, Gay-Escoda C, Bermejo B, Buenechea-Imaz R. Morphological study of the parotid lymph nodes. J Craniomaxillofac Surg. 1993;21(5):207–9.
11. Pisani P, Ramponi A, Pia F. The deep parotid lymph nodes: an anatomical and oncological study. J Laryngol Otol. 1996;110(2):148–50.
12. Attie JN, Sciubba JJ. Tumors of major and minor salivary glands: clinical and pathologic features. Chicago: Year Book Medical Publisher; 1981.
13. Werner JA. Patterns of metastasis in head and neck cancer. In: Leong SPL, editor. Cancer metastasis and the lymphovascular system: basis for rational therapy. Berlin: Springer; 2007.
14. Uren RF, Howman-Giles R, Thompson JF. Patterns of lymphatic drainage from the skin in patients with melanoma. J Nucl Med. 2003;44:570–82.
15. Vasconcelos L, Melo JC, Miot HA, Marques MEA, Abbade LPF. Invasive head and neck cutaneous squamous cell carcinoma: clinical and histopathological characteristics, frequency of local recurrence and metastasis. An Bras Dermatol. 2014;89(4):562–8.
16. O'Brien C, Pathak I. Neck dissection and parotidectomy. In: Balch CM, Sober AJ, editors. Cutaneous melanoma. St. Louis: Quality Medical Publishing; 2003. p. 419–38.
17. Vu A, Laub Jr D. Metastatic basal cell carcinoma. In: Madan V, editor. Basal cell carcinoma. Rijeka: InTechOpen; 2012.
18. Vazquez V, Serrano S, Capuzzo R. Advanced squamous cell carcinoma of the skin. In: Li X, editor. Squamous cell carcinoma. Rijeka: InTechOpen; 2012.
19. Dean NR, Sweeny L, Scott Magnuson J, Carroll WR, Robinson D, Desmond RA, et al. Outcomes of recurrent head and neck cutaneous squamous cell carcinoma. J Skin Cancer. 2011;2011:972497. doi:10.1155/2011/972497. Article ID 972497.

20. Verim A, Faruk Çalım Ö, Düzcı Yüksel Ö, Naiboğlu B, Tepe Karaca Ç. Parotid gland mass as the presenting symptom of nasopharyngeal carcinoma. Istanbul: Galenos Publishing; 2013. doi:10.4274/haseki.1436.
21. Pavlidis N, Briasoulis E, Pentheroudakis G. Cancers of unknown primary site: ESMO clinical practice guidelines for diagnosis, treatment and follow-up. Ann Oncol. 2010;21 Suppl 5:v228–31. doi:10.1093/annonc/mdq193.
22. Andreadis D, Poulopoulos A, Nomikos A, Epivatianos A, Barbatis C. Diagnosis of metastatic malignant melanoma in parotid gland. Oral Oncol Extra. 2006;42:137–9.

Extended Parotid Tumors with Origin in the Skin of the Head and Neck

4

Tatiana V. Taranu and Mihaela Paula P. Toader

Abstract

Skin cancer of the head and neck may involve the parotid gland or parotid lymph nodes either by direct invasion or by lymphatic/hematogenous spread.

The most common cutaneous malignancies that spread to the parotid gland are squamous cell carcinoma and malignant melanoma. Other tumors that potentially involve the parotid gland include basal cell carcinoma, Merkel cell carcinoma, mucinous carcinoma or malignant fibrous histiocytoma.

Parotid lymph node metastasis from cutaneous malignancy of the head and neck, though rare, has a high prognostic value, rendering clinical exam of the parotid and cervical lymph nodes mandatory in patients with high risk of developing regional metastases. Cases with metastatic spread to the lymph nodes benefit from aggressive surgical treatment.

4.1 Introduction

Most of the skin tumors of the head and neck that potentially involve the parotid gland are squamous cell carcinomas and malignant melanomas (80–85 % of all metastases of the major salivary glands) [1]. Rare cases of basal cell carcinoma and Merkel cell carcinoma with metastases or direct invasion of the parotid gland have also been reported.

Cancer metastasis counts for 10–15 % of malignant neoplasms of the parotid gland [1]. Parotid lymph nodes are an important group at risk for metastases from skin cancers of the head and neck. Involvement of the parotid may be a result of direct invasion (favored by an interconnected plexus of peri- and intraglandular lymph nodes), lymph node metastasis from an extraglandular tumor, and hematogenic spread from a distant primitive tumor.

4.2 Squamous Cell Carcinoma (SCC)

Cutaneous SCC is considered a multifactorial form of skin cancer that is rarely fatal but with an increasing incidence, leading to significant morbidity and being the fifth most costly malignancy [2].

T.V. Taranu, MD, PhD (✉) • M.P.P. Toader, MD, PhD
Department of Dermatology, "Grigore T. Popa" University of Medicine and Pharmacy, University Clinical Railways Hospital, Iasi, Romania
e-mail: toaderpaula@gmail.com

© Springer International Publishing Switzerland 2016
V.-V. Costan (ed.), *Management of Extended Parotid Tumors*, DOI 10.1007/978-3-319-26545-2_4

4.2.1 Epidemiology

SCC is the second most common skin cancer in Caucasians. Its rising incidence may be explained by the increasing percentage of elder population, increasing exposure to risk factors such as exposure to artificial UV, depletion of the ozone layer, and more effective detection methods. The incidence of cutaneous SCC varies according to the region. The highest incidence is reported in Australia (five times more than other cancers) [2, 3]. Seventy percent of SCC cases are located in the photoexposed areas of the head and neck [2, 3].

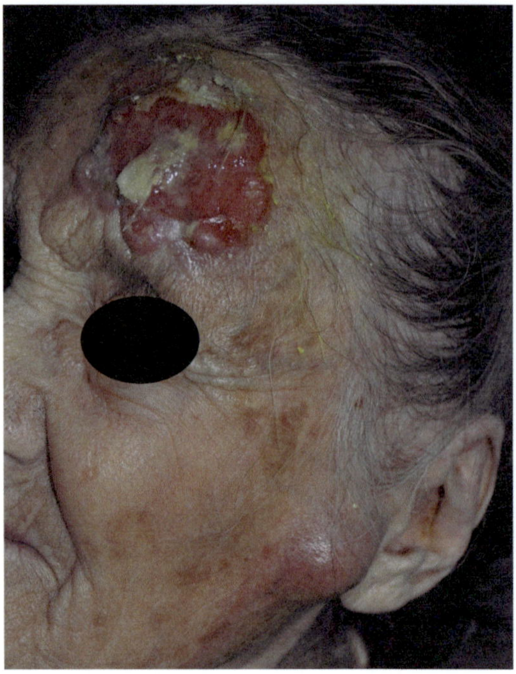

Fig. 4.1 Frontal ulcero-vegetant SCC, extended to the parotid gland

4.2.2 Etiopathogenesis

Cutaneous SCC results from the interaction between carcinogenetic-promoting factors and the host response. The most important carcinogenetic-promoting factor is chronic exposure to UV radiations (sunlight, artificial tanning, UV therapy). UV radiations are mutagenic and negatively influence the skin immune response. UV radiations determine DNA injury leading to pyrimidine dimers and a clonal expansion of keratinocytes with genetic defects. TP53 mutations are positive in more than 90 % of skin cancers in the USA but also in the premalignant lesions [2–4]. Other genetic anomalies involved in the pathogenesis of SCC are mutations of Bcl2 and RAS genes and alterations of EGFR and COX intracellular signaling transduction pathways [2]. Genetic factors contributing to SCC development are incompletely understood.

The markers of vulnerability to UV radiations are fair complexion, blue eyes, blond or red hair, albinism, and xeroderma pigmentosum.

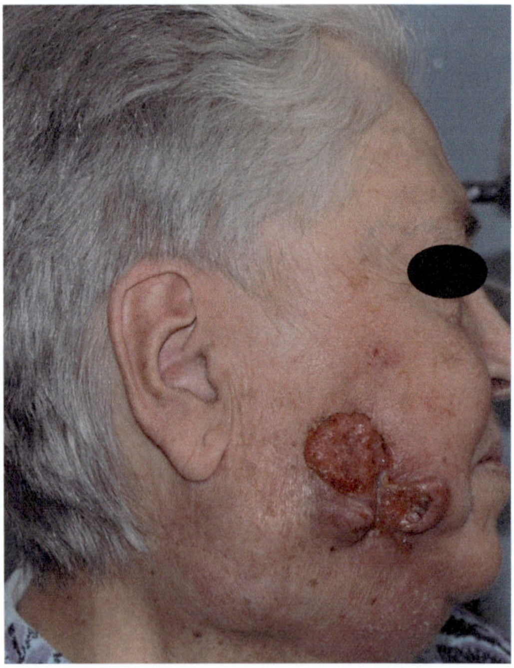

Fig. 4.2 Recurrent SCC extended to the parotid gland, with metastatic parotid and submandibular adenopathy

4.2.3 Clinical Presentation

Classical aspect of SCC is that of an ulceration with heaped-up edges, often covered by a plaque, on a sun-exposed area, with no tendency to heal (Figs. 4.1 and 4.2) or a firm, squamous bump on an erythematous base with elevated edges and insidious margins.

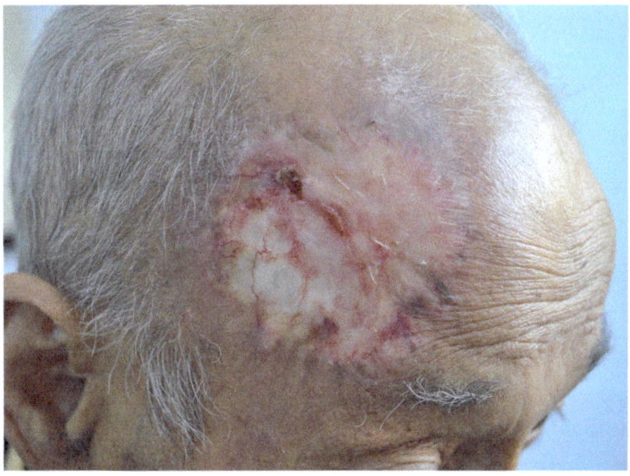

Fig. 4.3 Recurrent SCC developed on a chronic radiodermitis scar

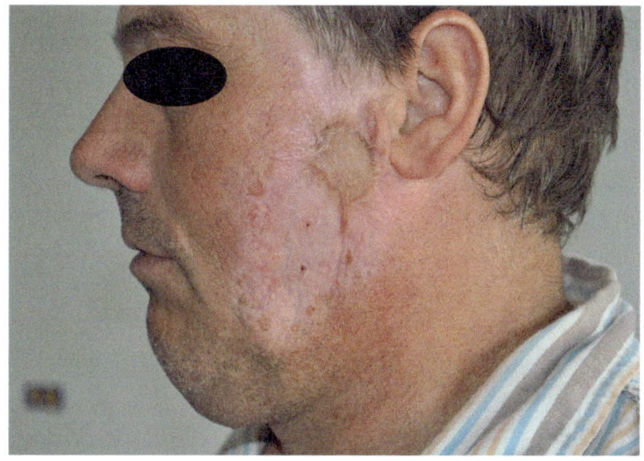

Fig. 4.4 Surgically removed SCC on an atrophic discoid lupus erythematosus scar

4.2.4 Diagnosis

Positive diagnosis is based on:

1. History and physical exam (evaluation of risk factors for SCC, growth rate, signs of nerve invasion – local pain, numbness, twitching or muscle weakness, regional invasion – preauricular, submandibular, cervical node enlargement).
2. Biopsy and pathology exam: according to nuclear and keratinocyte atypia SCC may be well differentiated (numerous nuclei with a normal aspect and keratin pearls at the periphery), moderately differentiated, or poorly differentiated (high grade of nuclear atypia, frequent mitoses, increased nuclear/cytoplasmic ratio, poor/absent keratinization). Other histologic variants include acantholytic (adenoid) SCC with pseudoglandular appearance and spindle cell SCC with atypical spindle-shaped cells.
3. CT scan for the evaluation of bone/nerve/lymph node invasion.
4. MRI for the evaluation of perineural invasion and orbital/intracranial extension.

There is an aggressive subset of SCC with a high risk of recurrence, local invasion, and metastasis and potentially fatal that can be appreciated on initial consultation according to intrinsic and extrinsic factors (Figs. 4.3 and 4.4) (Table 4.1).

If these factors are present (in less than 10 % of SCC of the head and neck), prophylactic treatment of the parotid and cervical lymph nodes is necessary [15]. Parotid involvement represents an independent prognostic factor for survival in patients with head and neck cutaneous SCC [12–16].

4.3 Malignant Melanoma (MM)

Most of the melanomas affecting the parotid gland are metastases of a primitive skin tumor of the head and neck. Cutaneous melanoma of the head and neck is a complex, aggressive condition that requires an elaborate treatment plan due to the intricate lymphatic draining system and to the tight proximity of the lesion to anatomical structures of functional and esthetic importance [17].

The incidence of malignant melanoma (MM) increased with 600 % in the last 50 years due to a better education level and to better skin screening leading to early diagnosis [18].

4.3.1 Etiopathogenesis and Risk Factors

The most important risk factor in MM is exposure to sunlight, which explains the relatively frequent location on the head and neck (one-third of primary

Table 4.1 Predictive factors for recurrence, local invasion, and metastasis of head and neck SCC

Intrinsic factors	Extrinsic factors
Location: columella, nasal vestibulum, ears, scalp, forehead, temporal area, eyelids [2, 3, 5–8]	*Organ transplantation*
Preexisting lesions: chronic ulcers, fistulas, radiodermitis, scars (discoid lupus, burns) (see Figs. 4.3 and 4.4)	*Hematologic malignancies*: chronic lymphatic leukemia and lymphoma [2, 3, 6, 9, 10]
Chronic inflammatory diseases: acne conglobata, dissecting cellulitis of the scalp [3, 6–8]	*Prolonged iatrogenic immunosuppression*
Tumor size: larger than 2 cm – increases the risk of local recurrence by twofold and of metastasis by threefold [2, 3, 6–8]	*HIV and AIDS* [2–4]
Histologic features: poorly differentiated SCC and spindle cell SCC [2, 3, 6–8]; rapid growth rate [3, 6]; tumor thickness: tumors with a thickness above 4–5 mm located near the parotid gland have a higher risk of metastasis [2, 6–8]	*Autoimmune disorders*: epidermolysis bullosa [11]
Recurrence after treatment [2, 3]	*Exposure to arsenic*
Perineural invasion is a sign of poor prognosis and a metastasis rate of up to 47 % if a major nervous branch is involved [2, 3]	*PUVA-therapy* [2, 3]

cutaneous MM) [19]. The frequency of sunburns, the age when these happened, and geographical latitude directly correlate with the development of a MM during lifetime. There appears to be a positive correlation between the number of melanocytic nevi (considered premalignant lesions) and the risk of developing MM in a person [20]. Other individual risk factors include fair complexion, genetic predisposition, and immune suppression. Individuals with dysplastic nevus syndrome and family history of MM have a 50 % risk of developing MM during their lifetime. Lentigo maligna melanoma located on the nose or cheeks is considered a melanocytic lesion with a 5–10 % risk of becoming invasive melanoma [19].

In 90 % of MM cases, mutations of CDKN2A, CDK4, Braf-kinase, PTEN, and cKIT-tyrosine kinase genes may be detected, but CDKN2A mutations carry the highest risk for MM development [17].

4.3.2 Clinical Aspect

The most frequent site for head and neck MM is the face, scalp, neck, and external ear. The location on the scalp renders the poorest prognosis [19, 20].

Clinical variants include superficial spreading Melanoma (SSM), nodular MM, lentigo maligna MM, in situ MM and desmoplastic MM. SSM is the most common type and usually arises on a nevus in younger patients. Desmoplastic MM, either amelanotic or pigmented, is the most rare type and usually develops on a premalignant lesion. It has a high rate of local recurrence after treatment, but a lower metastatic potential. It may spread through perineural involvement.

The presence of melanocytes in the glandular acinary and ductal cells suggests the possibility of a primitive parotid melanoma. The epicenter of a primitive parotid melanoma is the glandular tissue and does not include lymph nodes in the tumor mass [18].

In patients with MM on sun-exposed areas, spontaneous regression may occur in 0.22–0.27 % of cases [21]. Unidentified primitive MM is more common than parotid primitive MM. Patients with unidentified primitive MM appear to survive longer than those with known primitive MM [1].

In patients with head and neck melanoma, the rate of regional metastases correlates with tumor thickness. The rate of occult regional metastasis is 5 % for tumors with a thickness under 1 mm, 20 % for a thickness of 1 to 4 mm, and over 50 % for thickness over 4 mm [1].

4.4 Basal Cell Carcinoma (BCC)

BCC represents the most common malignancy in Caucasians, representing 80 % of all nonmelanoma skin cancers, with a very low risk for

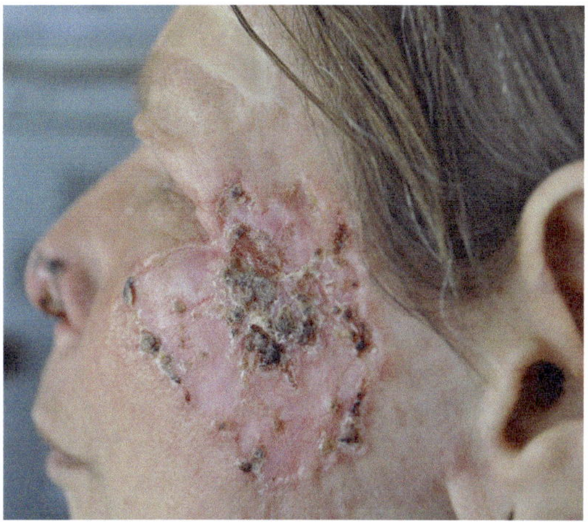

Fig. 4.5 Extended, ulcerated multiple, recurrent BCCs

metastasis, but locally aggressive and potentially involving the parotid gland by direct invasion [21]. Metastatic BCC is a rare entity, first documented in 1894 by Beadles. The incidence of metastatic BCC varies between 0.0028 and 0.55 % of the total BCC cases [22]. It mainly affects males (M:F=2:1) between the ages 20 and 60. There are only five reported cases in the black race [23].

4.4.1 Etiology and Predisposing Factors

Etiological factors are represented mainly by UV radiations and arsenic and genetic disorders (nevus sebaceous of Jadassohn, xeroderma pigmentosum, basal cell nevus syndrome, bazex syndrome, Rombo syndrome).

4.4.2 Clinical Aspects

The classical aspect of BCC is that of a papulonodular pearly lesion, with no tendency to heal, with an elevated border and telangiectasia on the surface, that may ulcerate and grows slowly (Fig. 4.5). Most of BCCs arise on sun-exposed skin areas: face, ears, neck, scalp, and the upper trunk.

Diagnosis of metastatic BCC (after Lattes and Kessler criteria in 1951) requires the existence of a primitive cutaneous tumor, distant dissemination of the primitive tumor (not by local invasion), similar pathological features of the disseminated tumor to the primitive tumor, and absence of SCC features in the metastatic tumor [24].

Predictive factors for aggressive BCC are age, location, and size of the primitive tumor, long evolution, multiple BCCs, tissue invasion, and extension to adjacent structures. The median age for the first signs of metastasis is 59 years [22]. The average interval between the primitive tumor and metastasis is around 9 years [22]. Most of BCC that metastasize (85 %) are located on the head and neck, and two-thirds of them are on the face [24]. The most critical areas are the center of the face (nasolabial folds, paranasal areas), retroauricular area, and internal canthus [21]. BCC on the area immediately above the superficial parotid has a risk for metastasis if it penetrates the deeper tissue. Tumors larger than 3 cm have a metastasizing risk of 2 %; it increases to 25 % in the case of tumors larger than 5 cm and to 50 % in tumors larger than 10 cm [21]. Tissue invasion and extension to adjacent structures increase the risk of metastasis.

Other factors that correlate with BCC spread are recurrence after treatment, history of radiotherapy for a large primitive tumor or for a recurrent tumor, immunosuppression, chromosome anomalies such as trisomy 6, and aggressive histological subtypes: morpheaform, infiltrative, and adenocystic; apparently the highest metastatic risk belongs to the metatypic variant (basosquamous cell carcinoma) (Fig. 4.6), with a metastasizing rate of 6 % [23]. Immunohistochemical markers for BCC aggression (p53, Ki67, Bcl2) do not indicate a risk for metastasis [24]. Recent studies showed that decreased expression of actin and increased expression of E-cadherin may contribute to the metastatic potential of BCC [25]. Perineural invasion is rare and bears a poor prognosis, especially for the retroauricular BCC and BCC on the cheek, when facial nerve and trigeminal nerve are involved. It is more frequent in recurrent lesions, and commonly 50 % of these patients underwent radiotherapy [23]. Thus, perineural invasion correlates both with the recurring character of the tumor and the metastatic potential increasing them both fivefold [24].

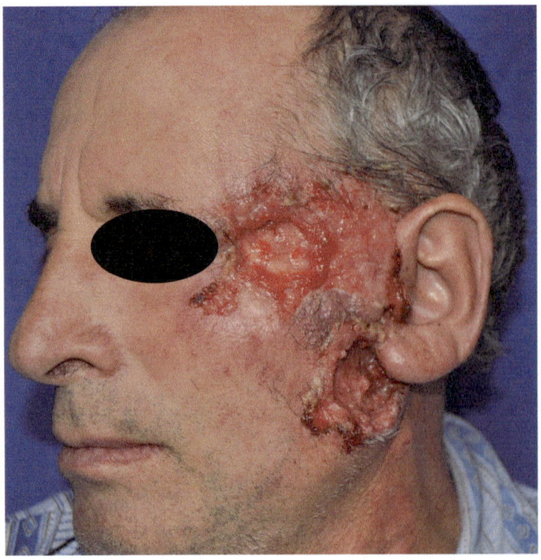

Fig. 4.6 Metatypic BCC extended to the parotid

Metastatic spread of a BCC is via hematogenous or lymphatic route, but parotid metastasis is usually the result of direct extension. Metastasizing path, time interval until the first signs of metastasis, age of the patient when metastasis is diagnosed, and sex of the patient do not correlate with survival. Parotid metastatic BCC has a poor prognosis, median rate of survival after the diagnosis being between 8 months and 3.6 years. Less than 20 % of the patients survive for 1 year, and approximately 10 % survive for 5 years [26].

Parotid metastasis must be differentiated from a basal cell adenocarcinoma (difficult distinction, both morphologically and immunohistochemically) [27].

4.5 Merkel Cell Carcinoma (MCC)

MCC is a rare neuroendocrine tumor of the skin that occurs more frequently in the head and neck area (50 % of cases), in Caucasians, elderly (over 65 years), and male patients [28].

4.5.1 Etiology and Risk Factors

MCC occurrence correlates with UV exposure and cutaneous infection with polyoma virus. MCC incidence rate increases mainly with sun exposure and immunosuppression (associated chronic lymphatic leukemia and organ transplant recipients). MCC often occurs in association with epithelial neoplasia [28].

4.5.2 Clinical Aspect

Usually MCC appears as a solitary pink asymptomatic nodule that may be easily mistaken both clinically and histopathologically for other carcinomas (such as small cell carcinomas). Electronic microscopy and immunohistochemistry are necessary for diagnostic confirmation. Clinical features of MCC may be summarized in an acronym: AEIOU (**a**symptomatic nodule, rapidly **e**xpanding, **i**mmune suppression, **o**lder than 50 years, **u**ltraviolet exposed site on a person with fair skin) [29]. Most often MCC in the parotid gland is the result of metastasis from a primitive cutaneous tumor of the head and neck (14 reported cases) or of local invasion from a cutaneous MCC in the retroauricular area.

MCC is an aggressive tumor. Despite surgical removal, radiation therapy, and medication, 25–35 % of the patients die [30].

There is a limited number of unidentified primitive MCC reported thus far, especially in elderly Caucasian males, with a better survival and a low risk of death due to the tumor [31]. The 5-year survival rate for head and neck MCC is between 40 and 68 % [28]. Factors that correlate with survival duration are tumor stage at the time of diagnosis and distant recurrence [28].

4.6 Rare Skin Malignancies That Spread to the Parotid Gland

4.6.1 Mucinous Carcinoma

Mucinous carcinoma (MC), also called adenoid cystic carcinoma, may occur in the breast, gastrointestinal tract, salivary glands, lacrimal glands, bronchi, ovaries, and skin. Cutaneous primitive MC frequently involves the eyelids, scalp, or other areas of the head and neck. It originates

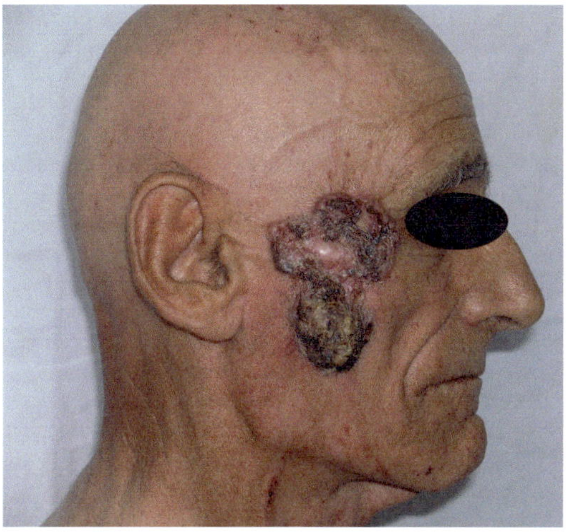

Fig. 4.7 Adenoid cystic carcinoma extended to the parotid gland and the malar bone

from the sudoral glands, but the exact source, whether the apocrine or the eccrine sudoral glands, is still debated [32].

Clinical aspect is that of an asymptomatic, slow growing nodule or ulcer that tends to expand rapidly [32–34] (Fig. 4.7). MC has a high rate of recurrence after surgical removal (30–40 %), but metastasis via hematogenous or lymphatic spread is very rare (only three cases of metastatic MC reported until 2005, one located on the scalp with parotid metastasis) [32]. Assessment of metastases is critical for the distinction between primitive cutaneous MC (rare entity) and secondary metastatic cutaneous MC with a poor prognosis. Pathology and immunohistochemistry do not render distinctive data.

Even though the usual evolution of a primitive cutaneous MC is slow, with asymptomatic lesions that rarely metastasize, the occurrence of multiple new lesions indicates a more aggressive tumor with a higher metastatic potential. All cases of cutaneous MC require systemic evaluation to exclude a skin metastasis from an occult visceral MC.

4.6.2 Malignant Fibrous Histiocytoma

Malignant fibrous histiocytoma (MFH) is the third most common soft tissue sarcoma, predominantly affecting male patients (two-thirds of cases) in the sixth and seventh decades of life [35]. The most frequent locations are the head and neck, trunk, extremities, and retroperitoneum. Precipitating factors include exposure to ionizing radiations, alterations of p53 genes, and activation of H- and K-ras genes. Radiation-associated MFH are often located on the neck or in the parotid gland [36, 37].

Clinical presentation is nonspecific, as superficial or subcutaneous painless, rapidly enlarging papules or nodules.

Histologically MFH are classified into superficial (confined to the dermis and subcutaneous tissue and associated with a higher rate of local recurrence) and deep (penetrate the subcutaneous fascia and reach the fascia and deeper tissue layers and associated with a higher mortality rate). MFH is an aggressive type of soft tissue sarcoma that requires further patient follow-up, to assess the degree of local invasion and distant metastasis [38].

References

1. Witt RL, editor. Salivary glands diseases: surgical and medical management. New York: Thieme; 2006. p. 141–71.
2. Goh RY, Bova R, Fogarty GB. Cutaneous squamous cell carcinoma metastatic to parotid – analysis of prognostic factors and treatment outcome. World J Surg Oncol. 2012;10:117.
3. Johnson TM, Rowe DE, Nelson BR, Swanson NA. Squamous cell carcinoma of the skin (excluding lip and oral mucosa). J Am Acad Dermatol. 1992; 26(3):467–84.
4. De Gruijl FR, Rebel H. Early events in UV carcinogenesis – DNA damage target cells and mutant p53 foci. Photochem Photobiol. 2008;84(2):382–7.
5. Barzilai G, Greenberg E, Cohen-Kerem R, Doweck I. Pattern of regional metastases from cutaneous squamous cell carcinoma of the head and neck. Otolaryngol Head Neck Surg. 2005;132:852–6.
6. Rowe DE, Carroll RJ, Day Jr CL. Prognostic factors for local recurrence, metastasis and survival rates in squamous cell carcinoma of the skin, ear and lip. Implications for treatment modality selection. J Am Acad Dermatol. 1992;26(6):976–90.
7. Brantsch KG, Meisner C, Schönfisch B, Trilling B, Wehner-Caroli J, Röcken M, et al. Analysis of risk factors determining prognosis of cutaneous squamous cell carcinoma: a prospective study. Lancet Oncol. 2008;9(8):713–20.

8. O'Bryen K, Sherman W, Niedt GW, Taback B, Manolidis S, Wang A, Ratner D. An evolving paradigm for the workup and management of high risk cutaneous squamous cell carcinoma. J Am Acad Dermatol. 2013;69(4):595–602.
9. Mehrany K, Weenig RH, Pittelkow MR, Roenick RK, Otley CC. High recurrence rates of squamous cell carcinoma after MOHS surgery in patients with chronic lymphocytic leukemia. Dermatol Surg. 2005;31(1):38–42.
10. Frierson Jr HF, Deutsch BD, Levine PA. Clinicopathologic features of cutaneous squamous cell carcinoma of the head and neck in patients with chronic lymphocytic leukemia, small lymphocytic lymphoma. Hum Pathol. 1988;19(12):1397–402.
11. Fine JD, Johnson LB, Weiner M, Li KP, Suchindran C. Epidermolysis bullosa and the risk of life-threatening cancers: the National EB registry experience, 1986–2006. J Am Acad Dermatol. 2009;60(2):203–11.
12. Ch'ng S, Maitra A, Lea R, Brash H, Tan ST. Parotid metastasis – an independent prognostic factor for head and neck cutaneous squamous cell carcinoma. J Plast Reconstr Aesthet Surg. 2006;59(12):1288–93.
13. Kihurana VG, Mentis DH, O'Brien CJ, Hurst TL, Stevens GN, Packham NA. Parotid and neck metastasis from cutaneous squamous cell carcinoma of the head and neck. Am J Surg. 1995;170(5):446–50.
14. Veness MJ, Porceddu S, Palme CE, Morgan GJ. Cutaneous head and neck squamous cell carcinoma metastatic to parotid and cervical lymph nodes. Head Neck. 2007;29(7):621–31.
15. Spriano G, Roselli R. Lymph node problem in cutaneous head and neck carcinomas. Acta Otorhinolaryngol Ital. 1995;15(3):159–62.
16. Bumpous J. Metastatic cutaneous squamous cell carcinoma to the parotid and cervical lymph nodes: treatment and outcomes. Curr Opin Otolaryngol Head Neck Surg. 2009;17(2):122–5.
17. Andrews GA, Myers JN. Head and neck melanoma in: head and neck cancer: multimodality management. New York: Springer; 2011. p. 533–6.
18. Lai SY, Weinstein GS, Chalian AA, Rosenthal DI, Weber RS. Parotidectomy in the treatment of aggressive cutaneous malignancies. Arch Otolaryngol Head Neck Surg. 2002;128:521–6.
19. Golger A, Young SD, Ghazarian D, Neligan CP. Epidemiological features and prognostic factors of cutaneous head and neck melanoma. A population-based study. Arch Otolaryngol Head Neck Surg. 2007;133:442–7.
20. Kienstra MA, Padhya TA. Head and neck melanoma. Cancer Control. 2005;12(4):242–7.
21. King M, Spooner D, Rowlands DC. Spontaneous regression of metastatic malignant melanoma of the parotid gland and neck lymph nodes: a case report and a review of the literature. Clin Oncol. 2001;13(6):466–9.
22. Lo JS, Snow SN, Reizner GT, Mohs FE, Larson PO, Hruza GJ. Metastatic basal cell carcinoma: report of 12 cases with a review of the literature. J Am Acad Dermatol. 1991;24:715–9.
23. Malone JP, Fedok FG, Belchis DA, Maloney ME. Basal cell carcinoma metastatic to the parotid: report of a new case and review of the literature. Ear Nose Throat J. 2000;79(7):511–5.
24. Vu A, Laub DJ. Metastatic basal cell carcinoma: a case report and review of the literature. Eplasty. 2011;11:ic8. PubMed PMC3088016.
25. Uzquiano MC, Prieto VG, Nash JW, Ivan DS, Gong Y, Lazar AJF, et al. Metastatic basal cell carcinoma exhibits reduced actin expression. Mod Pathol. 2008;21:540–3.
26. Farmer ER, Helwig EB. Metastatic basal cell carcinoma: a clinicopathologic study of 17 cases. Cancer. 1980;46:748–57.
27. Spates ST, Ramsey J, Mellette R, Fitzpatrick J. Metastatic basal cell carcinoma. Dermatol Surg. 2003;29:650–2.
28. Suarez C, Rodrigo JP, Ferlito A, Devaney KO, Rinaldo A. Merkel cell carcinoma of the head and neck. Oral Oncol. 2004;40(8):773–9.
29. Heath M, Jaimes N, Lemos B, Mostaghimi A, Vang LC, Peñas PF, Nghiem P. Clinical characteristics of Merkel cell carcinoma at diagnosis in 195 patients: the AEIOU features. J Am Acad Dermatol. 2008; 58(3):375–81.
30. Gillenwater AM, Hessel AC, Morrison WH, Burgess MA, Silva EG, Roberts D, et al. Merkel cell carcinoma of the head and neck. Effect of surgical excision and radiation on recurrence and survival. Arch Otolaryngol Head Neck Surg. 2001;127(2):149–54.
31. Tarantola TI, Vallow LA, Halyard MY, Weenig RH, Warschaw KE, Weaver AL, et al. Unknown primary Merkel cell carcinoma: 23 new cases and review. J Am Acad Dermatol. 2013;68(3):433–40.
32. Jih MH, Friedman PM, Kinuyai-Asadi A, Goldberg LH. A rare case of fatal primary cutaneous mucinous carcinoma of the scalp with multiple in-transit and pulmonary metastases. J Am Acad Dermatol. 2005; 52:s76–80.
33. Requena L, Kiryu H, Ackerman AB. Mucinous carcinoma in: neoplasm with apocrine differentiation. Philadelphia: Lippincott-Raven; 1998. p. 907–47.
34. Mendoza S, Helwig EB. Mucinous (adenocystic) carcinoma of the skin. Arch Dermatol. 1971;103:68–78.
35. Clark DW, Moore BA, Patel SR, Guadagnolo BA, Roberts DB, Sturgis EM. Malignant fibrous histiocytoma of the head and neck region. Head Neck. 2011;33:303–8.
36. Sakamoto A, Oda Y, Itakura E, Oshiro Y, Nikaido O, Iwamoto Y, et al. Immunosuppression of ultraviolet photoproducts and p53 mutation analysis in atypical fibroxanthoma and superficial malignant fibrous histiocytoma. Mod Pathol. 2001;14:581–8.
37. Satomi T, Watanabe M, Kaneko T, Matsubayashi J, Nagao T, Chiba H. Radiation-induced malignant fibrous histiocytoma of the maxilla. Odontology. 2011;99:203–8. Epub 2011 Apr 13.
38. Peiper M, Zurakowski D, Knoefel WT, Izbicki JR. Malignant fibrous histiocytoma of the extremities and trunk: an institutional review. Surgery. 2004;135: 59–66.

Parotid Tumours with Skin Extension

5

Felix P. Koch, Robert A. Sader, and Victor-Vlad Costan

Abstract

Tumours affecting the parotid gland and the external skin can evolve from the gland itself or infiltrate secondarily the parotid gland originating from the external skin or metastases. Due to the anatomy of the gland and its close relation to the facial and auriculotemporal nerve, these structures can be affected, either by the tumour itself or the resection.

The complete resection of these extended tumours requires the reconstruction of the skin, the nerve and sometimes even the mandibular bone as well. There are multiple ways to reconstruct the defects after resection by local flaps, myocutaneous flaps or free, microvascular flaps. This chapter focuses on the reconstruction by local flaps, such as skin rotation and transposition techniques of the neighbouring tissue, including large skin transpositions, e.g. the cervicofacial flap. Pedicled flaps like the submental island flap or the supraclavicular artery flap are alternative possibilities. A parotid resection could cause severe complications. The auriculotemporal syndrome accompanied with gustatory sweating can be prevented by an interpolation of a temporal muscle flap. A salivary fistula after surgery of the parotid gland can be addressed by a pressure bandage or infiltration of botulinum toxin A.

F.P. Koch, MD, DMD, MBA, PhD •
R.A. Sader, MD, DDS, PhD (✉)
Department of Oral, Cranio-Maxillofacial and Facial Plastic Surgery, University Hospital Frankfurt, Frankfurt, Germany
e-mail: r.sader@em.uni-frankfurt.de

V.-V. Costan, MD, DMD, PhD
Department of Oral and Maxillo-Facial Surgery, Faculty of Dental Medicine, "Grigore T. Popa" University of Medicine and Pharmacy, "St. Spiridon" University Hospital Iasi, Iasi, Romania
e-mail: victorcostan@gmail.com

5.1 Introduction

The parotid tumours may be primary or secondary, such as lymph node metastases from carcinomas that drain into intraparotid lymph nodes. During their progression, the tumours may extend to overlying skin or the external ear. As external skin tumours could involve the parotid gland, also spinalioma, basaloid cell carcinoma or malignant melanoma occur as secondary parotid gland tumours. Depending on the structure affected by the neoplasia and the size of the defect, the reconstructive

© Springer International Publishing Switzerland 2016

V.-V. Costan (ed.), *Management of Extended Parotid Tumors*, DOI 10.1007/978-3-319-26545-2_5

techniques may be simple or complex, especially when other tissues are resected, such as the bones, muscles or the facial nerve.

5.2 Anatomical Relation

The extension of the gland is variable and can reach the lateral pharyngeal wall, the internal jugular vein or internal carotid artery. The parotid gland is completely enclosed by the parotid fascia. The facial nerve defines a superficial and a deep parotid portion, which is not congruent to anatomical lobes. The seventh cranial nerve leaves the skull base through the stylomastoid foramen, which is found in between the styloid and mastoid processes. The surgeon could identify the main trunk by following the cartilaginous auditory meatus, freeing the parotid gland from the mastoid process to a formation called the triangular process. The main trunk is found 10 mm caudally in a fatty, connective tissue area and divides into two main trunks and within the gland in several, at least five, branches, which have connections to neighbouring nerves as the auriculotemporal branch of the fifth cranial nerve, the auricular nerve and the transverse cervical nerve. These anastomoses could cause a difficult resection of the gland. To avoid facial nerve injuries, no muscle relaxation should be applied and a nerve stimulation should be used. In case of a complete superficial parotidectomy, the nerve branches can be followed starting from the main trunk, dissecting the parotid tissue above the nerve fibres after blunt dissection.

Another important nerve is the greater auricular nerve providing sensory function to the lower and posterior part of the auricular lobe. It arises from the cervical plexus and is easily found at the McKinney point (crossing of a vertical line drawn from the tragus and the sternocleidomastoid muscle).

The auriculotemporal nerve, a branch of the trigeminal nerve, passes through the parotid gland arising from the pterygomaxillary fossa and follows the superficial temporal vessels anteriorly to the auditory external meatus. In case of its injury, anastomoses of the auriculotemporal nerve and the parasympathetic fibres cause the so-called auriculotemporal syndrome or Frey syndrome, associated with gustatory sweating.

Important blood vessels, which could cause heavy bleeding, are the maxillay and the carotid arteries in the very deep space. To avoid a damage to these vessels, a surgical approach starting caudally and following the vessels to the scull base should be chosen. Such extended surgeries cause a partial resection of the mandible to gain space and visual control.

For plastic reconstruction after extended resection, the superficial temporal artery, which is found anteriorly to the meatus acusticus externus, and the facial artery crossing the mandible anterior to the antegonial notch and following the nasolabial fold are important anatomical structures.

Finally, the parotid duct is an important structure leaving the gland at the anterior border through the masseter muscle. It enters the oral cavity at the level of the second upper molar.

5.3 Symptoms

Mainly patients present a slow growing preauricular mass which finally infiltrates the skin leading to induration, erythema and ulceration. In cases with secondary parotid tumours, we can find the primary neoplasia on the facial skin, scalp or sometimes even submandibularly or intraorally. In patients with skin carcinoma or melanoma that directly infiltrate the gland, we can observe a big infiltrative and exophytic tumour on the topography of the parotid. If the tumour infiltrates external ear, hearing problems may be encountered.

5.4 Treatment Plan/Principle of Treatment: Surgery, Irradiation and Neck Dissection

For solid tumours of the gland, surgical removal of the tumour en bloc with the infiltrated structures is the first choice. The extent of resection or additional neck dissection depends on the tumour entity and the stage of disease. If a neck dissection is necessary, the surgeon needs to keep the recon-

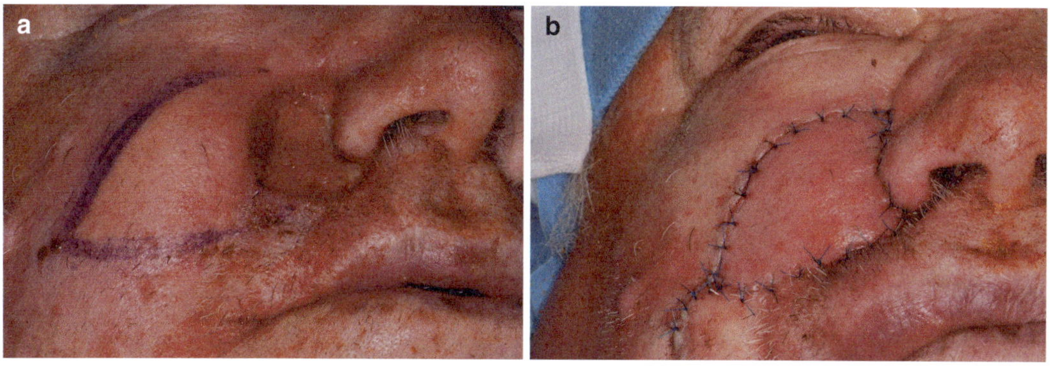

Fig. 5.1 (**a**, **b**) Example of local management of a small skin defect by a kite flap. The mobility is gained by an incision of the subcutaneous fat layer neighbouring the defect

struction in mind and plan the surgical access to the neck in a way that permits a sufficient blood supply and flap design.

Radiotherapy is applied in aggressive or inoperable tumours or in case the tumour was not removed completely. The indication for adjuvant radiotherapy depends on the histopathological characterizations of the tumour, as there are extracapsular spread and positive lymph node involvement. The reconstructive techniques depend on defect size and complexity as well as the general status of the patient. In cases with a general poor status, it is not recommended to perform complex covering operations, such as free flaps. The same consideration applies to nerve reconstruction if it was resected.

5.5 Reconstructive Options

The covering method must take into account the structures involved, the need for neck dissection or postoperative irradiation. Additional factors are the general health condition and the surgery time.

5.5.1 Tumours Extended to the Skin With or without the Involvement of the External Ear

In cases the tumour has infiltrated the external skin of the face, the reconstruction of the skin defect is necessary.

In general, local, regional and microvascular reconstructive techniques can be applied depending on the defect size and patient's general health situation and prognosis.

Local flaps can be distinguished in pivot, advancement and hinge flaps. The group of rotation, transposition, interpolated and island flaps belong to the group of pivot flaps. In case of nice soft tissue underlying the defect, a split skin graft is the easiest method to close the defect, but does not reconstruct the volume and has another skin texture. Local reconstruction techniques usually need less time to be performed and reduce the total anaesthesia time.

If the tumour infiltrates only the overlying skin and the defect is small, it can be closed primarily. One choice for the local reconstructive techniques is the *V/Y-flaps*. The blood is supplied by the underlying fat tissue. To mobilize the skin flap, the proximal part of the subcutaneous skin can be incised and the flap advanced (Fig. 5.1a, b).

Another local flap is the *bilobed flap*, taken from the cervical or even retroauricular region to cover the parotid region. First Esser described this technique 1918 to cover defects of the nose [1]. The axes of the lobes are designed with angulation 45° to each other but could also be modified and extended to 110° depending on the skin laxity. The height of the first lobe is defined by the bigger arch. The height of the second lobe should be twice that of the first lobe. The width of the first lobe corresponds to the defect size, and

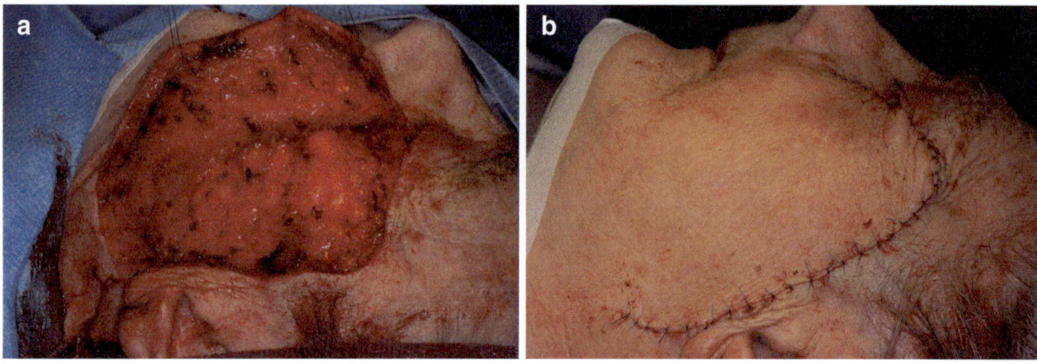

Fig. 5.2 (**a**, **b**) Larger defects of the cheek, the lower eyelid and the preauricular region can be reconstructed by a rotation of a cervicofacial flap. To prevent an ectropion in lower eyelid defects, the incision needs to be extended cranial to the lateral canthus

the width of the second lobe is slightly smaller than the first lobe. Alternatively, instead of a bilobed transposition flap, skin rotations could be applied. The decision from where to take the skin rotation is dependent on the region of defect; for defects near the lower jaw, a rotation from the cervical skin should be performed. For defects at the cranial part, rotations from the anterior cheek and the nasolabial fold could be applied. To avoid skin necrosis, the ratio of width and length of the flap should not exceed 1:2 or better, 2:3, especially if there was a neck dissection performed including a ligation of the facial vessels. The donor site usually can be closed primarily. To avoid "dog ears", a Burow triangle needs to be removed. For anterior/cranial defects of the cheek, the Esser cheek rotation is an approved technique (Fig. 5.2a, b). A preauricular defect could be closed by an advancement of the nasolabial skin. Another principle is the *transposition* of retroauricular skin to the preauricular region or region of the caudal parotid part. This technique provides quite thick skin coverage but also transposes hair from the head. The donor site can easily be covered by a split skin graft. Therefore, the transposition flap needs to be taken epiperiostal, so that the periosteum remains at retroauricular bone (Fig. 5.3). Instead of skin grafts, skin rotations of the scalp could be applied but could extend surgery time and often cause additional blood loss. As an alternative to flap rotations, a bilobed flap could be performed.

For regional flaps, the donor and recipient site are located at a significant distance from each other.

In severe cases with extended resections, the transposition of an *acromiopectoral flap*, supplied by the acromiopectoral vessels and taken from the upper chest and shoulder, is an effective and pretty simple technique to cover the defect. After 6 weeks, the flap could be repositioned to its former place. The remaining non-covered areas are reconstructed by free skin grafts. This flap, however, often suffers from venous insufficiency due to the flap's own weight. A dressing to lift the flap or single sutures could help to keep the flap elevated and prevent venous obliteration.

Other types of advancement flap are the cervicofacial or cervicopectoral flaps, techniques that advance and rotate the skin overlying the M. pectoralis major. The skin receives its blood supply from the medial part of the neck and the mammarial vessels at the thoracic part. Therefore, the median preparation needs to be performed with caution to prevent a damage to the vessels arising from the arteria mammaria interna. This flap could even be applied in combination with a musculocutaneous flap of the musculus pectoralis major, which is nutrited by the thoracoacromial vessels. First described in 1969 by Beare, the *cervicofacial flap* was modified by other surgeons, e.g. Mustarde, who applied it to cover orbital defects [2, 3]. The advantages are similar skin colour and texture to the facial skin. The scars can be easily hidden in the preauricular region.

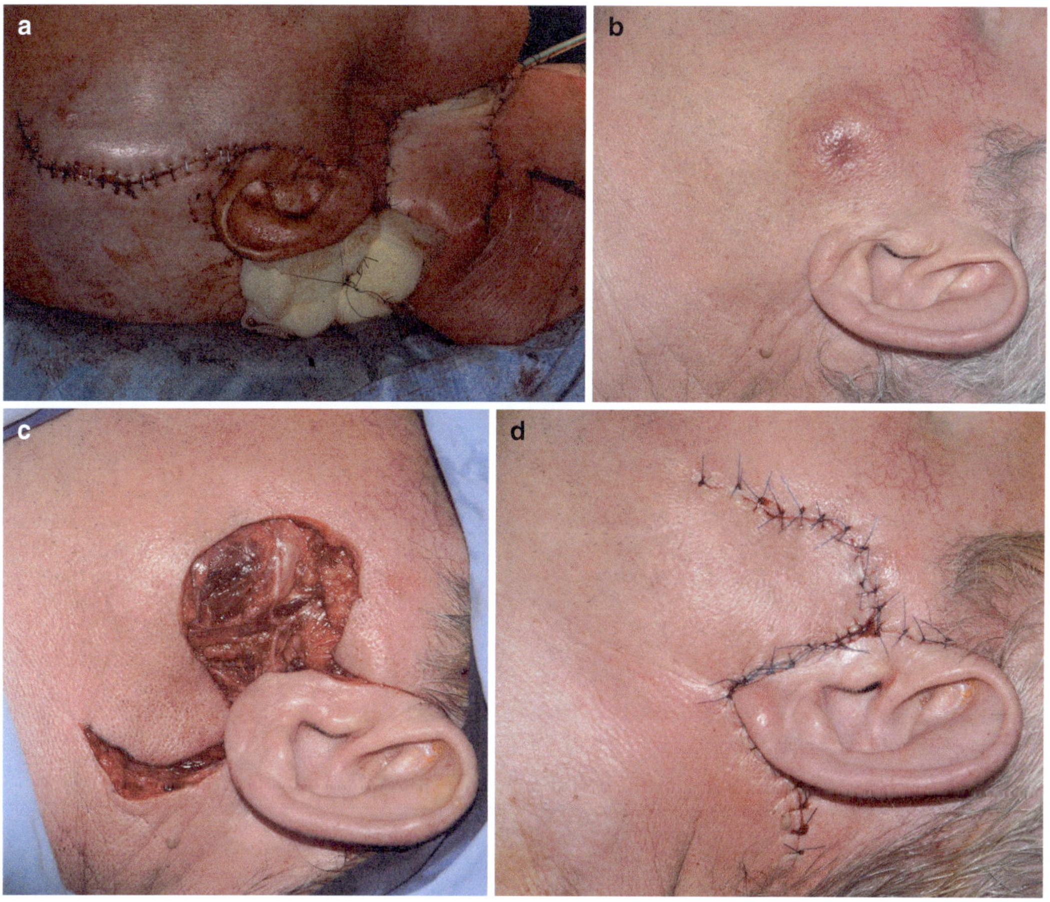

Fig. 5.3 (**a**) Transposition of skin from the retroauricular region to cover defects at the caudal pole of the parotid gland. The flap is harvested in a supraperiosteal layer to cover the donor site by a split skin graft. (**b–d**) Transposition of skin from the cervical region to cover a preauricular defect and direct closure of the donor site

Especially in elderly patients, this is technically easy to perform as the skin laxity allows good movement and the surgery time is limited. Attention has to be taken for the facial nerve, which is often resected in extended parotid gland tumours anyway. Another aspect emphasizes the venous congestion, as the flap is quite heavy and could compress its own veins. Therefore, some authors suggest an extension to the deeper superficial musculoaponeurotic system (SMAS) layer that, however, harms the facial nerve branches. For the coverage of the parotid region or cheek, the flap design should be extended higher than the lateral canthus, to prevent an ectropion. The flap is raised in the subcutaneous layer and in the cervical region as well as the face superficially to the SMAS. To support the heavy flap, additional sutures to release the tension can be applied. As already mentioned, this flap can be combined with the M. pectoralis major flap but also with free microvascular flaps. The donor site defect is usually closed primarily by undermining the surrounding tissue. If a primary closure is not possible, a free skin graft needs to be applied [4].

Defects of the orbit and the cheek could also be covered by a *scalping forehead flap*, which was first described by Converse in 1942 [5, 6]. By this approach, the skin of the forehead is transposed and rotated from the supraorbital region. The donor site needs to be covered by a skin graft. The advantage of this technique is the local approach and rather short surgery time. To

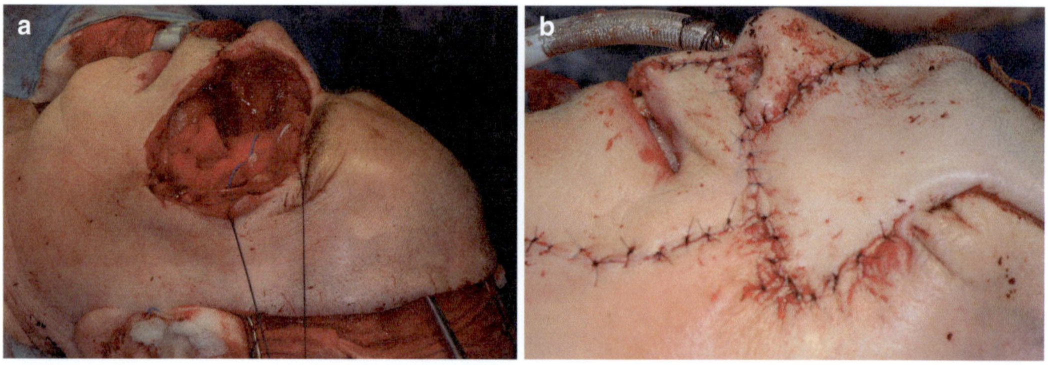

Fig. 5.4 This case of neuroendocrine carcinoma of the sinus maxillaris infiltrated the cheek as well as the eye and left a penetrating defect after resection (**a**). By a combination of a converse flap from the subraorbital region and a smaller rotation, the defect was closed (**b**) (Courtesy of Dr. H. Kuffner, University Medical Centre, Mainz)

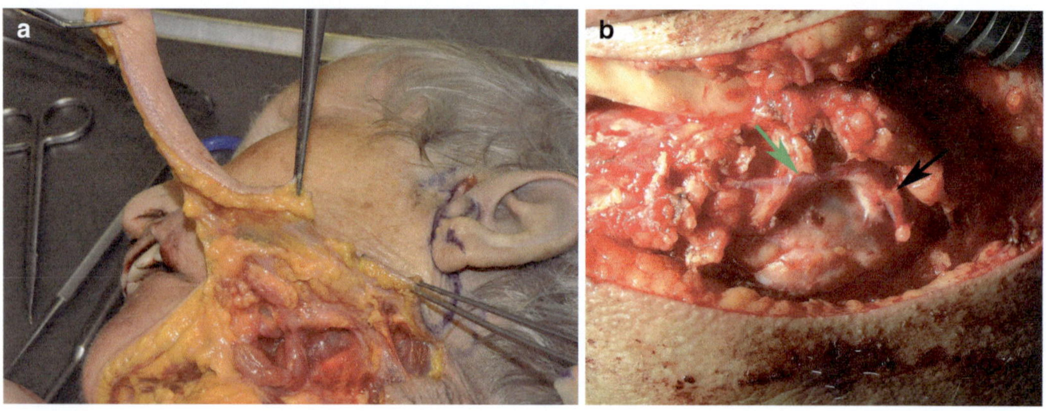

Fig. 5.5 The submental island flap reaches the caudal parotid pole and the preauricular region of the cheek as shown by this cadaver model (**a**). Care needs to be taken if a neck dissection is performed, as shown in (**b**), because the submandibular artery (*green arrow*) is easily damaged. It arises from the facial artery (*black arrow*) and is situated right to the submandibular gland (left submandibular neck region is shown)

achieve an acceptable aesthetic result, secondary correction could be necessary (Fig. 5.4a, b).

The *submental island flap* is another option to cover a defect ranging from the medial canthus to the zygomatic arch. The flap is pedicled by the submental artery, which arises from the facial artery (Fig. 5.5a, b). The flap preparation starts from the contralateral side after defining the amount of skin needed. In order not to damage the submental artery, the anterior digastric muscle is included in the flap. By nerve monitoring, the marginal branch of the facial nerve is preserved. The dissection of the submental artery to the facial artery permits a pedicle, long enough to cover defects of the cheek as well as intraorally at the ipsilateral side: a flap of up to 8 × 18 cm could be harvested.

The caudal part of the parotid gland can also be reconstructed by the *supraclavicular artery island flap*. This flap is supplied by the supraclavicular artery arising from the triangle of the musculus sternocleidomastoideus, clavicle and the external jugular vein. The two draining veins consist of a comitant vein and a second one, draining into the external jugular vein. The flap harvest starts at the deltoid region by an incision to the deltoid fascia, proceeding with a subfascial preparation towards the medial part until the middle of the clavicle is reached. Then a preparation in the subcutaneous layer continues to prevent

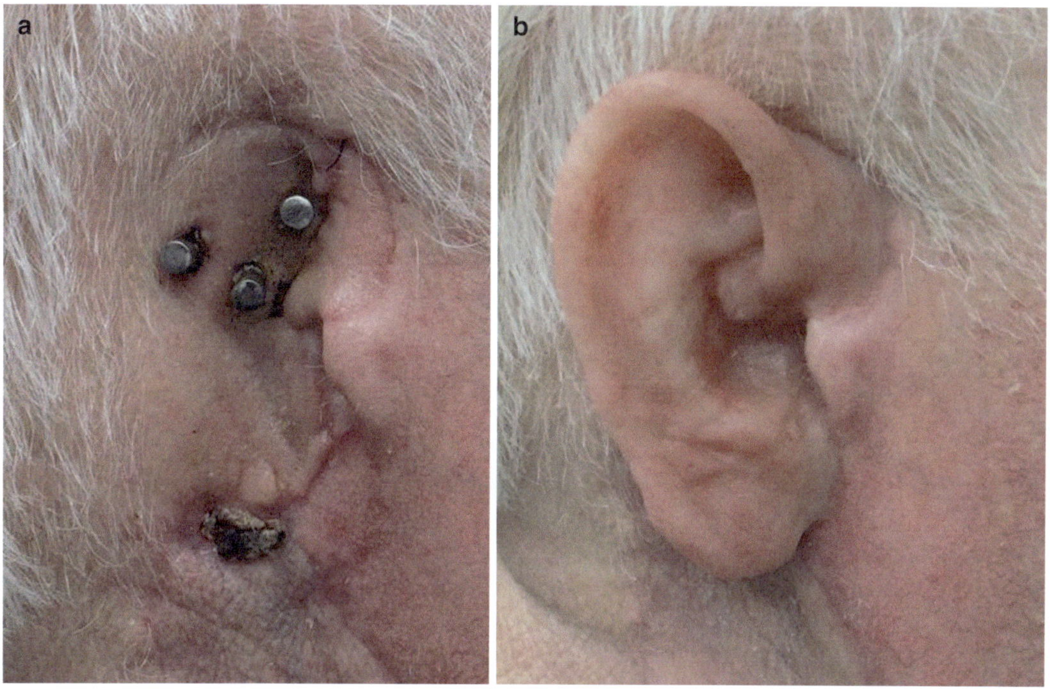

Fig. 5.6 Implant-supported magnets (**a**) to fix an external ear prosthesis (**b**) (Courtesy of Florian E. Raithel, Laboratory for Facial Prostheses)

any damage to the pedicle. After the flap harvest, it can be carefully rotated to cover the lower parts of the parotid region. The donor site can be closed primarily or by a split skin graft [7].

The external ear is usually reconstructed secondarily. For the transplantation of cartilage, good soft tissue coverage is necessary and is mostly performed by a two-stage approach. For cartilage donor site, the 8 to 10th costae are usually used by a small incision at the thoracic wall. The chest wall or pleura should not be damaged. In case the pleura is perforated, a thoracic Bulow drainage is applied. If just the thoracic wall is perforated, a close soft tissue closure is sufficient. To find a leakage, the wound is filled with NaCl water to check the appearance of bubbles. Alternatively, an ear prosthesis fixed by implants and magnets gives an uncomplicated and fast result with a good aesthetic outcome (Fig. 5.6).

Other common regional flaps are the M. trapezius flap, latissimus dorsi myocutaneous flap or the pectoralis major flap. These techniques, however, are described in other chapters of this book.

5.5.2 Tumours Involving Neighbouring Structures of the Bone and Muscle

During its evolution, the tumour may extend to bony structures, such as TMJ, mandible, temporal, sphenoid and malar bone, zygomatic arch, and to nearby muscles, such as sternocleidomastoid, massetericus, digastricus, external pterygoid and temporal muscles. In these cases, local flaps are not always enough, and we may need local regional or free flaps. If the skull base is involved, a myocutaneous flap would be recommended to seal the skull base and to protect from irradiation.

The application of myocutaneous flaps is discussed in other chapters of this book as there are the m. pectoralis major flap, the M. sternocleidomastoideus flap, the platysma flap, the M. trapezius flap and the M. latissimus dorsi flap.

The microvascular technique provides a variety of flaps to cover defects of different sizes ranging from latissimus dorsi or ALT flaps for big defects and lack of soft tissue to the radial forearm flap for smaller defects. Composite defects, including the reconstruction of the bone and skin, sometimes require even the application of a free fibula flap. At the recipient site, the A and V. temporalis superficialis or any other cervical vessels, preferably the facial artery with a rather long course or lingual artery could be used.

If the tumour involved the external ear, we may try to reconstruct it in a second operation using ear prothesis which can be fixed with adhesive or implants and magnets.

5.6 Complications

As a complication, the parotid gland surgery can be associated with gustatory sweating, known as auriculotemporal syndrome, described by Frey. It is associated with sweating in the region of the cheek and forehead and caused by the auriculotemporal nerve stimulating salivary secretion. The sweating usually occurs while eating. The auriculotemporal nerve in its course along the posterior aspect of the parotid gland carries parasympathetic fibres, which supply motor innervation of secretory function in the parotid gland, and sympathetic fibres, which innervate sweat glands in the skin. By an injury of the nerve, these fibres could get connected by a short circuiting of impulses. Therefore, the salivary stimulus, which would normally evoke secretion of saliva, results in sweating of the forehead and cheek skin. Another common complication after parotid gland surgery is a saliva fistula. The fixation of a bandage to bring pressure onto the fistula is the first aid in this case. If this does not help, the application of botulinum toxin type A prevents the production of saliva and closes the fistula.

Other common complications are facial paralysis, which could be addressed by an immediate nerve reconstruction or other techniques, like McLaughlin's (1952) or a microvascular free m. gracilis transfer [8]. Due to the lack of volume after tumour resection, a facial asymmetry could occur, which could be addressed by the choice of reconstruction. Secondarily, a free fat transfer helps to augment the soft tissue. An ectropion occurs due to scarring after resection, aggravated by radiotherapy. Also the paralysis of the facial nerve causes an ectropion. Additional tissue transfer, e.g. by a forehead flap, and in case of rotation flaps, the extension more cranially to the lateral canthus could help.

References

1. Esser JFS. Gestielte lokale Lappenplastik mit zweizipfeligen Lappen, Deckung des sekundären Defetes vom ersten Zipfel durch den zweiten. Dtsch Z Chir. 1918;143:385–90.
2. Beare R. Flap repair following exenteration of the orbit. Proc R Soc Med. 1969;62(11 Part 1):1087–90.
3. Mustarde JC. The use of flaps in the orbital region. Plast Reconstr Surg. 1970;45(2):146–50.
4. Fernandes R. Local and regional flaps in head and neck reconstruction. a practical approach. Hoboken: Wiley; 2015.
5. Converse JM. New forehead flap for nasal reconstruction. Proc R Soc Med. 1942;35:811.
6. Converse JM, McCarthy JG. The scalping forehead flap revisited. Clin Plast Surg. 1981;8(3):413–34.
7. Martin D, Pascal JF, Baudet J, Mondie JM, Farhat JB, Athoum A, et al. The submental island flap: a new donor site. Anatomy and clinical applications as a free or pedicled flap. Clin Plast Surg. 1993;92(5):867–73.
8. McLaughlin CR. Permanent facial paralysis; the role of surgical support. Lancet. 1952;2(6736):647–51.

Parotid Tumors with Muscle Extension

6

Orlando Guntinas-Lichius

Abstract

The diagnosis of a parotid tumors with muscle extension is usually and primarily established by clinical examination, ultrasonography and fine-needle aspiration cytology (FNAC). Ultrasonography is limited to clearly depict the tumor infiltration in or into the deep parotid lobe and to exhibit the exact muscle infiltration. As most of the tumors will muscle extension will be malignant, additional radiological imaging by MRI or CT is required to define the tumor extension and for tumor staging. Treatment of choice is complete surgical excision. Most frequently, total parotidectomy will be the starting approach or radical parotidectomy if parts of the facial nerve are infiltrated. Only these parts should be resected under control of frozen section. Best facial reanimation is achieved if facial nerve reconstruction surgery directly follows the tumor removal in the same surgical session. Any malignant tumor needs in addition a neck dissection. A wide approach, the parapharyngeal space, is necessary if muscle infiltration takes place in this area. All infiltrated muscle parts are radically resected. The muscle resection itself normally does not indicate special reconstructive surgery. In high-risk malignant tumors, surgery is followed by postoperative radiotherapy.

6.1 Introduction

Parotid tumors with muscle extension, i.e., a situation where the tumor has infiltrated a muscle in the neighborhood of the parotid gland space, let primarily think of a malignant parotid tumor and less of a benign salivary gland neoplasm [1, 2]. Multinodular recurrences of pleomorphic adenoma sometimes present with tumor spread also into muscles surrounding the parotid space. Benign salivary gland neoplasms are relatively common, whereas malignant salivary gland tumors are rare. The parotid gland is the most frequent site of benign (80 % are pleomorphic adenomas) and also of the malignant tumors [3].

The parotid gland is located between the posterior border of the mandible and the mastoid process of the temporal bone. The deep layer is attached to the mandible and the temporal bone at

O. Guntinas-Lichius, MD
Department of Otorhinolaryngology,
University Hospital Jena, Jena, Germany
e-mail: orlando.guntinas@med.uni-jena.de

© Springer International Publishing Switzerland 2016

V.-V. Costan (ed.), *Management of Extended Parotid Tumors*, DOI 10.1007/978-3-319-26545-2_6

the tympanic plate and styloid and mastoid processes. The superficial surface of the parotid gland is covered with skin and platysma muscle. Therefore, a parotid tumor can extend into the platysma. Normally, this does not lead to any specific symptoms. Anteriorly, the gland lies over the masseter muscle and the posterior border of the mandible. The masseter may be infiltrated by large parotid tumor with anterior extension. The parotid duct emerges from the anterior border of the parotid gland and passes horizontally across the masseter muscle. This is the reason why salivary duct carcinoma of the parotid may also infiltrate the masseter muscle. As the gland wraps around the ramus, it is related to the medial pterygoid muscle at its insertion onto the deep aspect of the angle. Here, a tumor can invade the pterygoid muscles. Posteriorly, the parotid is molded around the styloid process and the styloglossus, stylohyoid, and stylopharyngeus muscles from below upwards causing the next possibilities of muscle extensions. Behind this, the parotid lies on the posterior belly of the digastric muscle and the sternocleidomastoid muscle. These two muscles can also be infiltrated. In summary, the most frequent sites of a muscles extension of a parotid tumor are masseter muscle, pterygoid muscles, digastric muscle, sternocleidomastoid muscle, styloglossus, stylohyoid, and the stylopharyngeus muscles.

6.2 Symptoms

Clinical features of parotid tumors are presented in more detail in Chap. 10. Benign salivary gland tumors normally grow slowly and over a long time. They often become obvious, more or less by chance, only as a new palpable or visible lump anterior or inferior to the ear. Later, as large tumors, they can create a cosmetically unattractive mass on the face. As the tumor increases in size, it can affect swallowing and breathing, depending on its location. Infiltration of the masseter or of the pterygoid muscles can cause pain and functional limitations when clenching the teeth. A trismus, i.e., a spasm of the muscles of mastication, can occur and might lead to reduced opening of the jaws. Infiltration of the sternocleidomastoid muscle may be noticed by limited head rotation. Other muscle infiltrations (digastric, styloglossus, stylohyoid, and stylopharyngeus) normally do not cause specific symptoms. Infiltration of muscles can come along with a skin infiltration (Fig. 6.1).

6.3 Diagnostics

The diagnostics are presented in detail in Chaps. 10 and 11. The diagnosis is usually established by clinical examination, ultrasonography, and fine-needle aspiration cytology (FNAC). If FNAC is not available, frozen section is the worse alternative because detailed surgical planning knowing in advance to be faced with a malignant tumor is not possible. Open biopsy is normally not recommended because of the risk of tumor cell spreading, except for a situation of a tumor with skin infiltration. As many of the parotid tumors with muscle extension refer to malignant tumors, additional staging is necessary: magnetic resonance imaging (MRI) for the staging of the primary tumor and simultaneously of the neck is first choice (Fig. 6.2) [4]. Computed tomography (CT) is the alternative if MRI is not available. In advanced malignant tumors (stages III and IV), an additional CT of the chest is recommended to rule out lung metastasis. Further imaging is complied with individual symptoms.

6.4 Surgery

Surgery is the standard treatment for all benign parotid tumors and for all resectable malignant parotid tumors. Radiation alone has not proved to be curative in larger series, especially not for parotid tumors with muscle extension. The aim of surgery is to completely remove the tumor and to preserve the facial nerve if not infiltrated. If the nerve is tumor infiltrated, partial or total nerve resection is necessary. Final histology and histological risk criteria are necessary to decide if postoperative radiotherapy is indicated. Chemotherapy normally is reserved of palliative cases. Benign

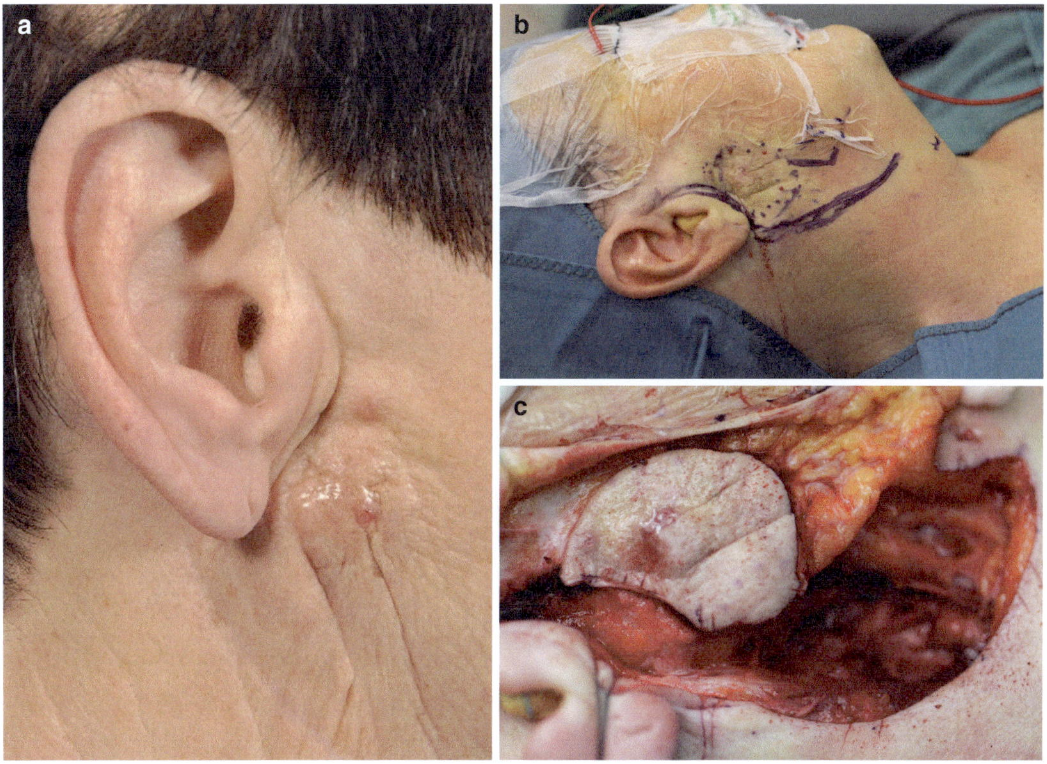

Fig. 6.1 Clinical and intraoperative situs of the same patient. (**a**) Tumor recurrence with skin infiltration. (**b**) Resection lines and intraoperative facial monitoring. (**c**) Skin resection area resected in toto with the underlying tumor

parotid tumors with muscle extension are normally large as first the parotid space will be filled in by the tumor before the muscle infiltration or extrusion starts. Therefore, most benign parotid tumors with muscle extension will need a total parotidectomy. In cases with exclusive muscle extrusion, this will be sufficient. Only in case of muscle infiltration (that might be the result of a secondary inflammation rather than by a direction tumor infiltration) additional resection of the involved muscle will be necessary. The standard surgical procedure for parotid cancer will almost always be a total parotidectomy. Lateral parotidectomy may be sufficient only for small, superficial, low-grade malignant tumors with no evidence of lymph node metastasis and/or nerve invasion, particularly if the tumor is located in the inferior parotid portion – but such tumors normally do not show a muscle infiltration. If the patient has a facial palsy and facial nerve infiltration is confirmed during surgery, radical parotidectomy is indicated.

6.4.1 Preparation of Surgery

Informed consent discussing the surgical steps, its complication, and information about therapeutical alternatives is mandatory. Surgery is usually performed in general anesthesia. Facial nerve monitoring may be helpful. Using an operating microscope is recommend to detect or rule out facial nerve infiltration and if facial nerve resection and reconstruction is necessary. In general, parotid surgery should always be performed using a microscope or loupe magnification.

6.4.2 Superficial Parotidectomy

Superficial parotidectomy means the complete removal of the parotid tissue lateral to the facial plexus [5]. Thereby, it implies a complete dissection of the facial nerve and its plexus. In most cases a standard preauricular-submandibular inci-

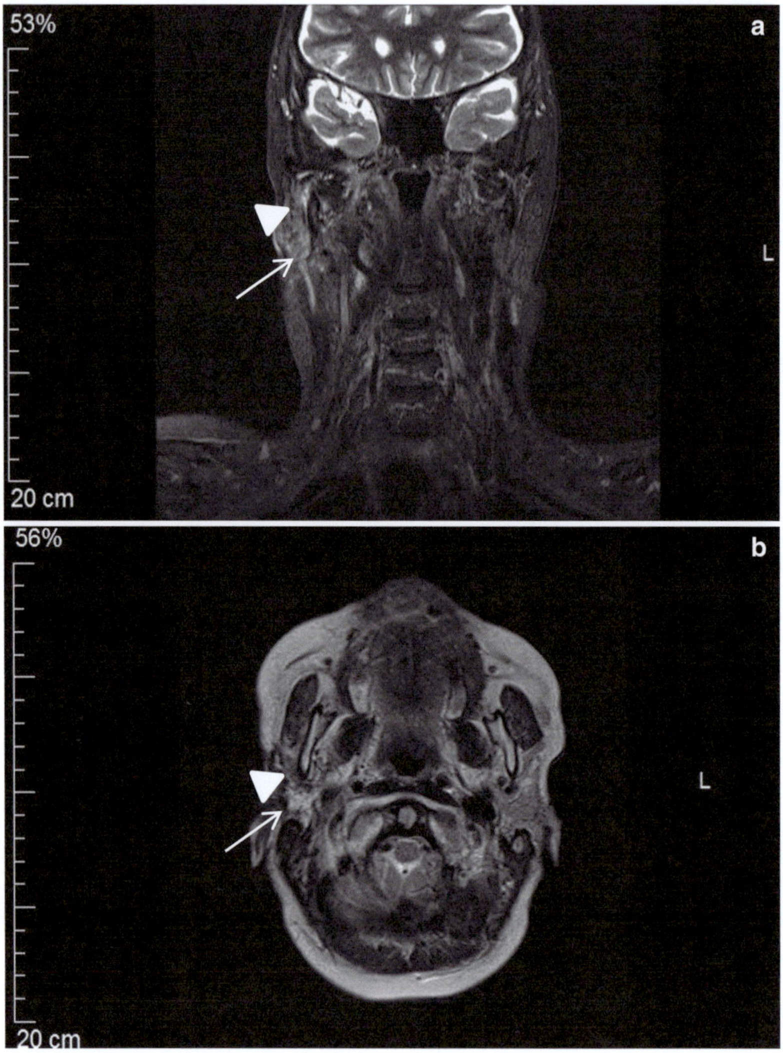

Fig. 6.2 MRI showing a deep lobe recurrence of a adenocarcinoma of the right parotid with infiltration of the masseter muscle in the same patients as in Fig. 6.1. (**a**) Sagittal view. (**b**) Axial view. *Arrow* parotid cancer, *Arrrowhead* masseter muscle infiltration

sion is used. Standard approach to expose is an anterograde approach exposing the main trunk of the facial nerve in the preauricular region [6]. In large tumors filling the preauricular region, this may not be possible. In these cases, and if the facial nerve is enclosed in the tumor close to its trunk or bifurcation, it may be necessary to change the surgical approach from an anterograde to a retrograde approach to identify the facial nerve [7]. The dissection of the facial nerve is primarily directing the surgery and not the tumor itself. When using an anterograde approach, each peripheral branch of the facial nerve is dissected from proximal to distal until it leaves the parotid space. Depending on the tumor localization, the preparation starts superior with the frontal branch inferior with the ramus colli or with marginal mandibular branch. Sometimes, in cases with larger extended tumors, it might be necessary to switch back and force between superior and interior preparation. Finally, the plane of the facial nerve is completely freed and thereby automatically the lateral parotid. If the tumor is part of the lateral parotid, it is resected, too. When using a retrograde approach, the frontal branch of the facial nerve can be located and identified in the first third of a line between the tragus and the lateral canthus. The subcutaneous fat on the zygomatic arch is spread perpendicularly until the frontal branch becomes visible. The facial nerve is then dissected retrogradely toward the bifurcation until the next branch becomes visible and so on. Finally, the superficial parotid gland lobe is dissected as a whole, as it would be with an anterograde approach.

6.4.3 Total Parotidectomy

Total parotidectomy is defined as complete dissection of the facial nerve and removal of all parotid gland tissue lateral to the facial nerve in combination with a resection of the deep lobe [8–10]. Total parotidectomy including resection of the intraparotid gland lymph nodes will be the minimal approach in most parotid tumors with muscle extension. Surgery starts with lateral parotidectomy (see Sect. 6.4.2). Thereafter, the facial plexus and the peripheral facial nerve branches lifted gently as far as needed to resect the deep lobe (Fig. 6.3). The borders of the dissection of the deep lobe (the extension of the tumor might need to cross some of these borders) are as follows: cranially, the ear cartilage and skull base define the border of the resection area; at the other end, caudally, the cervical lymph nodes, depending on the extent of neck dissection (see Sect. 6.4.8), mark the border of resection; dorsally, the border is the sternocleidomastoid muscle; and ventrally, the surgeon respects the ascending mandible and adjacent muscles (masseter and pterygoid muscles) as surgical margins. Larger vessels like the maxillary artery and retromandibular vein have to be ligated. Finally, the retromandibular space is limited medially by the styloid process.

6.4.4 Radical Parotidectomy

Radical parotidectomy is defined as resection of all parotid gland tissue with complete or incomplete sacrifice of the facial nerve [11]. Once more, it has to be emphasized that nowadays the strategy is to preserve that facial nerve if not infiltrated. From an oncological point of view, it is not justified to resect an intact facial to guarantee wide surgical margins. The results with such a traditional, antiquated approach are not better than with nerve-preserving surgery. To spare as much healthy nerve branches as possible, the resection should be performed under the microscope and accompanied by frozen section until tumor-free nerve stumps are obtained.

6.4.5 Approaches to the Parapharyngeal Space

Most extended parotid rumor located in or invaded into the parapharyngeal space can be resected with either a parotid or a transcervical approach [12]. A transoral approach normally is not an alternative. A transoral approach does not allow a resection in safe margins, especially in cases with muscle infiltration and in patients with extended parotid tumor. In patients with parotid tumors with muscle extension, especially into the deep pterygoid muscles, a parotid or a transcervical approach does not provide adequate access to the parapharyngeal space. In these cases, an open midline mandibulotomy approach might be necessary [13, 14]. After the total parotidectomy, the posterior belly of the digastric is exposed. The carotid artery and the cranial nerves of the area, the vagal, the accessory, and the hypoglossal nerve are followed toward the base of the skull. The tumor is dissected the parapharyngeal space, if possible by blunt dissection. Dividing the stylomandibular ligament will help to widen the approach. The tumor is mobilized step by step. The mass must be frequently controlled to ensure that all of the tumor and directions of its infiltration are inside the tumor margins. The standard cervical incision, placed in an upper neck crease, from the parotidectomy and upper neck dissection is extended medially to the mental foramen region. From here, the skin incision is extended on the chin using a broken line technique to ensure favorable cosmetic results. The soft tissue of the chin, as well as the floor of the mouth with

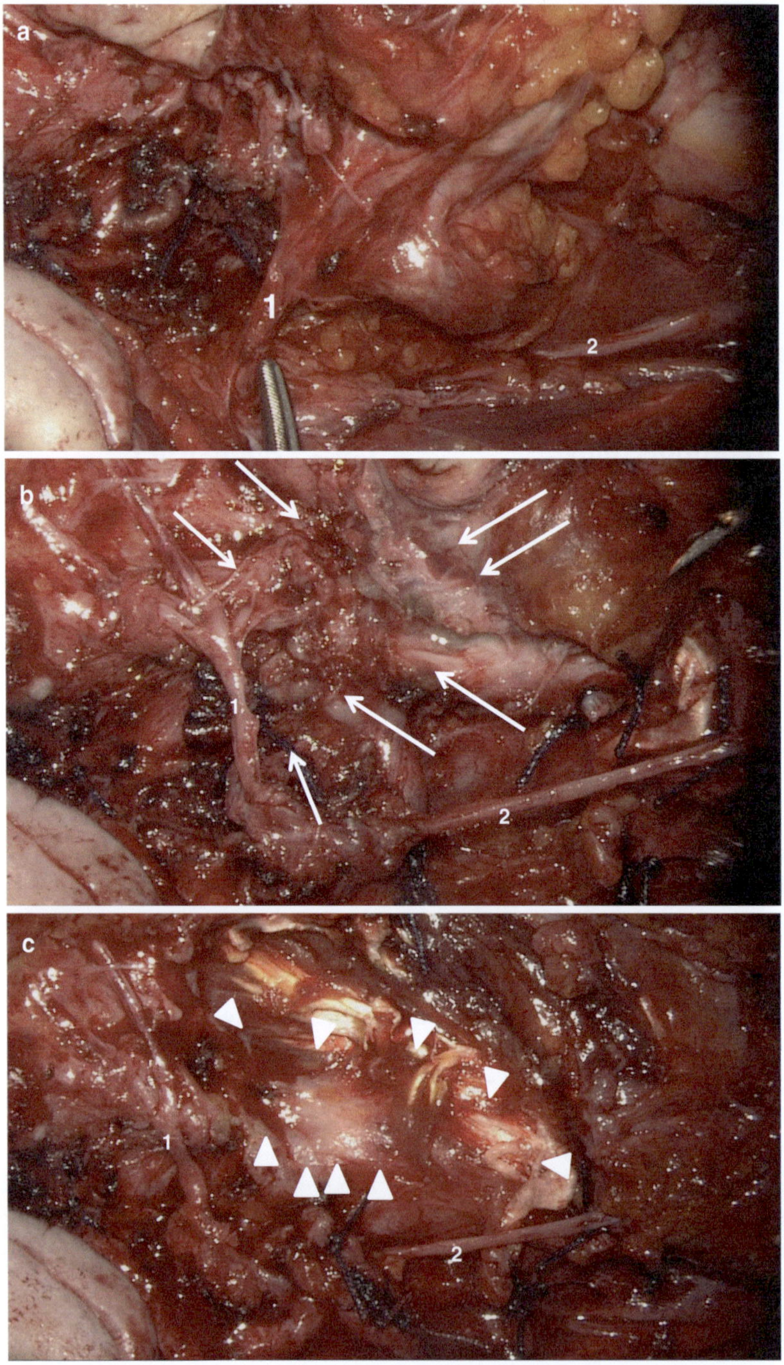

Fig. 6.3 Intraoperative situs of the same patient as in Figs. 6.1 and 6.2. (**a**) Situs after total parotidectomy. (**b**) Exposition of the tumor in the retromandibular space with masseter muscle infiltration. (**c**) Situs after tumor resection including partial resection of the masseter muscle. *1* temporofacial main branch of facial nerve, *2* cervicofacial main branch of facial nerve, *Arrows* tumor infiltration of the parapharyngeal space and the masseter muscle, *Arrowheads* area of the masseter muscle resection

the mylohyoid muscle and the digastric muscle is transected. The anterior osteotomy starts at the inferior edge of the mandible. To avoid damage to adjacent tooth roots, the osteotomy is performed perpendicularly in the symphysis. The mandible is rotated laterally and cranially and opens wide, providing an overview of the parapharyngeal space and the tumor invasion into the area. The complete pterygoid fossa and the skull base with the descending vessels and nerves can be optimally observed. This surgery ends after tumor removal with the osteosynthesis of the mandible using compression miniplates to allow precise adjustment of the mandible parts preventing malocclusion.

6.4.6 Surgery of the Tumor Extension into the Musculature

In cases of parotid tumors with muscle extension, an extended parotidectomy approach is necessary as the involved muscle parts have to be resected. This may include the resection of the masseter muscle or parts of the ascending portion of the mandible. To reach the area, a transzygomatic approach to the infratemporal fossa and cranial base is an option. Using this way, an involvement of the pterygoid muscles in the infratemporal fossa is also possible. Hereby, this larger approach has also the advantage to have a better view into the situs to ensure that the internal carotid artery, the hypoglossal, and other cranial nerves are not damaged. Patients with masseter muscle infiltration are likely to require extended-type procedures for complete tumor clearance. Therefore, an additional approach is normally not necessary. After total parotidectomy, the masseter is completely exposed, and infiltrated parts can be resected. The resection of infiltrated muscles itself, be it the masseter, pterygoid, sternocleidomastoid, digastric, styloglossus, stylohyoid, or the stylopharyngeus muscle, normally do not need special measures of reconstructive surgery.

6.4.7 Facial Nerve Reconstruction

The facial nerve is topic of Chap. 21. Briefly, facial nerve resection is only recommended for patients with preoperative facial palsy and tumor infiltration of the facial nerve [15]. If only one or some branches of the facial nerve are involved, it is recommended to resect those that are infiltrated, leaving the main stem and the unaffected branches intact. This makes the reconstruction much easier and results in better functional outcome. In tumors that completely infiltrate the facial plexus, nerve grafts, hypoglossal-facial jump nerve suture, or a combination of these techniques (combined approach) are methods of choice for facial nerve rehabilitation [16]. If branches of the facial nerve have to be removed, immediate reconstruction will give the best functional results. Nerves grafting using the great auricular nerve or sural nerve are the method of choice in the majority of patients. Closure of the eye can be restored at the same time or later at best by implanting an upper eye lid weights (details in Chap. 22). The angle of the mouth can be alternatively restored with dynamic muscle palsy or a static suspension plasty with fascia.

6.4.8 Neck Dissection

In case of malignant tumors with muscle extension, a neck dissection is mandatory. Because of the muscle extension, most often the patients have to be classified as high-risk patients. That means that even in a clinical N0 situation, a radical-modified neck dissection is indicated as it is in all clinical N+ cases [17]. If muscles of the neck (primarily the sternocleidomastoid muscle) are infiltrated, a radical neck dissection is indicated. It might be better to start surgery with the neck dissection before approaching the primary parotid tumor, because this will help to identify the large neck vessels and cranial nerve for their later preservation at the base of the skull.

6.5 Nonsurgical Treatment

Indications for radiotherapy and chemotherapy are presented in Chaps. 24 and 25. Briefly, post-operative radiotherapy is indicated to improve local and regional control of disease in patients with extended parotid cancer. Chemotherapy is reserved for palliative care in metastatic disease or locoregional recurrence that is not amenable to further surgery or radiotherapy.

References

1. Shah K, Javed F, Alcock C, Shah KA, Pretorius P, Milford CA. Parotid cancer treatment with surgery followed by radiotherapy in Oxford over 15 years. Ann R Coll Surg Engl. 2011;93(3):218–22. PubMed.
2. Ch'ng S, Ashford BG, Gao K, McGuinness J, Clark JR. Reconstruction of post-radical parotidectomy defects. Plast Reconstr Surg. 2012;129(2):275e–87. PubMed.
3. Carlson ER, Webb DE. The diagnosis and management of parotid disease. Oral Maxillofac Surg Clin North Am. 2013;25(1):31–48. v. PubMed.
4. Friedman ER, Saindane AM. Pitfalls in the staging of cancer of the major salivary gland neoplasms. Neuroimag Clin N Am. 2013;23(1):107–22. PubMed.
5. Tweedie DJ, Jacob A. Surgery of the parotid gland: evolution of techniques, nomenclature and a revised classification system. Clin Otolaryngol. 2009;34(4):303–8. PubMed.
6. O'Regan B, Bharadwaj G, Elders A. Techniques for dissection of the facial nerve in benign parotid surgery: a cross specialty survey of oral and maxillofacial and ear nose and throat surgeons in the UK. Br J Oral Maxillofac Surg. 2008;46(7):564–6. PubMed.
7. Yu GY. Superficial parotidectomy through retrograde facial nerve dissection. J R Coll Surg Edinb. 2001;46(2):104–7. PubMed.
8. Guntinas-Lichius O, Klussmann JP, Wittekindt C, Stennert E. Parotidectomy for benign parotid disease at a university teaching hospital: Outcome of 963 operations. Laryngoscope. 2006;116(4):534–40. PubMed.
9. Jouzdani E, Yachouh J, Costes V, Faillie JL, Cartier C, Poizat F, et al. Prognostic value of a three-grade classification in primary epithelial parotid carcinoma: result of a histological review from a 20-year experience of total parotidectomy with neck dissection in a single institution. Eur J Cancer. 2010;46(2):323–31. PubMed.
10. Olsen KD, Moore EJ. Deep lobe parotidectomy: clinical rationale in the management of primary and metastatic cancer. Eur Arch Otorhinolaryngol. 2014;271: 1181–5.
11. Guntinas-Lichius O, Klussmann JP, Schroeder U, Quante G, Jungehuelsing M, Stennert E. Primary parotid malignoma surgery in patients with normal preoperative facial nerve function: outcome and long-term postoperative facial nerve function. Laryngoscope. 2004;114(5):949–56. PubMed.
12. Kanzaki S, Nameki H. Standardised method of selecting surgical approaches to benign parapharyngeal space tumours, based on pre-operative images. J Laryngol Otol. 2008;122(6):628–34. PubMed.
13. Kolokythas A, Eisele DW, El-Sayed I, Schmidt BL. Mandibular osteotomies for access to select parapharyngeal space neoplasms. Head Neck. 2009;31(1): 102–10. PubMed.
14. Jungehuelsing M, Guntinas-Lichius O, Klussmann JP, Eckel HE, Stennert E. Modifications of the midline mandibulotomy for access to the parapharyngeal space. Laryngoscope. 2010;120(8):1557–62. PubMed.
15. Guntinas-Lichius O. The facial nerve in the presence of a head and neck neoplasm: assessment and outcome after surgical management. Curr Opin Otolaryngol Head Neck Surg. 2004;12(2):133–41. PubMed.
16. Volk GF, Pantel M, Guntinas-Lichius O. Modern concepts in facial nerve reconstruction. Head Face Med. 2010;6:25. PubMed Epub 2010/11/03.
17. Stennert E, Kisner D, Jungehuelsing M, Guntinas-Lichius O, Schroder U, Eckel HE, et al. High incidence of lymph node metastasis in major salivary gland cancer. Arch Otolaryngol Head Neck Surg. 2003;129(7):720–3. PubMed.

7 Parotid Tumors with Bone Extensions

Constantin-Cătălin Ciocan-Pendefunda, Marius Dabija, and Victor-Vlad Costan

Abstract

Parotid tumors may extend during their evolution to the surrounding soft tissues but also to bone structures. Due to anatomical relations of the gland, the most often infiltrated bones are temporal mandibular joint, mandible (ascending ramus or angle), malar bone, and zygomatic arch and rarely temporal bone, mastoid, styloid process, and sphenoid. Surgery is the first option for all resectable parotid tumors with bone involvement. In order to get free margins, the resection specimen must include en bloc the parotid tumor and infiltrated subjacent bone. The reconstructive necessities must take into consideration the status of the patients, the complexity of the defect, and, depending on the histological diagnose and preoperative clinical and paraclinical examination, the need to perform an additional neck dissection. An option to achieve an optimal result is the use of bony free flaps or grafts to reconstruct bone defects. The missing soft tissues may be addressed with local, regional, or microsurgical flaps in order to reestablish facial symmetry. There are cases where the reconstruction of bone defects is not mandatory, such as sphenoid or temporal bone resection, and only bringing enough soft tissue is enough to achieve a good esthetic and functional outcome. In patients where, due to poor general status, a free flap is not possible, pedicle myocutaneous flaps, such as major pectoralis flap, are the method of choice. Latissimus dorsi or other

C.-C. Ciocan-Pendefunda, MD, DMD, PhD (✉)
Department of Oral and Maxillofacial Surgery, Fachklinik Hornheide Münster, Nordrhein-Westfalen, Germany
e-mail: catalinciocan2004@yahoo.com

M. Dabija, MD, PhD
Department of Neurosurgery, Faculty of General Medicine, "Grigore T. Popa" University of Medicine and Pharmacy, Iasi, Romania
e-mail: mariusdabija2003@yahoo.com

V.-V. Costan, MD, DMD, PhD
Department of Oral and Maxillo-Facial Surgery, Faculty of Dental Medicine, "Grigore T. Popa" University of Medicine and Pharmacy, "St. Spiridon" University Hospital Iasi, Iasi, Romania
e-mail: victorcostan@gmail.com

© Springer International Publishing Switzerland 2016

V.-V. Costan (ed.), *Management of Extended Parotid Tumors*, DOI 10.1007/978-3-319-26545-2_7

myocutaneous, either pedicle or microsurgical, flaps are very useful for defects which involve the skull base, preventing cerebral fluid leakage. Postoperative complications and sequelae depend directly on the type of bone resected and reconstruction technique.

7.1 Introduction

Over the last decades, there has been significant improvement in treatment of extended parotid tumors despite their involvement in nearby structures, large postoperative defect, and subsequent sequelae.

These tumors can involve tissues such as the temporal and mandibular bone, skin, muscles, external and middle ear, zygomatic arch, and malar bone [1].

Postoperative sequelae, like facial paralysis, paralytic lagophtalmos, ectropion, facial asymmetry, and the loss of the sensibility of the ear lobe, are very common after tumor resection and are difficult to treat [2]. If we do not reconstruct these complex defects as good as possible for each case, the risk of invalidating functional and esthetic sequelae for patients is very high [3, 4].

Another problem in these cases is the age of the patients. Extended parotid tumors are more often seen in elderly people with many general diseases, such as diabetes, high blood pressure, and other heart diseases. All these comorbidities have a big impact when choosing the best reconstructive technique.

Extended parotid tumors can arise from glandular tissue (primary tumors), or they can be secondary after direct invasion of the gland from carcinoma or malignant melanoma of the skin, or after involvement of parotid lymph nodes from nearby skin or oropharynx malignant tumors [5], and also from primary thyroid and renal malignancies. From our experience, we have noticed that the intraparotid lymph node metastases tend to extend more often to bone than to skin.

Extended parotid tumors with bone involvement are rare and mainly malignant. Due to anatomical relations of the gland, these malignancies may infiltrate the mandible (ascending ramus or angle), temporal mandibular joint (TMJ), malar bone, and zygomatic arch and more rarely in their evolution temporal bone, sphenoid, mastoid, and styloid process.

The reconstruction technique aims to reestablish mainly function and facial symmetry. There are cases, such as zygomatic, temporal, or sphenoid bone resection, in which the symmetry is obtained without bone augmentation, but only with soft tissue covering and filling techniques and combined later with lipofilling. In the last two cases, it is very important to seal watertight the skull base to prevent cerebral fluid leakage and subsequent complications, such as meningitis or fistulas. In patients with temporal mandibular joint involvement, after the removal of the tumor en bloc with TMJ, no special reconstruction technique for bony defect is required.

7.2 Anatomy

The parotid lies itself behind the ascending ramus of the mandible, between mastoid and external ear conduct. Superiorly it is delimitated by zygomatic arch, but in evolution the tumors may come into relation with malar bone, styloid process, temporal bone, and temporal mandibular joint, and when the deep lobe is involved, the neoplastic process may reach to sphenoid bone.

7.3 Symptoms

Clinical features depend on the type of tumor (primary or secondary) and the structures involved.

Commonly, a primary parotid or a lymph node metastatic tumor presents as a hard rapid growing mass anterior, inferior, or posterior to the ear, which is fixed to surrounding tissues. The differential diagnosis between these two is made by the presence in anamneses of a primary neoplasm, from skin or oropharynx, which could drain into the parotid lymph nodes.

In cases with secondary tumors after direct invasion from skin carcinomas, patients present an ulcerative and infiltrative lesion in the parotid region that extends to underlying structures.

In evolution, these tumors may involve the bones leading to specific clinical manifestations.

Patients with the involvement of temporal mandibular joint or ascending ramus of the mandible present a parotid tumor associated with a limited mouth opening and in late phases may associate pathological fractures of the mandible. Infiltration of the inferior alveolar nerve determines sensitivity problems of the lip.

The infiltration of temporal bone and mastoid may determine hearing loss, headache, facial numbness [6], vestibular problems, and tinnitus [7].

In evolution, all these tumors may present pain and may lead to facial paralyses and asymmetry, breathing problems, and dysphagia. In late phases of the disease, the carcinomas may infiltrate the whole malar bone and, in advanced stadiums, the orbit.

7.4 Diagnosis

Usually the diagnosis is established by clinical and paraclinical examination, such as contrast CT and in some cases PET scan, very useful in parotid masses with unknown primary tumor, known as CUP syndrome. When possible, fine-needle aspiration cytology (FNAC) is recommended before the operation in order to have a histological confirmation of a malignancy. In the absence of preoperative FNAC, we could use frozen section during the operation.

Biopsy of the parotid is normally not recommended because of the risk of damaging the facial nerve and of tumor cell spreading. As an exception, we can perform a biopsy in situation of a tumor with skin infiltration or a carcinoma of the skin which infiltrates the parotid.

Before operation, an additional staging is necessary. For primary tumor and neck, contrast CT is recommended [8], and in order to rule out lung or abdominal metastasis, an additional CT for thorax and abdomen is useful.

7.5 Treatment

Surgery is the first option for all resectable parotid tumors with bone involvement. The reconstructive technique depends on the status of the patients, the complexity of the defect, and, depending on the histological diagnose and preoperative clinical and paraclinical examination, the need to perform an additional neck dissection. Performing the neck surgery depends on the histological diagnose, and it facilitates the preparation of vessels for microsurgical anastomosis.

Postoperative radiotherapy depends on the histological result, and it is recommended in positive neck and in residual and/or highly aggressive tumors.

Primary irradiation is reserved for inoperable patients or patients who refuse surgery.

Chemotherapy is palliative for unresectable relapses, patients who cannot undergo radiotherapy and for those with distant metastases.

7.6 Reconstruction Techniques

When we have to manage an extended parotid tumor with bone extension, the reconstruction method depends on the bone and soft tissues resected in order to achieve clean margins. The best outcome is achieved when we try to replace like with like. To reestablish the facial symmetry and optimal functional and esthetical results, we may use bony grafts (iliac crest) or free flaps (fibula, with or without skin paddle, or deep circumflex iliac artery) in defects involving the mandible. There are cases in which the tumor infiltrates zygomatic arch, malar, or temporal bone, and for these the lining of the defect only with soft tissue, such as local or microsurgical flaps, without bone reconstruction, leads to a satisfactory esthetic result. The same attitude we adopt in patients with deep lobe parotid masses extended along the neck vessels to the skull base up to the sphenoid bone. Its resection does not need any reconstruction method, except the lining of the defect in order to prevent cerebral liquid fistulas and to reestablish facial symmetry.

In late phases of the disease, the neoplasia may extend to the orbit so, in order to have free margins, we need to perform exenteration leading to an invalidating outcome for patients. A viable option is to cover the defect using magnetic fixed epithesis. The advantages are permanent good control of tumor follow-up, possibility to reconstruct big defects involving orbita and the cheek, no big reconstructive techniques are needed, and, not the least, the esthetic outcome is very good. As an alternative to epithesis, we may cover the defect using local (lateral pedicle forehead or parietal – temporal flaps) or free flaps, such as radial or anterolateral thigh flap. The disadvantages are: complex operations are needed, local tumor control is not very good, and the esthetic result is doubtful.

The parotid tumors may involve the bone, but it is not necessary to extend also to the facial nerve. In cases where possible, we have to preserve it. If the nerve cannot be dissected due to tumor infiltration, after its resection, we have to perform facial reanimation, static or dynamic, or we may try, depending on the site where it was interrupted, to use nerve grafts in order to reestablish its function. But this subject is treated in another chapter.

From our experience, the mandible (ascending ramus and temporal mandibular joint) is the most frequent bone involved by the neoplastic process, mainly due to its anatomical relation with the parotid gland. After tumor resection en bloc with the mandibular ramus, the chin deviates toward the affected side leading to loss of occlusion. In these patients, we have to reconstruct, when possible, the skeletal structure and also the soft tissues. An option to achieve an optimal result is the use of free flaps and grafts [3, 4, 9].

In cases where, due to poor general status, a free flap is not possible, pedicle myocutaneous flaps, such as major pectoralis flap, are, in our opinion, the method of choice. In patients with mandibular or total malar bone defects, iliac crest grafts are very useful, especially if, due to histological grading and type, or clear margins, postoperative irradiation isn't planned. The postoperative functional and esthetical outcomes are very good.

The use of free flaps requires the presence of an experienced team and a longer operation time.

Bone grafts continue to play an important role in head and neck reconstruction, being useful in the management of small (<4 cm) defects of the mandible for which vascularized osteocutaneous free tissue transfer is neither required nor justified [10]. In our experience we have successfully used iliac crest graft also after resection of half of the mandible with good and stable functional outcome. There are literature data which show an improving of the outcome of osseous grafts [11], the limitation of these techniques being postoperative irradiation.

The reconstruction of soft tissues is not the aim of this chapter. If necessary, to cover the skin defects, there are a lot of flaps available: the lateral arm free flap with or without the harvesting of the posterior cutaneous nerve for facial nerve reconstruction [12]; major pectoralis, with the possibility to harvest it as a composite pedicle flap with a rib for mandible reconstruction [3]; anterolateral thigh (ALT) and fascial radial forearm and lateral arm free flaps [13]; latissimus dorsi free flap and perforator flaps from the flank area [14]; and parascapular flap [15].

The reconstruction of mandible after extended parotidectomy may be performed at the same time with the tumor resection and covering of soft tissue, or in a secondary stage. These depend on the type of tumor, the need of irradiation, general status of patients, and local reconstruction option. In some cases, due to severe comorbidities, we cannot address the mandible restoration, despite all the subsequent sequelae such as occlusion problems and facial asymmetry.

Some authors recommend the lateral thoracic wall as donor site for mandible defects after extended parotidectomy [3, 4]. A composite free flap composed by latissimus dorsi cutaneous perforator flap, the thoracodorsal nerve graft and a rib can be used to reconstruct the mandibular condyle and ascending ramus.

Another option to reestablish bony continuity is a fibula free flap [16, 17], with or without skin paddle [18–21]. If we need also soft tissue and a fibula composite flap is not possible due to risk of necrosis, we may combine the fibula as a bone flap with other techniques for skin reconstruction.

If preoperative angiography, angio-IRM, or eco-Doppler contraindicates the use of the fibula, we may change to deep circumflex iliac artery (DCIA) flap to reestablish the mandible continuity [22–24]. Because there is a high amount of bone, future prosthetic rehabilitation using dental implants may be achieved without problems, transforming DCIA flap in the first choice for functional masticatory reconstruction of the mandible [25]. Myocutaneous vessels provide blood to the overlying skin of the iliac crest [26], making possible to include also a cutaneous paddle [25, 27] in order to reconstruct complex defects after extended parotidectomy, without needing other flap.

The intraoperative fixation of the bone flap is made using a titanium reconstruction plate, which can be associated with osteosynthesis plates.

Because of anatomical relations, extended parotid tumors may involve also the zygomatic arch and malar bone. Resection of these, partial or completely, may lead to facial asymmetry. But the use of local flaps, such as scalp rotation, cervico-facial and platysma myocutaneous flap, or local regional flaps, such as major pectoralis, or free flap for the skin defect, such as fore arm or latissimus dorsi, associated later with lipostructure may resolve this problem. If we plan to reconstruct the bony defects, we may use DCIA flap or fibula flap, composite or combined with other cutaneous covering techniques. Another option to reestablish facial symmetry is the use of CAD-CAM or Medpor implants, but they require a very good vascularized overlying tissue and very often they are associated with infections at the recipient site. The postoperative irradiation increases the risk of complications for these technics.

In evolution parotid tumors may extend to temporal and sphenoid bone. In the past, when a parotid tumor involved the skull base or infratemporal fossa, it used to be considered inoperable, but nowadays, with the development of surgical techniques, especially microsurgery, and intensive care, these patients can undergo surgical procedures in mixed teams, with neurosurgeons and with good survival and decent quality of life. Reconstruction method should provide enough soft tissue to seal the skull base and to ensure a good protection against radiation therapy.

If the temporal bone or sphenoid is involved by the parotid tumor (Fig. 7.1), its resection accompanies the surgical management of the parotid tumor, and latissimus dorsi is the best choice to cover the defect. In cases where, due to general factors, a free flap is not possible, major pectoralis is a good and reliable alternative to cover the defect and to seal the skull base. Beside the risk of necrosis, another disadvantage is the important muscle atrophy, leading to a significant facial asymmetry.

The medial extension of tumor establishes the type of resection: lateral temporal bone resection and subtotal or total temporal bone resection [28]. When the parotid mass infiltrates the skull base, lateral or subtotal temporal bone resection is enough in order to get free margins, and the specimen must include en bloc the parotid tumor and infiltrated subjacent bone. The dissection of the infratemporal and parapharyngeal spaces may be facilitated through the resection of the mandibular condyle and zygomatic root, allowing performing a more accurate and tumor free surgery [28].

After specimen removal, we can cover the defect using a latissimus dorsi free flap.

The first description of this flap was made by Tansini in 1896, and its first use for head and neck defects was performed by Quillen in 1978 [21]. The blood supply originates from thoracic dorsal artery [21]. The flap has a long pedicle and constant anatomy and good quantity and quality of soft tissues with good blood supply [21], appropriate to seal the skull base if the tumor involved temporal bone, preventing cerebral fluid leakage.

The morbidity of donor site is low. This flap allows facial dynamic reanimation after extended parotidectomy associated with nerve VII resection.

Sometimes the flap is too bulky, with subsequent facial asymmetry, and needs additional corrective procedure. There is a difference of color and texture compared to facial skin. Because of its weight and gravity, it can lead to ectropion and some wound healing problems. But we can reduce the risk of ectropion by using some nonresorbable suspension sutures onto zygoma or lateral wall of the orbit.

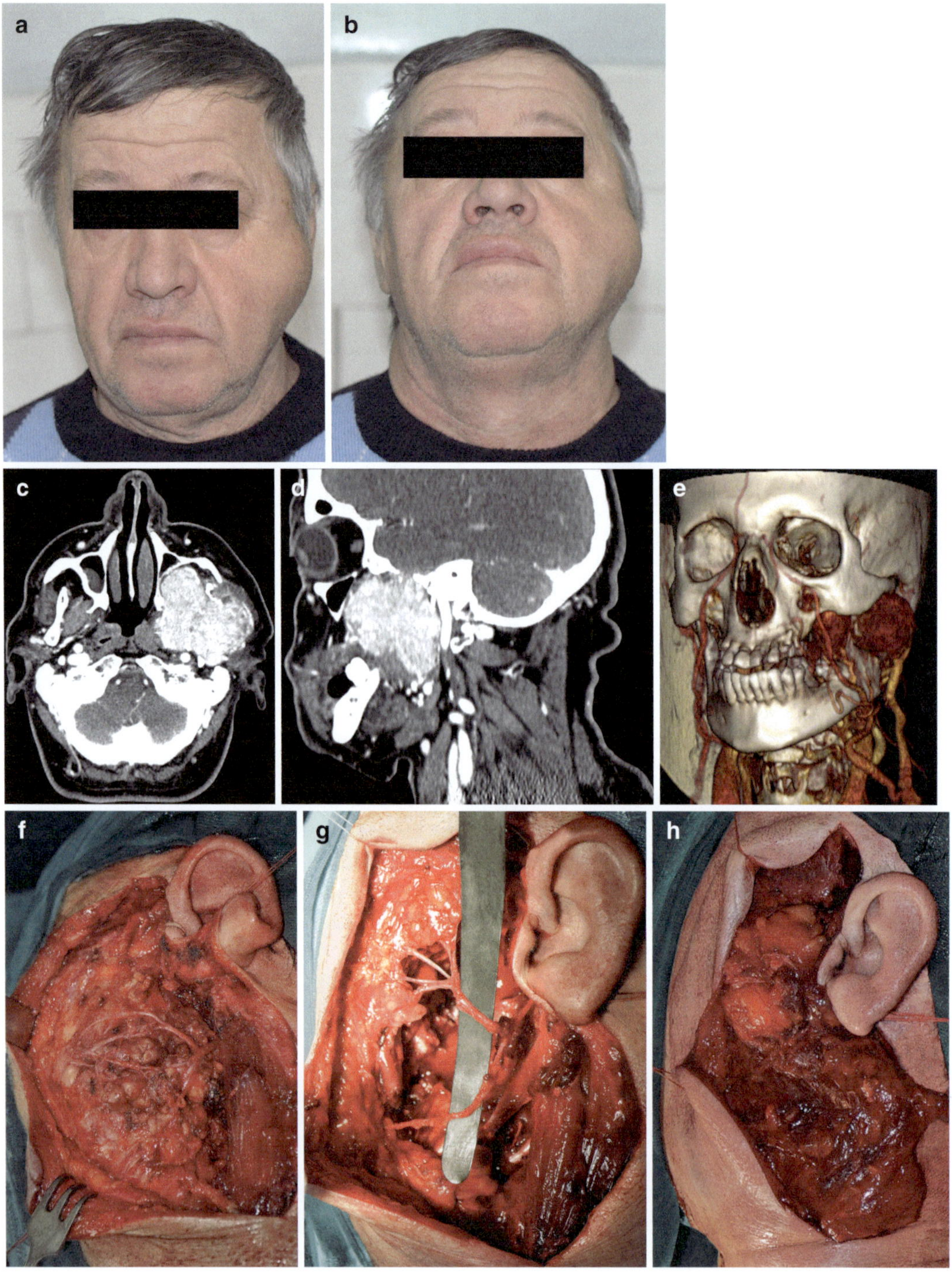

Fig. 7.1 (**a**) Patient with intraparotid metastatic lymph node from a primary papillary thyroid carcinoma operated 2 years before with total thyroidectomy. After 1 year after the resection of the primary tumor, the patient noticed a slow-growing parotid mass (**b**). The FNAC revealed a secondary parotid tumor: infiltration with papillary carcinoma. The tumor extended to the skull base, great wing of sphenoid bone (**c**, **d**), and ascending ramus and condyle of the mandible (**e**). Intraoperatively, the neoplastic process invaded also the deep lobe of the parotid, but without facial nerve paralysis (**f**, **g**). After the extended parotidectomy en bloc with a part of temporal and sphenoid bones, and ascending mandibular ramus and the condyle, the defect was lined using a major pectoralis muscle flap (**h**). The postoperative scars are barely visible, and the esthetic and functional outcomes 2 years postoperative are very good (no facial paralysis or asymmetry, satisfactory occlusion), despite the fact that the patient refused other corrective operations (**i–k**)

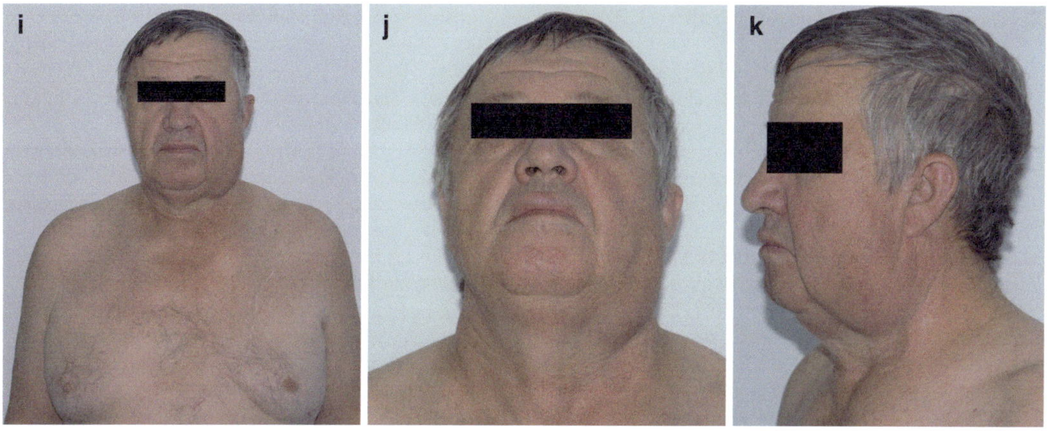

Fig. 7.1 (continued)

7.7 Complications and Sequelae

Postoperative complications and sequelae depend directly on the structures involved by tumor, such as facial nerve, type of bone resected, and reconstruction technique.

The most common are permanent facial paralyses, paralytic lagophtalmos, ectropion, and facial asymmetry due to failing of soft tissues, which can be corrected using Coleman technique, but also to facial paralyses. Reconstruction of facial nerve and correction of ectropion are subjects of other chapters.

If the mandible or temporal mandibular joint is resected and it's not reconstructed, the patients will present occlusion problems and facial asymmetry due to deviation of the chin toward the affected side.

In cases where zygoma or malar bone where resected, facial paralyses and asymmetry, and also ectropion, due to traction, gravity, and healing process, are very common.

As an immediate complication after skull base resection, meningitis is very severe. Sequelae after temporal bone resection can be important, with lower cranial nerve lesions. Postoperative patients may present equilibrium (when internal ear is involved), swallowing, voice, and speech problems. Rehabilitation of voice and swallowing dysfunction demands a team approach for the best outcome [29].

References

1. Myers NE, Ferris RL, Clark J, Sneddon L, O'Brien C, Laramore GE, et al. Salivary gland disorders. New York: Springer; 2007. p. 237–57, 257–76, 378–90, 436–92.
2. Hoff SR, Mohyuddin N, Yao M. Complications of parotid surgery. Oper Tech Otolaryngol. 2009;20:123–30.
3. Ioannides C, Fossion E. Reconstruction of extensive defects of the parotid region: experience with the pectoralis major and free latissimus dorsi flaps. J Craniomaxillofac Surg. 1997;25:57–62.
4. Biglioli F, Pedrazzoli M, Rabbiosi D, Colletti G, Colombo V, Frigerio A, et al. Reconstruction of complex defects of the parotid region using a lateral thoracic wall donor site. J Craniomaxillofac Surg. 2013;41:265–9.
5. Shah J. Head and neck surgery and oncology. 3rd ed. New York: Mosby; 2006.
6. Leonetti JP, Smith PG, Anand V, Kletzker GR, Hartman JM. Subtotal petrosectomy in the management of advanced parotid neoplasms. Otolaryngol Head Neck Surg. 1993;108:270–6.
7. Kuhel WI, Hume CR, Selesnick SH. Cancer of the external auditory canal and temporal bone. Otolaryngol Clin North Am. 1996;29(5):827–52.
8. Friedman ER, Saindane AM. Pitfalls in the staging of cancer of the major salivary gland neoplasms. Neuroimaging Clin N Am. 2013;23(1):107–22.
9. Ioannides C, Fossion E, Boeckx W. Serratus anterior muscle in composite head and neck flaps. Head Neck. 1992;14:177–82.
10. Foster RD, Anthony JP, Singer MI, Kaplan MJ, Pogrel MA, Mathes SJ. Reconstruction of complex midfacial defects. Plast Reconstr Surg. 1997;99:1555–65.
11. Lalikos JF, Mooney MP, Janosky J, Losken A, Losken HW. Bacterial exposure required to induce rabbit calvarial bone graft infection by superficial contamination. J Craniofac Surg. 1994;5:247–52.

12. Teknos TN, Nussenbaum B, Bradford CR, Prince ME, El-Kashlan H, Chepeha DB. Reconstruction of complex parotidectomy defects using the lateral arm free tissue transfer. Otolaryngol Head Neck Surg. 2003;129:183e191.
13. Cannady SB, Seth R, Fritz MA, Alam DS, Wax MK. Total parotidectomy defect reconstruction using the buried free flap. Otolaryngol Head Neck Surg. 2010;143:637–43.
14. Kim JT. Two options for perforator flaps in the flank donor site: latissimus dorsi and thoracodorsal perforator flaps. Plast Reconstr Surg. 2005;115:755–63.
15. Biglioli F, Autelitano L. Reconstruction after total parotidectomy using a deepithelialized free flap. J Craniomaxillofac Surg. 2007;35:364e368.
16. Chen ZW, Yan W. The study and clinical application of the osteocutaneous flap of fibula. Microsurgery. 1983;4:11.
17. Hidalgo DA. Fibula free flap: a new method of mandible reconstruction. Plast Reconstr Surg. 1989;84:71.
18. Flemming AFS, Brough MD, Evans ND, Grant HR, Harris M, James DR, et al. Mandibular reconstruction using vascularised fibula. Br J Plast Surg. 1990;43:403.
19. Taylor GI, Miller G, Ham F. The free vascularized bone graft: a clinical extension of microvascular technique. Plast Reconstr Surg. 1975;55:533.
20. Wei FC, Seah C, Tsai Y, Liu S, Tsai M. Fibula osteoseptocutaneous flap for reconstruction of composite manibular defects. Plast Reconstr Surg. 1994;93:294.
21. Wolff KD, Herzog K, Ervens J, Hoffmeister B. Experience with the osteocutaneous fibula flap: an analysis of 24 consecutive reconstructions of composite mandibular defects. J Craniomaxillofac Surg. 1996;24:330.
22. Acland RD. The free iliac flap. Plast Reconstr Surg. 1979;64:30.
23. Bitter K, Danai T. The iliac bone or osteocutaneous transplant pedicled on the deep circumflex iliac artery. I. Anatomical and techniqueal considerations. J Maxillofac Surg. 1983;11:195.
24. Taylor GI. Reconstruction of the mandible with free composite iliac bone grafts. Ann Plast Surg. 1982; 9:361.
25. Riediger D. Restoration of masticatory function by microsurgically revascularized iliac crest bone grafts using enosseous implants. Plast Reconstr Surg. 1988; 81:861.
26. Sanders R, Mayou BJ. A new vascularized bone graft transferred by microvascular anastomoses as a free flap. Br J Plast Surg. 1979;36:787.
27. Urken ML, Vickery C, Weinberg H, Buchbinder D, Biller HF. The internal oblique-iliac crest osseomyocutaneous microvascular free flap in head and neck reconstruction. J Reconstr Microsurg. 1989; 5:203.
28. Manolidis S, Pappas Jr D, Doerslen P, Jackson CG, Glasscock 3rd ME. Temporal bone and lateral skull base malignancy: experience and results with 81 patients. Am J Otol. 1998;19(16 Suppl):S1–15.
29. Myers NE, Ferris RL, Clark J, Sneddon L, O'Brien C, Laramore GE, et al. Temporal bone resection. Salivary gland disorders. New York: Springer; 2007. p. 393–405.

8 Parotid Tumors Extended to the Skull Base

Bogdan F. Iliescu and Ion Poeata

Abstract

Cranial involvement in parotid malignancies is rare and more common for certain types of tumors (e.g., adenoid cystic carcinoma). The spread of the parotid tumor to the skull base and intracranial may happen either by direct extension of the tumor and erosion of the bone or through perineural and endoneural invasion. Consequently, the clinical picture has the potential of becoming very complex (depending on the skull base and intracranial structures involved), and the management has to include a thorough neurosurgical assessment and interventional planning. These tumors pose particular management challenges due to their relative rarity and the lack of a unified extended experience, deep location, close proximity to critical neurovascular structures, and the extension beyond classical anatomic, surgical, and specialty landmarks. The outcome in the management of this particular type of tumors is improved significantly when their treatment is thought and carried out in a multidisciplinary fashion, using the knowledge and the therapeutical resources of various medical, surgical, and radiotherapy specialists. In this chapter we overview the patterns of skull involvement of parotid tumors and the clinical manifestations of cranial extension, and we look at the particularities of imaging and surgical planning and principles in this event.

8.1 Epidemiology

Malignant salivary gland neoplasms are relatively rare. They represent less than 0.5 % of all malignancies diagnosed yearly in the United States [1]. They account for 3–7 % of all head and neck cancers having an annual incidence of approximately 2.5–3.0 cases per 100,000 individuals [1].

B.F. Iliescu, MD, PhD (✉)
Department of Neurosurgery, "Prof. Dr. Nicolae Oblu" Clinical Emergency Hospital, Iasi, Romania
e-mail: bogdan.iliescu@gmail.com

I. Poeata, MD, PhD
Department of Neurosurgery, "Grigore T. Popa" University of Medicine and Pharmacy, Iasi, Romania

© Springer International Publishing Switzerland 2016

V.-V. Costan (ed.), *Management of Extended Parotid Tumors*, DOI 10.1007/978-3-319-26545-2_8

Most patients who develop malignant salivary gland tumors are in the sixth or seventh decade of life [2]. Approximately 80–85 % of salivary gland tumors arise in the parotid glands and only up to 20 % of these tumors are malign [3, 4].

A particular case is that of the adenoid cystic carcinoma that has a particular feature in its propensity for perineural invasion (50–70 % of the cases) [3], even in the early stage. It can spread centripetally through the skull base and peripherally along both named and unnamed nerves.

It is important to note that no matter which staging system we use for malignant parotid tumor the spread to the skull and intracranial places the patient in a T4b stage ("tumor invades skull base and/or pterygoid plates and/or encases carotid artery" – TNM classification of salivary glands carcinomas, same in AJCC staging system).

8.2 Spread Patterns

It is a well-documented fact that the cranial base is one of the noncontiguous regions where parotid tumors can metastasize along neural pathways (Fig. 8.1). Perineural and endoneural tumor extension along the mandibular division of the trigeminal nerve passing through the foramen ovale gains access into the middle cranial fossa and can involve the cavernous sinus. The presenting signs and symptoms will therefore be related to the involvement of the third, fourth, first, and second branches of the fifth and sixth cranial nerves as they run their course through the cavernous sinus.

Perineural tumor extension along the facial nerve passing through the stylomastoid foramen, facial canal, and internal acoustic meatus gains access into the posterior cranial fossa and grows in the cerebellopontine angle. The presenting signs and symptoms therefore will be related to the involvement of the seventh and eight cranial nerves, which pass through the internal acoustic meatus, and the 9th, 10th, and 11th cranial nerves, which pass through the jugular foramen. Patients also will experience occipital headaches and cerebellar dysfunction depending on the size of the lesion (vide infra) (Fig. 8.2).

When patients with a prior history of head and neck malignancies develop signs and symptoms of cranial nerve palsies, it is important to recognize the possibility of neurotropism and carry out appropriate diagnostic procedures.

Several different pathways exist which allow tumors to spread from one branch of the trigeminal nerve to the other. As mentioned above, tumors that gain access to the pterygopalatine

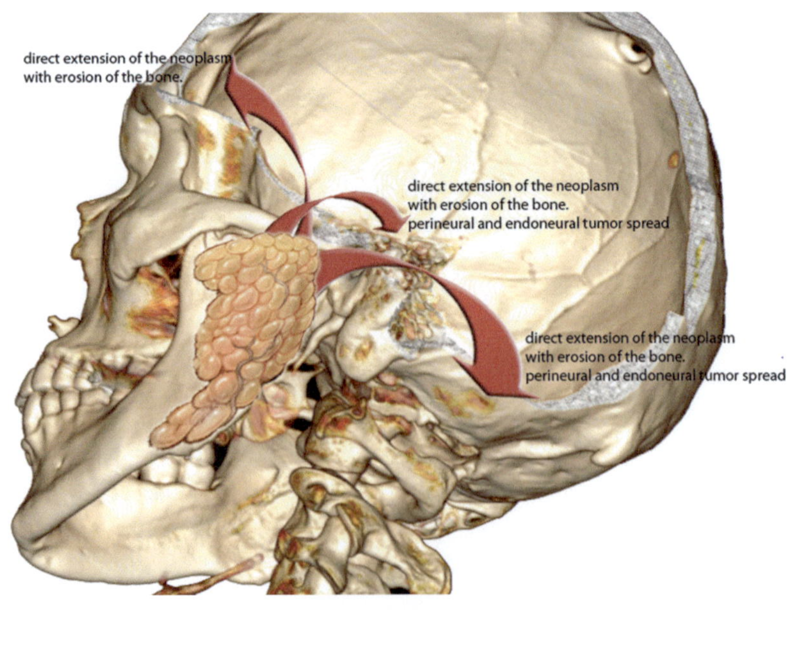

Fig. 8.1 Intracranial spread patterns for parotid tumors

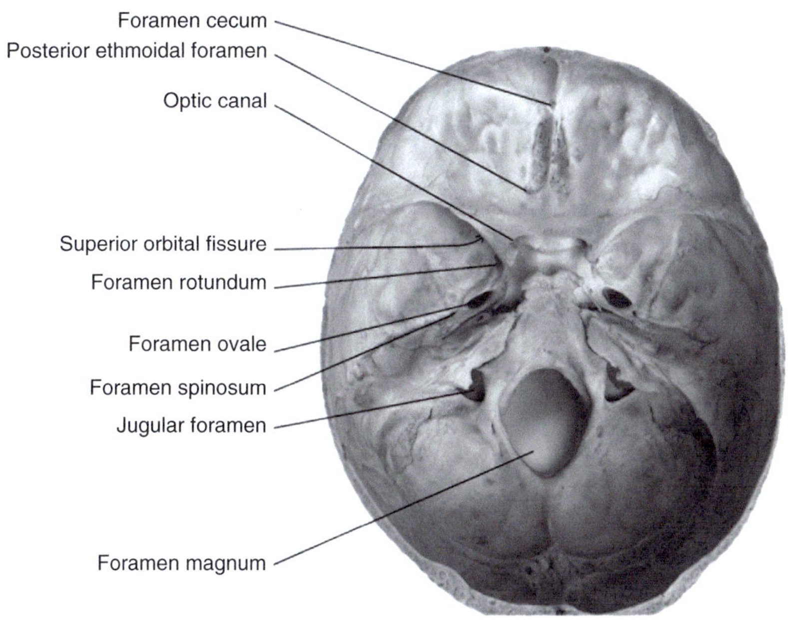

Fig. 8.2 Main anatomical landmarks of the skull base

fossa can spread to different branches of the trigeminal nerve and even the facial nerve.

Lesions in the parotid gland can spread via the auriculotemporal nerve to the mandibular nerve and thus up to the foramen ovale. From these nerves, tumor can ascend to the pterygopalatine fossa.

Peripheral spread is less common. Lesions that involve the pterygopalatine fossa can spread into the cheek region along the infraorbital groove or into the orbit via the inferior orbital fissure. Tumors may involve the cisternal portion of the trigeminal nerve and may spread antegrade into the Meckel cave and then to either the pterygopalatine fossa via the pterygoid canal or downward through the foramen ovale to the masticator space. Tumors may exit the pterygopalatine fossa to the cavernous sinus via the foramen rotundum or to the greater superficial petrosal nerve via the pterygoid canal.

From the cavernous sinus, tumors can spread to the Meckel cave and then along the cisternal portion of the trigeminal nerve to the lateral aspect of the pons or the trigeminal nuclei. From the greater superficial petrosal nerve and geniculate ganglion, tumors can spread either to the IAC/CPA region or into the middle ear cavity and eventually down the vertical facial nerve canal to the stylomastoid foramen. To date, no report exists of antegrade spread down the pharyngeal canal to the oropharynx.

The primary access point to the facial nerve is at the stylomastoid foramen at the skull base. Thus, the most common tumors to access the facial nerve are squamous cell carcinomas (SCCs) of the external ear/skin or tumors of the parotid gland. The most common lesion of the parotid gland to spread in a perineural fashion is adenoid cystic carcinoma, followed by acinic and mucoepidermoid carcinoma. Once in the vertical facial canal, tumor can then ascend to the middle ear cavity and exit either via the eustachian tube or out from the geniculate ganglion along the greater superficial petrosal nerve, which becomes the pterygoid nerve. Thus, tumor accessing the facial nerve could spread to the pterygopalatine fossa along the pterygoid nerve and thus the pterygopalatine ganglion of the maxillary nerve.

Tumors can also follow the course of the facial nerve past the geniculate ganglion to the fallopian canal and exit from the IAC into the CPA region and eventually into the cranial nuclei of the facial nerve within the medulla. Very rarely, tumor within the temporal fossa can access the geniculate ganglion through the hiatus along the anterior petrosal ridge from which the greater superficial nerve exits. From the geniculate ganglion, tumor can then access the middle ear cavity and even extend down the vertical portion of the facial canal.

Tumors arising within the petrous bone involving the facial nerve can spread anterograde along the greater superficial petrosal nerve and then the pterygoid nerve to the pterygopalatine fossa and its ganglion.

Adenoid cystic carcinoma (ACC) is a relatively uncommon malignancy in the head and neck but has a well-documented propensity for perineural invasion. It generally has a very slow growing, indolent course with frequent recurrences and late metastasis. It is found more often in minor salivary glands than major, although the latter has a higher association with perineural invasion. This has been attributed to proximity of nerves to the major salivary glands. Interestingly, studies have shown that perineural invasion does not always portend a worse prognosis in ACC. It did, however, correlate with positive margin status and therefore higher recurrence rates. Controversy also exists regarding the correlation of perineural invasion and distant metastasis.

Depending on the reported series, the facial nerve will be involved in 50 % of the cases when the pterygopalatine fossa is involved by tumor. Again, the two most important connections between the trigeminal and facial nerves are the pterygoid nerve joining the second division of the trigeminal nerve to the greater superficial petrosal nerve of the facial nerve and the parotid gland joining the third division of the trigeminal nerve to the facial nerve. Another potential communication could be from the facial nerve via the chorda tympani branch of the facial nerve to the lingual nerve, which arises from the third division of the trigeminal nerve. Therefore, if perineural tumor spread involving the trigeminal nerve is noted, careful examination of the facial nerve should be performed for signs of tumor spread.

8.3 Signs and Symptoms in Cranial Involvement

Invasion of the skull base and the intracranial structures results in a variable and often complex clinical picture. Nonspecific symptoms ranging from increased intracranial pressure, frontal lobe dysfunction, and visual changes to pituitary hypo- or hyperfunction, optic neuropathy (nerve and chiasm), cavernous sinus syndrome, and dysmetria, ataxia, brainstem signs, and suboccipital neck pain are possible, depending on the pattern of invasion and the particular fossa affected.

However, as with any lesion involving the skull base, assessment of the cranial nerve function is essential. A comprehensive preoperative examination of the cranial nerves that are involved by the tumor and/or are at risk during the surgical approach is mandatory in order to assess all preoperative deficits that may either become aggravated or require special attention during the patient's recovery. Understanding the existent and potential neurological deficit and its effect on the patient's quality of life (cosmetically or functionally) and a proper education of the patient and the caregiver(s) prior to surgery will allow for a real informed consent and decisions regarding the patient's care. Although commonly overlooked and undiagnosed preoperatively, anosmia and ageusia can be associated with significant quality of life issues following surgery, for both the patient and his family.

8.3.1 Cranial Nerves II, III, IV, and VI

Loss of vision is extremely traumatic for the patient, especially if manifest preoperatively. Many of the patients with this kind of tumor will require some form of radiotherapy postoperatively. As a result further diminution of vision over time is a possible outcome and must be assessed in the context of the patient's life expectancy and the potential expected benefit from sacrificing the optic function. A formal visual field examination should be performed preoperatively to identify deficits that the patient can be unaware of. Ocular motility deficits can be a significant and a source of major concern for the patient. It raises the question of preserving a good optic function in the affected eye as it can be of little benefit and, in some cases, even detrimental to the patient.

8.3.2 Cranial Nerve V

Trigeminal nerve involvement in the pathologic process is apparent in many cases from the initial examination. These cases of malignancies involving the trigeminal complex present with neuralgia with the typical characteristics. Nonetheless some of the patients will have as initial complaint hypesthesia of different degrees with a facial distribution suggesting the affected ramus/rami and masticatory muscle weakness/atrophy. Some cases may present with no deficit at all. In all tumors invading the middle cranial fossa, the implications of this symptomatology either generated by the pathological process or as a possible complication of the intervention must be explained and discussed with the patient. In most cases recognition of a trigeminal nerve deficit and early intervention can minimize the functional deficit.

8.3.3 Cranial Nerves VII and VIII

Although not of vital interest, the loss of the facial nerve function can have a tremendous impact on the patient's quality of life. As is the case with the other cranial nerves, preoperative weighting of the benefit of a structure's sacrifice against the benefit of the patient's survival and quality of life must be thoroughly performed preoperatively. The implications of facial nerve loss, cosmetic and functional, including oral incontinence and eye lesions all the way to vision loss due to exposure keratitis, should be addressed early on in the patient's recovery. Exposure keratitis might be an even more imperious problem when both trigeminal and facial nerves are damaged concomitantly. Early gold weight implantation and lower lid tightening procedures should be carried out. Nerve repair during the initial surgery, whether by primary anastomosis, cable graft, or transposition (hypoglossal–facial), should be considered when the sacrifice of the nerve cannot be avoided.

The anastomosis can be considered and performed 12–18 months later if the nerve remains paralyzed but it is known to be structurally intact. An alternative for facial reanimation is temporalis or masseter muscle transpositions. The initial examination assessment of the facial nerve should be complemented by electromyography which can help identify subtle disturbances in facial nerve function.

The sacrifice of the cochlear–vestibular complex, if necessary, is usually well tolerated. In most cases the loss is unilateral and can be easily compensated for if the contralateral complex is functional. An objective assessment of the cochlear-vestibular system can be done preoperatively with audiogram and electronystagnogram.

8.3.4 Cranial Nerves IX, X, XI, and XII

A thorough preoperative examination of the lower cranial nerves is essential in all patients in whom potential involvement of these structures is suspected or foreseen. Lesions to the lower cranial nerves are a common finding when there is involvement of the temporal bone or lateral skull base. The functional status of these neural structures can be assessed through direct visualization of the vocal cords and, in certain cases, through barium radiological study. Special care should be taken in those cases at risk for lower cranial nerve paresis in discussing with the patient and family the eventuality of a feeding tube and tracheostomy. In cases with considerable lower cranial involvement risk due either to the surgical approach or to planned sacrifice, the tracheostomy and/or feeding tube placement can be performed simultaneously.

Contents of the jugular foramen, i.e., cranial nerves from IX to XII, petrosal sinus, sigmoid sinus, and carotid artery with the sympathetic

Table 8.1 Summary of various jugular foramen syndromes

Nerve	Symptom and signs	Syndrome					
		Vernet	Collet-Sicard	Villaret	Tapia	Jackson	Schmidt
IX	Loss of taste in posterior one-third of the tongue	•	•	•			
X	Paralysis of the vocal chords and palate, anesthesia of the pharynx and larynx	•	•	•	•	•	•
XI	Weak trapezius and SCM	•	•	•	±	•	•
XII	Tongue paralysis and atrophy		•	•	•	•	
Sympathetics	Horner's syndrome			•	±		

plexus at their entrance in the carotid canal can be affected, and the specific symptoms are classically grouped in certain syndromes (see Table 8.1 for a summary of various jugular foramen syndromes).

8.4 Radiologic Evaluation

Being usually a complex surgical entity, a parotid tumor extended to the skull base requires a detailed and careful imagistic evaluation. Computed tomography and magnetic resonance imaging pre- and postcontrast enhancement should be performed including angiography. The availability of CT and MRI has greatly improved the ability to diagnose the primary parotid tumor, its extension, and the relationships of the tumor with the skull base and intracranial structures. Although CT is accurate in detecting bony lesions and pathological processes in the cerebellopontine angle and the cavernous sinus, it cannot detect small lesions in the trigeminal cisterna or slight destruction of the bony basal foramina or the actual involvement of the nerves themselves. Magnetic resonance imaging has shown superior contrast resolution and will more accurately depict tumor soft tissue margins. The characteristics of perineural tumor spread include smooth isointense thickening of V3 and mild concentric enlargement of the foramen ovale. Cavernous sinus and ganglionic involvement should be considered in those cases where the hypointensity normal for the trigeminal cisterna is replaced by an isointense mass with lateral involvement of the cavernous sinus and visible dural membranes [5].

The capabilities of both imaging modalities are well known; however, a specific instance of the infiltrating parotid tumor has to be discussed. The particular phenomenon of perineural invasion might be asymptomatic, hence the increased importance of careful radiologic evaluation in suspicious cases. Published data that analyzed retrospectively images from cases with histologically confirmed perineural invasion underlined this concept. Imaging from 30 out of 38 patients (78 %) in whom invasion could be seen on retrospective analysis had no mention in preoperative reports. In addition, the remaining eight patients had no evidence of perineural invasion on imaging, although they were confirmed histologically.

In the evaluation of perineural spread, both CT and MRI play a role; nonetheless MRI has become the imaging modality highly due to its ability to accurately differentiate normal tissue from tumor. MRI sensitivity in perineural spread detection has been reported to be 95 %. T1-weighted images with contrast enhancement provide valuable information regarding the fat tissue surrounding the foramina. T2-weighted images are useful in differentiating inflammatory changes versus tumoral bone erosion, the former being hyperintense on T2. For example, MRI would be useful in differentiating inflammatory changes from neoplasm in the case of a differential diagnoses between a perineural tumor spread to the mastoid and benign inflammatory changes associated with Eustachian tube obstruction.

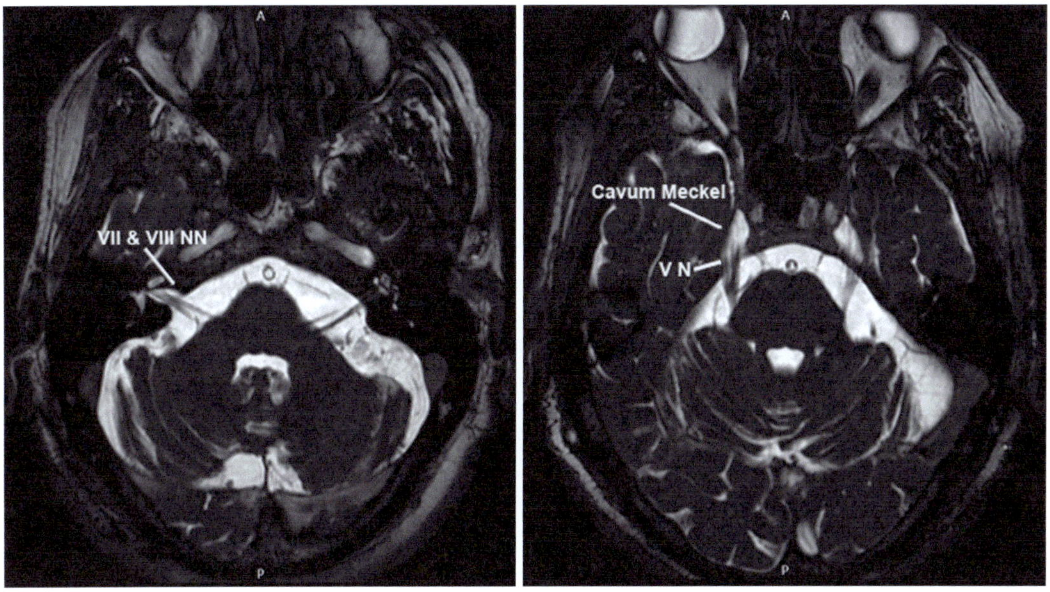

Fig. 8.3 MRI CISS images depicting the seventh and eighth (*left*) and fifth and cavum Meckel (*right*)

Examples of direct evidence of perineural spread on MRI would be enlargement and enhancement along the course of a cranial nerve. Disappearance of the fat tissue at the nerve exit is a key element in detecting perineural spread. Evaluation of the most common areas and foramina typically involved in tumor spread should be routine in assessing head and neck malignancies. These include the supraorbital foramen, pterygopalatine fossa, foramen rotundum, pterygoid canal, palatine foramen, foramen ovale, mandibular foramen, and stylomastoid foramen. Another important imagistic finding is the replacement of CSF in the cavum Meckel with enhancing tissue. In specific cases the nerves should be explored using the special MRI nerve sequence (3D Fiesta or equivalents; see Fig. 8.3).

One last remark has to be made regarding the presence of a venous plexus accompanying the facial nerve on its course at the anterior genu, tympanic, and mastoid segments. This plexus can be mistaken for neoplasm or perineural invasion and such attention should be paid in observing the facial nerve on MRI.

Although the MRI is the main imaging method for tumor assessment including its extension and perineural spread, the CT still plays a role in the evaluation of these cases. A major advantage of CT is that it is less expensive and is less dependent on patient status. The value of CT in depicting the perineural invasion is dependent on its superior imaging power of bony structures. CT findings include but are not limited to expansion of bony canals, pathological fissures, foramina deformities, or even frank destruction of these structures by mass lesion.

Preoperative assessment of the involvement of the cerebrovascular structures in this area in the tumor extension is paramount. One form of angiography at least should be performed. In most cases MR angiography (arterial and venous) is enough and should be readily available during the discussed imaging protocol. This technique is preferred due to its noninvasiveness as well; however, in those cases in which vascular involvement is very complex and information about flow, assessment of the patency and adequacy of the circle of Willis is necessary, or when it is clear that a preoperative embolization of the tumor is necessary, standard percutaneous angiography of the head and neck is mandatory.

Another particular case, although still a matter of debate, is the case of a planned CA ligature. In this case a balloon test occlusion in conjunction with a Xe-CT or positron emission tomography scan is helpful in establishing the tolerance to ischemia and to identify the patients at risk for vascular insufficiency. Even so if sacrifice of the internal CA is necessary, vascular reconstruction should be considered [6–9, 10], taking into consideration those 3–8 % of the patients pass successfully the preoperative test that will develop still an ischemic stroke.

On a different plane, identifying hypervascular tumors and their vascular supply pedicles and their subsequent embolization may significantly reduce the perioperative blood loss and associated complications. The relationship of the major cerebrovascular structures to the tumor is a very important aspect in the planning of the surgery, regarding the extent of tumor resection and identifying those patients in who sacrifice of the vessel is necessary. As a consequence, the interventional neuroradiologist should be an indispensable member of the multidisciplinary team necessary to manage these tumors.

8.5 Treatment

Prior to the mid-1950s, lateral skull base malignancies were primarily treated by radical mastoidectomy combined with radiotherapy [11, 12]. In 1954, the en bloc total temporal bone resection was described by Parsons and Lewis [13]. In 1974 Lewis [14] popularized single-stage total temporal bone resection in reporting a series of 100 cases. In that series, the overall 5-year survival rate was 27 %. Since the advancement of lateral skull base surgery began in the early 1970s, postresection survival rates have been improving as complete tumor excision has become more common [15]. In some series, the combination of radiotherapy and resection has resulted in increased survival rates [16, 17]. Consequently, some authors have advocated this combined intervention in most if not all cases. Unfortunately, successful treatment remains difficult. Even with combined-modality treatment, 5-year survival rates range from 20 to 58 % in the best of series [18, 19].

The surgical approach is chosen taking into account multiple factors, starting with the involved part of the cranial base and the intracranial extent, the vital structures that have to be monitored and controlled during surgery, the tumor characteristics (its vasculature, as discussed above, and the relationship with other important structures), the availability of various intraoperative technologies (neuronavigation, monitoring, ultrasonic aspirator, and so forth), and the surgical team experience [20].

We'll overview below the possibilities of surgical approaches depending on the cranial fossa involved by tumoral extension.

8.5.1 Anterior Skull Base

The anterior skull base can be approached intracranial, extracranial, or combined. Intracranial approaches to the anterior skull base typically include a bifrontal, unilateral subfrontal, or fronto-orbito-zygomatic craniotomy as the basis for the approach. The subfrontal approach includes osteotomies of the superior orbital rim(s) and/or nasion [21, 22]. These osteotomies can be performed in a one-piece manner with the craniotome (see Fig. 8.2) or as separate osteotomies. The subfrontal approach allows wider exposure of the anterior skull base, as well as the clival region, while limiting the amount of retraction of the frontal lobes of the brain. The dura acts as a barrier to the spread of the tumor in the intracranial space. In the cases with limited dural involvement, but without progression into the cerebral space, the dura should be excised and this usually provides an adequate oncological margin. On the other hand, if there is tumor progression in the intradural compartment, the prognosis worsens significantly [23, 24].

In those where dura has not been intentionally penetrated, its integrity should be evaluated carefully. Inspection of any CSF leak should be performed using tests with increasing intracranial pressure such as a moderate Valsalva maneuver. In case there is any violation of the dura, a meticulous watertight closure should be performed. This can be done primarily or with the addition of dural substitute grafts. The use of "sutureless" dural grafts is to be avoided in this area, as the risk of failed reconstruction with resulting CSF leak and concomitant contamination of the intradural space is high. The reconstruction of the skull in this area is controversial as any prosthetic material increases the risk of infection due to the vicinity of the frontal sinus

8.5.2 Lateral Skull Base

Choosing the appropriate approach for removal of the tumors involving the lateral skull base depends on the anatomical location of the tumor and its extension and the need to gain easy and rapid access to vascular structures both proximally and distally.

Tumors with progression into the temporal bone or jugular foramen can be approached by a postauricular incision that is extended inferiorly along the anterior border of the sternocleidomastoid. As the infratemporal fossa is part of the surgical approach, a neck dissection to gain access to the vascular structures should be performed. The extent of temporal bone drilling is dependent on the tumor origin (i.e., temporal bone, jugular foramen, endolymphatic sac, etc.) and its extent. Although the preservation of hearing is of utmost importance, when planning an extensive resection of a malignant neoplasm in this area, the appropriate amount of drilling should not be limited.

The involvement of cranial nerves in tumor progression makes continuous intraoperative neurophysiological monitoring mandatory in most of the approaches for lateral skull base resections [18, 17].

Facial nerve monitoring through electromyography of the orbicularis oculi and oris should be performed. In cases where hearing preservation is planned, auditory brainstem-evoked potentials are continuously monitored to assess both hearing and brainstem function at the level of the cochlear nuclei. The vagal nerve is monitored using either a specialized endotracheal tube or direct electrode recording into the vagus supplied muscles. Direct electromyography recording of the trapezius muscle and the tongue should be in place for monitoring cranial nerves 11 and 12, respectively [25].

The resection of these lateral skull base tumors is usually burdened by the formation of a significant dead-space cavity. Additionally, intradural extension of the tumor and/or dissection may also induce a direct CSF fistula usually with insufficient dural material to ensure a watertight closure. Therefore, a complete spectrum of grafts, dural substitutes, free tissue transfers, free vascularized soft tissue flaps, and pedicle flap transfers should be available to close the surgical planes. Evidently, the need for their use and availability should be assessed thoroughly and planned preoperatively.

As the outcome is directly dependent on the extent of tumor removal, lateral skull base malignancies should be treated aggressively through an extended surgical procedure. A lateral temporal bone resection is combined with local excision of the involved portion of the temporal bone. When possible, the tumor is removed en bloc with a margin of healthy bone. If it is not possible to perform a complete removal, the en bloc resection should be as large as possible. The remaining margins affected by the tumor are then excised using aggressive skull base dissection until a clear margin is obtained. Infiltrated bone margins are drilled until clear, while invaded cranial nerves are resected as well as the involved dura with intracranial extension. Involved neurovascular structures are aggressively resected and immediately reconstructed when possible.

In the immediate perioperative period, there are a number of various rehabilitative interventions directed at the resected cranial nerves, which include hypoglossal–facial nerve anastomosis, cable nerve grafts, and eyelid cosmetic procedures. Facial reanimation and maintenance of laryngeal competence are the main priorities in postoperative period.

Postoperative radiotherapy should follow all surgical procedures. The cases where postoperative radiotherapy is indicated are: subtotal temporal bone resection and subtotal tumor resection (positive margin); involvement of CA, venous sinus or jugular bulb, cranial nerve(s); and nodal metastasis, intracranial tumor extension, and advanced skull base involvement.

In the particular cases in which surgery follows preoperative radiotherapy, the surgical procedure of total en bloc temporal bone resection should be performed Lewis [14, 26]. In this procedure the entire temporal bone is removed en bloc. The CA, sigmoid sinus, jugular bulb, internal jugular vein, and dura should be preserved if possible. The first step is temporal craniotomy. Extradural dissection is performed to the petrous ridge and superior petrosal sinus.

The sigmoid sinus is dissected posteriorly and followed in an inferior and anterior direction all the way to the jugular bulb. Anteriorly, the parotid gland is dissected, the distal facial nerve is divided, the mandibular condyle is mobilized or resected, and the petrous portion of the internal CA is dissected through the infratemporal fossa. Following proximal and distal arterial and venous control, the temporal bone resection is completed with remaining medial attachments separated, including dural attachments, CA and jugular bulb attachments, and proximal division of the cochleovestibular and facial nerves.

References

1. Speight PM, Barrett AW. Salivary gland tumours. Oral Dis. 2002;8(5):229–40.
2. Wahlberg P, Möller T, Perfekt R. Carcinoma of the parotid and submandibular glands – a study of survival in 2465 patients. Oral Oncol. 2002;38(7):706–13.
3. Harrison LB, Sessions RB, Hong WK, editors. Head and neck cancer: a multidisciplinary approach, vol. 1. 3rd ed. Philadelphia: Lippincott Williams and Wilkins; 2009. p. 1002.
4. Lalwani AK. Current diagnosis and treatment in otolaryngology: head and neck surgery. New York: McGraw-Hill; 2008.
5. Laine FJ, Braun IF, Jensen ME, Nadel L, Som PM. Perineural tumor extension through the foramen ovale: evaluation with MR imaging. Radiology. 1990; 174:65–71.
6. Erba SM, Horton JA, Latchaw RE, Yonas H, Sekhar L, Schramm V, et al. Balloon test occlusion of the internal carotid artery with stable xenon/CT cerebral blood flow imaging. AJNR. 1988;9:533–8.
7. Eskridge JM. Xenon-enhanced CT: past and present. AJNR. 1994;15:845–6.
8. Gonzalez CF, Moret J. Balloon occlusion of the carotid artery prior to surgery for neck tumors. AJNR. 1990;11:649–52.
9. Goodwin WJ, Jesse RH. Malignant neoplasms of the external auditory canal and temporal bone. Arch Otolaryngol. 1980;106:675–9.
10. Lorberboym M, Pandit N, Machac J, Holan V, Sacher M, Segal D, et al. Brain perfusion imaging during preoperative temporary balloon occlusion of the internal carotid artery. J Nucl Med. 1996;37:415–9.
11. Boland J, Paterson R. Cancer of the middle ear and external auditory meatus. J Laryngol Otol. 1955;69: 468–78.
12. Ward GE, Loch WE, Lawrence Jr W. Radical operation for carcinoma of the external auditory canal and middle ear. Am J Surg. 1951;82:169–78.
13. Manolidis S, Pappas Jr D, Von Doersten P, Jackson CG, Glasscock 3rd ME. Temporal bone and lateral skull base malignancy: experience and results with 81 patients. Am J Otol. 1998;19 Suppl 6:S1–15.
14. Lewis JS. Temporal bone resection. Review of 100 cases. Arch Otolaryngol. 1975;101:23–5.
15. de Vries EJ, Sekhar LN, Horton JA, Eibling DE, Janecka IP, Schramm Jr VL, et al. A new method to predict safe resection of the internal carotid artery. Laryngoscope. 1990;100:85–8.
16. Barrs DM. Temporal bone carcinoma. Otolaryngol Clin North Am. 2001;34:1197–218.
17. Spector JG. Management of temporal bone carcinomas: a therapeutic analysis of two groups of patients and long-term follow-up. Otolaryngol Head Neck Surg. 1991;104:58–66.
18. Kartush JM, Bouchard KR. Intraoperative facial nerve monitoring: otology, neurotology, and skull base surgery. In: Kartush JM, Bouchard KR, editors. Neuromonitoring in otology and head and neck surgery. New York: Raven Press; 1992. p. 99–120.
19. Prasad S, Janecka IP. Efficacy of surgical treatments for squamous cell carcinoma of the temporal bone: a literature review. Otolaryngol Head Neck Surg. 1994;110:270–80.
20. Pensak ML, Gleich LL, Gluckman JL, Shumrick KA. Temporal bone carcinoma: contemporary perspectives in the skull base surgical era. Laryngoscope. 1996;106:1234–7.
21. Raveh J, Laedrach K, Speiser M, Chen J, Vuillemin T, Seiler R, et al. The subcranial approach for fronto-orbital and anteroposterior skull-base tumors. Arch Otolaryngol Head Neck Surg. 1993;119:385–93.
22. Sekhar LN, Nanda A, Sen CN, Snyderman CN, Janecka IP. The extended frontal approach to tumors of the anterior, middle, and posterior skull base. J Neurosurg. 1992;76:198–206.
23. Lund VJ, Howard DJ, Wei WI, Cheesman AD. Craniofacial resection for tumors of the nasal cavity and paranasal sinuses—a 17-year experience. Head Neck. 1998;20:97–105.
24. Shah JP, Kraus DH, Bilsky MH, Gutin PH, Harrison LH, Strong EW. Craniofacial resection for malignant tumors involving the anterior skull base. Arch Otolaryngol Head Neck Surg. 1997;123:1312–7.
25. Lanser MJ, Jackler RK, Yingling CD. Regional monitoring of lower (ninth through twelfth) cranial nerves. In: Kartush JM, Bouchard KR, editors. Neuromonitoring in otology and head and neck surgery. New York: Raven Press; 1992. p. 131–50.
26. Parsons H, Lewis JS. Subtotal resection of the temporal bone for cancer of the ear. Cancer. 1954;7: 995–1001.

Part II

Diagnostic Criteria for Extended Parotid Tumors

Pathological Variety of Extended Parotid Tumors

9

Mihai Danciu and Dan Ferariu

Abstract

Extended parotidectomy is a surgical procedure that removes the entire parotid gland and the adjacent structures (adipose tissue, temporal or mandibular bone, nerves, vessels, and skin). It is performed in advanced stages of parotid malignant tumors or when the parotid gland is affected by extrinsic or metastatic tumors. We present the pathological gross and microscopic features of the main tumors of the parotid glands. Whenever specific and useful for differential diagnosis, the immunohistochemical pattern is also described. Although rare, compared with benign tumors, malignant tumors of the parotid glands represent the main reason for extended parotidectomy; therefore, we focus on these tumors, following the World Health Organization histological classification of the salivary glands.

9.1 Introduction

The parotid gland may present intrinsic, extrinsic, and metastatic tumors, which due to size, extension, and infiltrative growth pattern, necessitate extended parotidectomy.

Intrinsic tumors may be benign or malignant. Extrinsic tumors include regional tumors which extend into the parotid gland, while metastatic tumors represent distant tumors that metastasized in the parotid. Generally, parotid tumors are similar to salivary gland tumors. Morphology is variable depending on histogenesis, the main categories being epithelial, mesenchymal, and lymphoid (Table 9.1) [1].

M. Danciu, MD, PhD (✉)
Pathology Department, "Grigore T. Popa" University of Medicine and Pharmacy, Iasi, Romania
e-mail: mihai.danciu@umfiasi.ro

D. Ferariu, MD, PhD
Department of Pathology, Regional Institute of Oncology, Iasi, Romania

9.2 Acinic Cell Carcinoma (ICD-O Code: 8550/3)

9.2.1 Definition

Acinic cell carcinoma is an epithelial malignant tumor developed from proliferation of acinic and ductal cells, at least some of which contain cytoplasmic PAS-positive granules of zymogen.

The vast majority (80 %) of acinic cell carcinomas of the salivary glands are located in the parotid gland [1].

© Springer International Publishing Switzerland 2016

V.-V. Costan (ed.), *Management of Extended Parotid Tumors*, DOI 10.1007/978-3-319-26545-2_9

Table 9.1 WHO histological classification of salivary glands tumors [1]

Malignant epithelial tumors	
Acinic cell carcinoma	Oncocytic carcinoma
Mucoepidermoid carcinoma	Salivary duct carcinoma
Adenoid cystic carcinoma	Adenocarcinoma, not otherwise specified
Polymorphous low-grade adenocarcinoma	Myoepithelial carcinoma
Epithelial-myoepithelial carcinoma	Carcinoma ex pleomorphic adenoma
Clear cell carcinoma, not otherwise specified	Carcinosarcoma
Basal cell adenocarcinoma	Metastasizing pleomorphic adenoma
Sebaceous carcinoma	Squamous cell carcinoma
Sebaceous lymphadenocarcinoma	Small cell carcinoma
Cystadenocarcinoma	Large cell carcinoma
Low-grade cribriform cystadenocarcinoma	Lymphoepithelial carcinoma
Mucinous adenocarcinoma	Sialoblastoma
Benign epithelial tumors	
Pleomorphic adenoma	Canalicular adenoma
Myoepithelioma	Sebaceous adenoma
Basal cell adenoma	Warthin tumor
Lymphadenoma	Ductal papillomas
Sebaceous	Inverted ductal papilloma
Nonsebaceous	Intraductal papilloma
	Sialadenoma papilliferum
Oncocytoma	Cystadenoma
Soft tissue tumors	**Hematolymphoid tumors**
Hemangioma	Hodgkin lymphoma
	Diffuse large B-cell lymphoma
	Extranodal marginal zone B-cell lymphoma
Secondary tumors (metastases)	

9.2.2 Macroscopy

The average size of acinic cell carcinoma is 1–3 cm. At the moment of diagnosis, the tumor presents itself as a well- or ill-defined solid nodule, usually solitary, firm to rubbery. When recurrent, it may be multifocal. On the cut surface it is lobular, light brown to red [1, 2].

9.2.3 Microscopy

Histological aspect is variable, depending on cellular types and architectural pattern; however, the common feature is the presence of cells with serous differentiation. Architecture might be solid, lobular, microcystic, papillary cystic, or follicular (Fig. 9.1). Tumor cells with serous differentiation represent the characteristic component and may or may not be mixed with clear (Fig. 9.2), vacuolar, or glandular cells and ducts. Acinar serous cells are large, round/polygonal, with characteristic basophilic, PAS-positive, diastase-resistant cytoplasmic granules [1, 3]. Nuclei are monomorphous, round, hyperchromatic, and located peripherally. The stroma is delicate, containing many vessels, sometimes with hemorrhage, hemosiderin deposits, and psammoma bodies. Aggregates of lymphoid infiltrate are also common.

9.3 Mucoepidermoid Carcinoma (ICD-O Code 8430/3)

9.3.1 Definition

Mucoepidermoid carcinoma is a malignant epithelial tumor composed mainly of mucous, intermediate, and epidermoid cells.

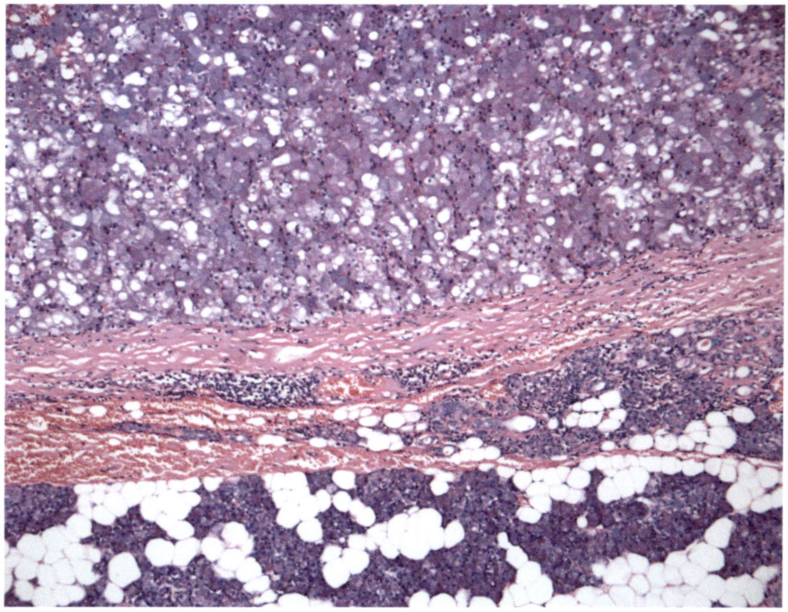

Fig. 9.1 Acinic cell carcinoma with solid architecture (*up*) and parotid gland (*bellow*) (HE, ×100)

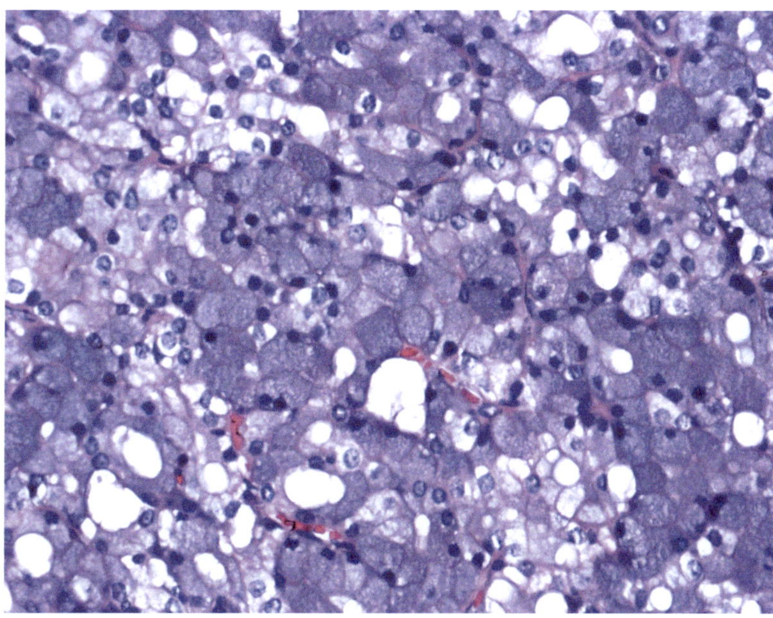

Fig. 9.2 Acinic cell carcinoma: serous cells and clear cells (focally) (HE, ×400)

About 45 % of mucoepidermoid carcinomas of the salivary glands occur in the parotid glands [1].

9.3.2 Macroscopy

It presents itself as a well-defined area (sometimes ill-defined infiltrative, in high-grade tumors), sized between 1 and 12 cm, is firm and white-grayish, and may often be cystic.

9.3.3 Microscopy

Tumor cells may form cysts, ductal structures, sheets, or solid nests. One may see epidermoid (squamoid), mucus-producing and intermediate cells, admixed with clear, columnar, and rarely oncocytic cells (Figs. 9.3 and 9.4) [2, 4]. Epidermoid cells are polygonal, with abundant eosinophilic cytoplasm and ovoid, vesicular nuclei, usually containing no keratin. The mucus-producing cells lining the cystic spaces are large, with light basophilic cytoplasm, positive for mucus staining, and eccentrically located nuclei. Intermediate cells found in the solid component are cuboidal or ovoid, small to medium sized, with pale cytoplasm and hyperchromatic nuclei. Mucin stainings are negative. Anaplasia and mitosis are uncommon. Stroma may contain focal sclerosis and inflammation adjacent to the extravasated mucus.

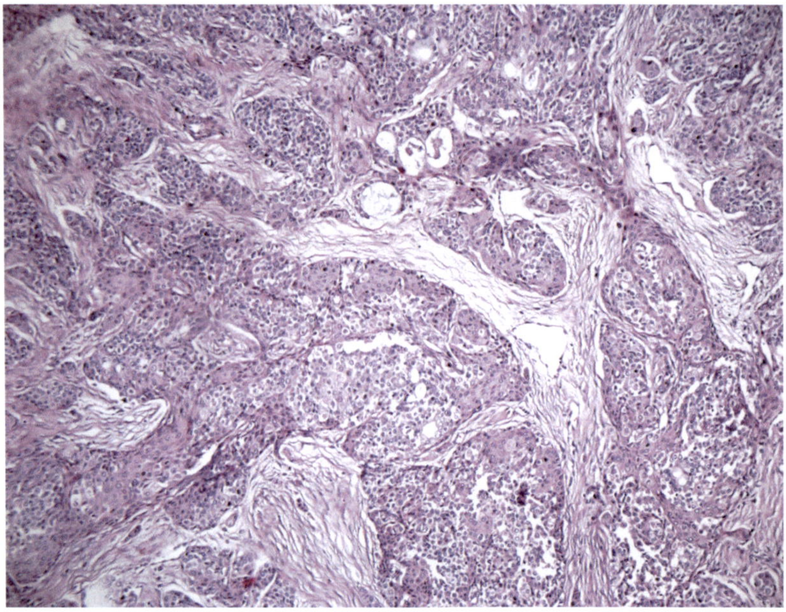

Fig. 9.3 Mucoepidermoid carcinoma with squamous and intermediate cells (predominant), and isolated microcysts with mucin (HE, ×100)

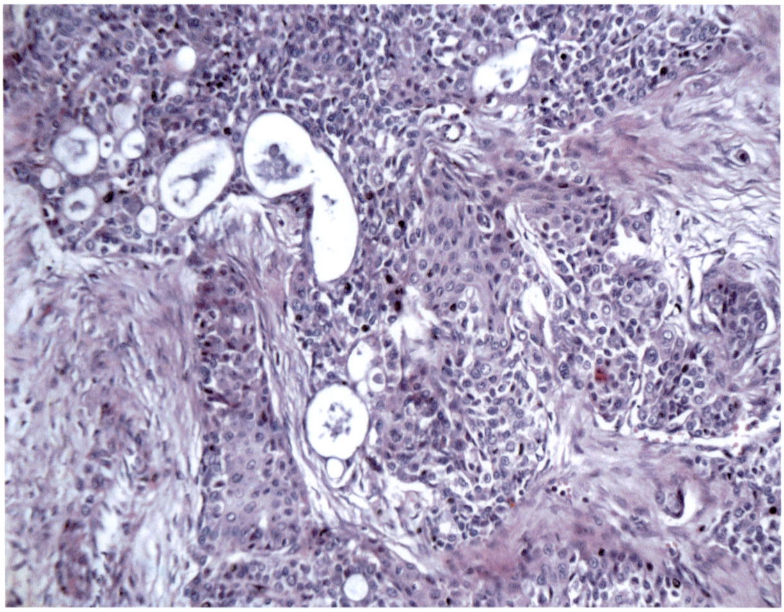

Fig. 9.4 Mucoepidermoid carcinoma (detail) (HE, ×200)

9.4 Adenoid Cystic Carcinoma (ICD-O Code 8200/3)

9.4.1 Definition

Adenoid cystic carcinoma is a malignant tumor composed of basaloid epithelial and myoepithelial cells.

Among the salivary glands, the parotid gland is the most frequent localization of adenoid cystic carcinoma. It represents less than 10 % of all epithelial tumors of the salivary glands.

9.4.2 Macroscopy

Adenoid cystic carcinoma is a firm, well-circumscribed, often unencapsulated, light red-brown, tumor.

9.4.3 Microscopy

Three main architectural types (cribriform, tubular, and solid) and two cell types (luminal ductal and myoepithelial) are described (Fig. 9.5). In the cribriform type, the most often observed, the luminal ductal cells, delineate round microcysts filled with mucoid or hyaline material (positive for low-molecular-weight keratins, carcinoembryonic antigen, c-kit, and epithelial membrane antigen) (Fig. 9.6) [2]. In the periphery of these cylindromatous nests are the myoepithelial tumoral cells, with monomorphic, hyperchromatic nuclei and sparse, amphophilic or clear cytoplasm. Immunohistochemistry shows positivity for myoepithelial markers (S100 protein, calponin, smooth muscle actin) (Fig. 9.7) [2]. The same distribution of cells is observed in the tubular pattern. In the solid pattern, the myoepithelial cells are prominent, with necrosis and mitosis being common. The stroma is hyalinized and, in sclerosing variant, may be extensive. Adenoid cystic carcinoma is an infiltrative tumor, locally aggressive toward adjacent tissues including the bone, with perineural or intraneural invasion, but which rarely metastasizes [1, 3, 5].

9.5 Polymorphous Low-Grade Adenocarcinoma (ICD-O Code 8525/3)

9.5.1 Definition

Polymorphous low-grade adenocarcinoma is a malignant epithelial tumor characterized by "cytologic uniformity, morphologic diversity, an infiltrative growth pattern, and low metastatic potential" [1].

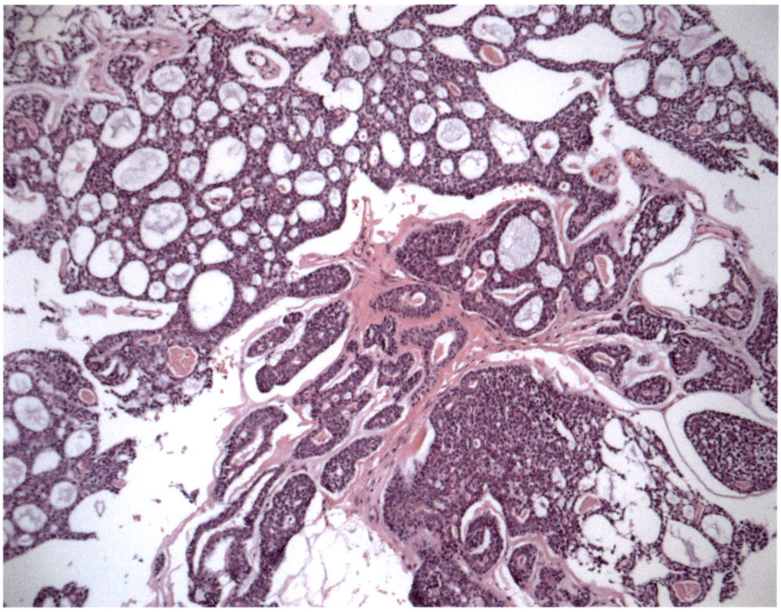

Fig. 9.5 Adenoid cystic carcinoma with cribriform, solid, and focally tubular architecture (HE, ×100)

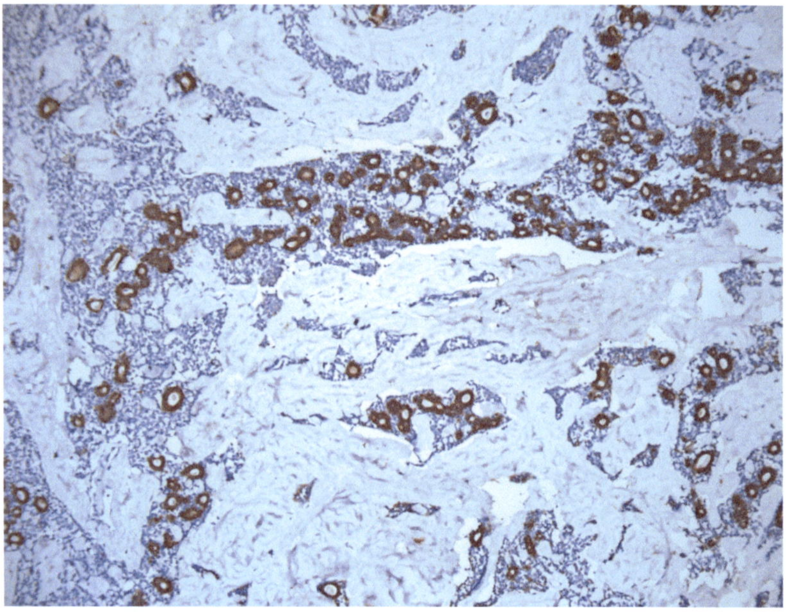

Fig. 9.6 Adenoid cystic carcinoma: cytokeratin 8 positive in luminal cells (IHC, CK8, ×100)

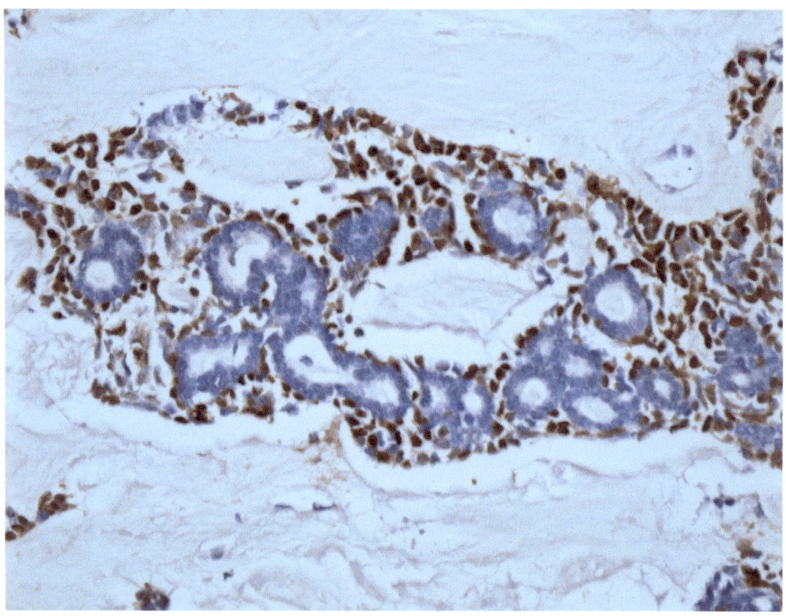

Fig. 9.7 Adenoid cystic carcinoma: S100 protein positive in myoepithelial cells (IHC, S100, ×400)

It is rarely found in the parotid gland compared to minor salivary glands.

9.5.2 Macroscopy

It is a well-circumscribed, unencapsulated, firm nodule, varying in size between 1 and 3 cm. On cut surface it is lobulated, gray to pale brown.

9.5.3 Microscopy

The main histological feature is the variety of the tumor patterns, as one may observe lobular, papillary, papillary cystic, tubular, cribriform, trabecular, or solid arrangements of the cells [1, 3, 6]. Tumor cells are uniform, small or medium sized, with round to oval pale nuclei. On immunohistochemistry, they are positive for cytokeratins, S100 protein, vimentin, galectin-3, and bcl-2

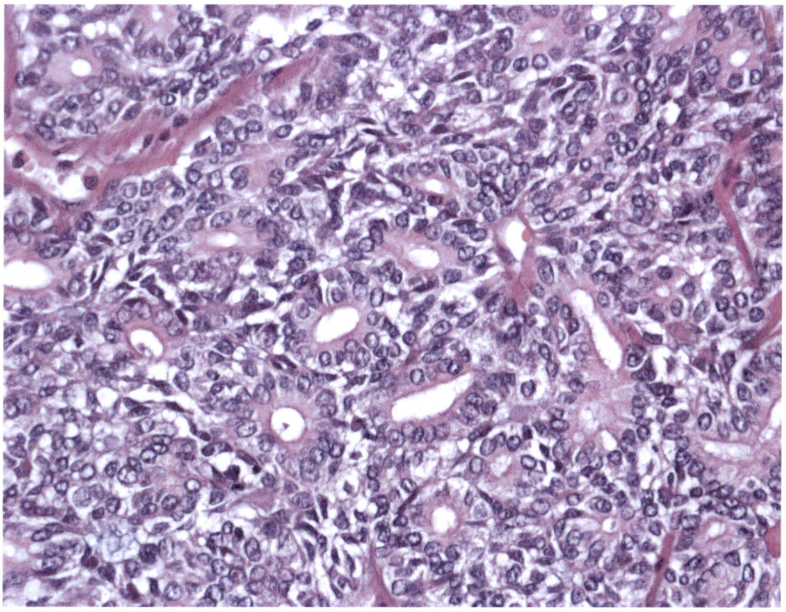

Fig. 9.8 Epithelial-myoepithelial carcinoma with tubular architecture (HE, ×400)

[1]. Mitosis and necrosis are rarely observed. Stroma is hyalinized or mucoid.

9.6 Epithelial-Myoepithelial Carcinoma (IDC-O Code 8562/3)

9.6.1 Definition

Epithelial-myoepithelial carcinoma is a malignant tumor composed of two main cell types: epithelial ductal cells and myoepithelial cells [1–3].

Although rare (less than 1 % of salivary glands tumors), almost 70 % of them are located in parotid glands [1].

9.6.2 Macroscopy

Epithelial-myoepithelial carcinomas are multinodular, unencapsulated tumors, growing in an expansive fashion.

9.6.3 Microscopy

The architecture of the tumor is tubular or solid, but papillary or cystic areas may be found. In the tubular pattern, the inner layer is represented by a single layer of epithelial tumor cells which are cuboidal, with dense eosinophilic cytoplasm and round, basal or central nuclei. Myoepithelial tumor cells around epithelial cells are single or multiple layered and have polygonal shape, clear cytoplasm and vesicular, eccentric nuclei (Fig. 9.8). On immunohistochemistry, luminal cells are positive for low-molecular-weight keratins (Fig. 9.9) and c-kit, while myoepithelial cells are positive for p63, S100 protein, smooth muscle actin (SMA) (Fig. 9.10), calponin, vimentin, and glial fibrilar acidic protein (GFAP) [1, 2]. The stroma is dense and fibrotic and, around ductal structures, one may observe a dense, hyaline, PAS-positive membrane-like material. Mitoses are rare (less than 2 mitoses/10 HPF) [1–3, 7].

9.7 Basal Cell Adenocarcinoma (IDC-O Code 8147/3)

9.7.1 Definition

Basal cell adenocarcinoma is a malignant epithelial tumor with basaloid epithelial cells, infiltrative growth, and metastatic potential [1].

It is a rare tumor, more than 90 % of basal cell adenocarcinomas of the salivary glands being located in parotid glands [1, 3].

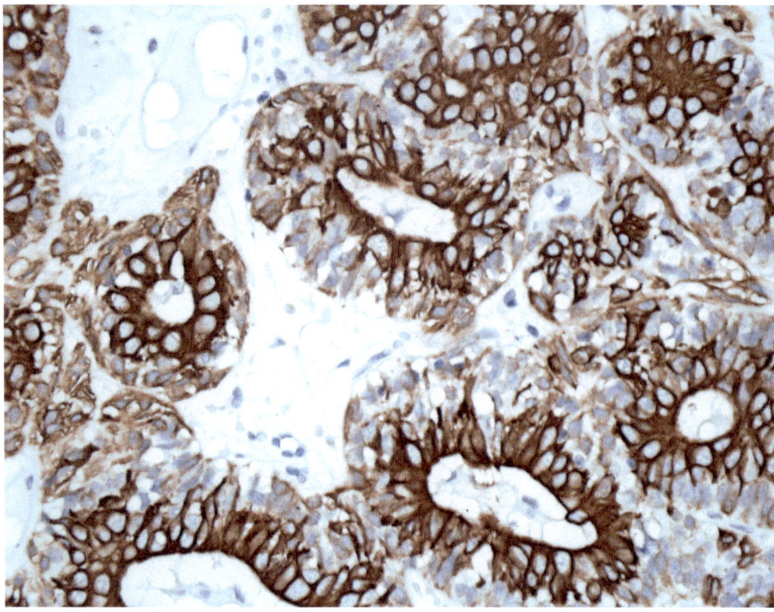

Fig. 9.9 Epithelial-myoepithelial carcinoma: cytokeratin 7 intense positive in luminal cells and mild positive in myoepithelial cells (IHC, CK7, ×400)

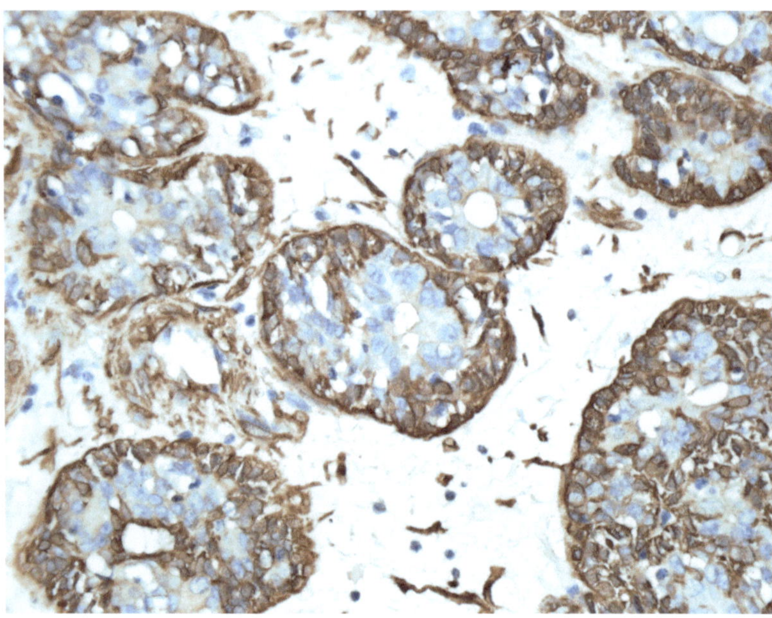

Fig. 9.10 Epithelial-myoepithelial carcinoma: SMA positive in myoepithelial cells and negative in luminal cells (IHC, SMA, ×400)

9.7.2 Macroscopy

At gross examination, basal cell carcinomas appear as non-encapsulated, tan, firm masses, sometimes with infiltrative margins. The size ranges from 0.7 to 7 cm [2].

9.7.3 Microscopy

Architecturally and cytologically, basal cell adenocarcinoma looks like basal cell adenoma and might be solid, trabecular, membranous, or tubular [1]. The solid pattern is the most frequent and consists of small and larger cells. The small cells are basaloid and dark, while the larger ones have pale cytoplasm. Nuclei are palisading at the periphery of the tumor nests, around which the stroma contains hyalinized, eosinophilic membrane-like material. Cytological and nuclear pleomorphism is reduced. Mitotic figures are more than 4/10 HPF [2]. Immunohistochemistry shows positivity for cytokeratin, and focally for epithelial membrane antigen (EMA), and carcinoembryonic antigen (CEA). Myoepithelial markers are positive in cells at the periphery [1, 2]. Necrosis and vascular and perineural invasion are common [7]. Usually, the tumor invades the parotid gland and the adjacent structures (skin, surrounding fat tissue and skeletal muscle), thus helping differentiate the basal cell carcinoma from basal cell adenoma [7].

9.8 Sebaceous Carcinoma (IDC-O Code 8410/3)

9.8.1 Definition

Sebaceous carcinoma is a malignant epithelial tumor composed of cells with sebaceous differentiation.

It is a very rare tumor in salivary glands, most of them (90 %) arising in parotid gland [1, 2].

9.8.2 Macroscopy

Sebaceous carcinoma is usually well circumscribed, sometimes with incomplete capsule, measuring up to 8 cm in greater diameter. The color is yellow, white, pink, or pale brown [1, 2].

9.8.3 Microscopy

Tumor cells grow in solid nests. The degree of cellular pleomorphism is variable, but at least some of the cells have sebaceous differentiation, with clear or eosinophilic cytoplasm, containing microvacuoles with lipids positive in Sudan III staining [1, 7]. At the periphery of the tumor nests, cells present basaloid aspect. Perineural invasion, necrosis, and fibrosis are often seen [1–3].

9.9 Cystadenocarcinoma (IDC-O Code 8440/3)

9.9.1 Definition

Cystadenocarcinoma is a malignant epithelial tumor with cystic growth, with intracystic papillary projections [1].

It is a rare tumor in salivary glands, less than 65 % occurring in the parotid gland [1].

9.9.2 Macroscopy

At gross examination, cystadenocarcinoma is a multicystic tumor containing mucin and less than 6 cm in size. It is well circumscribed and unencapsulated, invading the adjacent salivary tissue [1, 2].

9.9.3 Microscopy

The microscopical examination reveals cysts lined by cuboidal cells and, frequently, branched papillary projections lined by columnar cells [1, 2]. Also, ductal structures or solid nests might be seen. Mitotic activity is low and nuclear pleomorphism is, usually, mild.

9.10 Oncocytic Carcinoma (IDC-O Code 8290/3)

9.10.1 Definition

Oncocytic carcinoma is a malignant epithelial tumor with malignant oncocytes and architecture similar to an invasive adenocarcinoma [1, 2].

It is a rare tumor in salivary glands, over 80 % occurring in the parotid gland [1].

9.10.2 Macroscopy

Oncocytic carcinoma appears as a tan or grey, firm, non-encapsulated, single or multiple mass.

9.10.3 Microscopy

Tumor cells are arranged in solid nests or sheets, occasionally with ductal differentiation. Malignant oncocytes are large, polygonal, with central nuclei, dispersed chromatin, and macronucleoli [1]. Characteristically, the cytoplasm is intensely eosinophilic and fine granular (due to the numerous mitochondria). Mitotic activity is moderate, Ki-67 labeling providing help in differentiating benign from malignant oncocytomas [2]. Necrosis might be present. Unencapsulated, oncocytic carcinoma invades the surrounding tissues, vessels, and nerves.

9.11 Salivary Duct Carcinoma (IDC-O Code 8500/3)

9.11.1 Definition

Salivary duct carcinoma is an extremely aggressive malignant epithelial tumor with morphology similar to invasive ductal carcinoma of the breast [1, 3, 8].

The majority of them occur in parotid glands.

9.11.2 Macroscopy

It appears as an infiltrative grey to tan, rarely circumscribed, solid and cystic mass.

9.11.3 Microscopy

Architecture may vary from ductal, cribriform, or papillary (in intraductal and/or invasive component) to solid and trabecular [1, 7, 8]. Tumor cells harbor pleomorphism and high mitotic activity, resembling tumor cells of invasive breast ductal carcinoma. Sometimes, it may associate areas of pleomorphic adenoma. On immunohistochemistry, tumor cells express epithelial markers (cytokeratins, EMA, CEA), androgen receptor, HER-2/neu protein, gross cystic disease fluid protein-15 (focal), mitochondrial antigen (focal), and prostate-specific antigen (variable) [1, 2].

9.12 Adenocarcinoma, Not Otherwise Specified (NOS) (IDC-O Code 8140/3)

9.12.1 Definition

Adenocarcinoma, NOS, is a malignant epithelial tumor with ductal differentiation, without any morphological features belonging to other specific adenocarcinomas of the salivary glands.

9.12.2 Macroscopy

Adenocarcinoma, NOS, presents as a gray-whitish, solid mass, infiltrative in the surrounding tissues, including adjacent skin.

9.12.3 Microscopy

It is characterized by ductal and glandular structures admixed in variable proportions with solid, trabecular, papillary, cribriform, and cystic areas [1, 2]. Tumor cells are usually cuboidal, polyhedral, or ovoid. Clear cells and oncocytes might also be present [1, 2, 9]. Pleomorphism and mitotic activity may vary from mild in low-grade adenocarcinomas to prominent in high-grade adenocarcinomas [1]. Necrosis, hemorrhage, and invasiveness in vessels and nerves are commonly seen.

9.13 Myoepithelial Carcinoma (IDC-O Code 8982/3)

9.13.1 Definition

Myoepithelial carcinoma is a rare malignant tumor composed of "almost exclusively tumor cells with myoepithelial differentiation" [1].

9.13.2 Macroscopy

At gross examination, myoepithelial carcinomas are gray or white, solid, multinodular, well-defined, unencapsulated masses. The tumor may be large up to 10–20 cm, but the average size is about 3.5 cm [2].

9.13.3 Microscopy

Architecture and cytology in myoepithelial carcinoma is variable. The multilobulated aspect may contain areas of solid, trabecular, and reticular pattern, with central necrosis or myxoid degeneration [1, 2]. Tumor cells might be epithelioid, spindle, clear, plasmacytoid, or stellate. Usually, one tumor may associate different architectural and cytological features. Cellular pleomorphism and mitotic activity is common in most myoepithelial carcinomas. On immunohistochemistry, tumor cells express cytokeratin markers and one of the following myoepithelial markers (SMA, GFAP, CD10, calponin) [1, 2]. The tumor invades the adjacent structures.

9.14 Carcinoma Ex Pleomorphic Adenoma (IDC-O Code 8941/3)

9.14.1 Definition

Carcinoma ex pleomorphic adenoma results from a pleomorphic adenoma in which the epithelial component undergoes malignant [1].

It usually develops in parotid glands.

9.14.2 Macroscopy

Carcinoma ex pleomorphic adenoma is a large tumor, up to 25 cm. It is usually ill defined, infiltrating the surrounding tissues.

9.14.3 Microscopy

Most carcinoma ex pleomorphic adenomas present variable areas of preexisting pleomorphic adenoma which associates poorly differentiated adenocarcinoma, ductal type or NOS, or undifferentiated carcinoma [1, 2, 7, 9]. Sometimes, areas of mucoepidermoid carcinoma, polymorphous low-grade adenocarcinoma, clear cell myoepithelial carcinoma, or adenoid cystic adenocarcinoma may be present [1].

Malignancy can be stated due to infiltrative and destructive behavior, associated with variable cytological pleomorphism, obvious mitotic activity, and presence of necrosis. According to the invasiveness, there are three subtypes, noninvasive (carcinoma in situ ex pleomorphic adenoma), minimally invasive (less than 1.5 mm beyond the capsule), and invasive (more than 1.5 mm beyond the capsule) [1].

9.15 Metastasizing Pleomorphic Adenoma (IDC-O Code 8940/1)

9.15.1 Definition

Metastasizing pleomorphic adenoma is a "histological benign pleomorphic adenoma that inexplicably manifest local or distant metastasis," most frequent in the bone, lung, and lymph nodes [1].

9.15.2 Macroscopy

The tumor is well circumscribed.

9.15.3 Microscopy

Both the primary tumor and the metastases have a benign histology with epithelial and mesenchymal components.

Carcinosarcoma, *squamous cell carcinoma*, *small cell carcinoma*, *large cell carcinoma*, *lymphoepithelial carcinoma*, and *clear cell carcinoma not otherwise specified* (*NOS*) are very rare tumors each accounting for less than 1 % of the salivary glands' tumors. Their common feature is the invasiveness growth pattern in the adjacent tissues, implying extended parotidectomy.

Among benign tumors of the parotid glands, only the *pleomorphic adenoma* sometimes

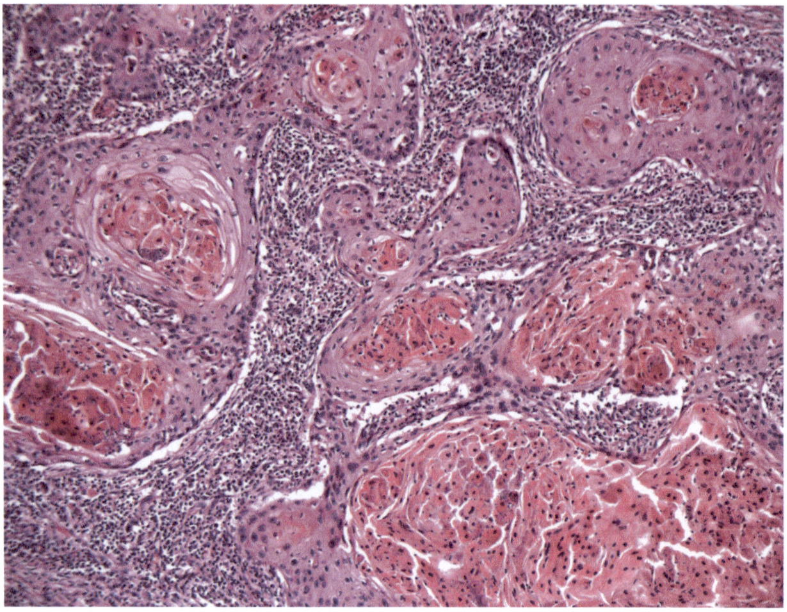

Fig. 9.11 Intraparotid lymph node metastasis of squamous cell carcinoma (HE, ×200)

necessitates extended parotidectomy. This is the case of large, neglected tumors or recurrences after superficial parotidectomies. Recurrences are more frequent after enucleation or superficial parotidectomy with incomplete pathological excision, rupture of the capsule during surgery, favored by multinodular tumors, satellite nodules beyond the capsule, or localization of the tumor in the immediate vicinity of the main tract or branches of the facial nerve [1, 10, 11].

Pleomorphic adenoma (*ICD-O code 8940/0*) is a benign tumor with architectural and cellular pleomorphism, comprising epithelial and myoepithelial cells admixed in variable proportions with mucoid, myxoid, and/or chondroid tissue [1]. Capsulation is variable, sometimes thin, dehiscent, with satellite nodules.

9.16 Vicinity Tumors Invading Parotid Glands

Malignant tumors of the skin may directly infiltrate the parotid glands (i.e., basal cell carcinoma) or metastasize in peri- or intraparotid lymph nodes (commonly, squamous cell carcinoma) (Fig. 9.11), in advanced stages. In these cases, excision of the skin tumor implies extended parotidectomy.

9.17 Secondary Tumors of the Parotid Glands

Parotid glands and intra- or periglandular lymph nodes may receive metastases, mainly from head and neck tumors (about 80 %; squamous cell carcinomas, in our experience), and, rarely, from lung, kidney, and breast carcinomas. The morphology of these metastases resembles the original tumor. In 10–15 % of the cases, the primary tumor cannot be identified.

References

1. Barnes L, Eveson JW, Reichart P, Sidransky D. World Health Organization classification of tumours. Pathology and genetics. Head and neck tumours. Lyon: IARC Press; 2005.
2. Eveson JW, Nagao T. Diseases of the salivary glands. In: Barnes L, editor. Surgical pathology of the head and neck. 3rd ed. New York: Informa Healthcare; 2009. p. 475–648.
3. Barnes L, Chiosea SI, Seethala RR. Head and neck pathology (consultant pathology). New York: Demos Medical Publishing; 2010.
4. Chen AM, Lau VH, Farwell DG, Luu Q, Donald PJ. Mucoepidermoid carcinoma of the parotid gland treated by surgery and postoperative radiation therapy: clinicopathologic correlates of outcome. Laryngoscope. 2013;123(12):3049–55.

5. Godge P, Sharma S, Yadav M. Adenoid cystic carcinoma of the parotid gland. Contemp Clin Dent. 2012;3(2):223–6.
6. Krishnamurthy A, Vaidhyanathan A, Majhi U. Polymorphous low-grade adenocarcinoma of the parotid gland. J Cancer Res Ther. 2011;7(1):84–7.
7. Gnepp DR, Henley JD, Simpson RHW, Eveson J. Salivary and lacrimal glands. In: Gnepp D, editor. Diagnostic surgical pathology of the head and neck. 2nd ed. Philadelphia: Saunders; 2009. p. 413–564.
8. Kallianpur A, Yadav R, Shukla NK, Deo S, Muduly DK. Locally advanced salivary duct carcinoma of the parotid gland. Ann Maxillofac Surg. 2012;2(2):178–81.
9. Staniceanu F, Streinu-Cercel A, Zurac S. Patologia glandelor salivare. Bucharest: Medical Publishing House; 2004.
10. Redaelli de Zinis LO, Piccioni M, Antonelli RA, Nicolai P. Management and prognostic factors of recurrent pleomorphic adenoma of the parotid gland: personal experience and review of the literature. Eur Arch Otorhinolaryngol. 2008;265(4):447–52.
11. Wittekindt C, Streubel K, Arnold G, Stennert E, Guntinas-Lichius O. Recurrent pleomorphic adenoma of the parotid gland: analysis of 108 consecutive patients. Head Neck. 2007;29:822–8.

10 Clinical Diagnosis of Extended Parotid Tumors

Orlando Guntinas-Lichius

Abstract

The clinical examination forms the fundament for decision making in a patient with an extended parotid tumor. The examination starts with an elaborate interview of the patients looking for clinical hints for a malignant disease. The clinical examination comprises a complete head and neck examination including an investigation of all major salivary glands. Thereafter, ultrasound is the first-choice imaging technique for an immediate assessment of the parotid tumor. If available, fine-needle aspiration cytology (FNAC) continues the diagnostic workup. FNAC will determine whether the parotid tumor process is malignant. Core-needle biopsy or an open biopsy may offer an additional effective diagnostic tool in cases in which FNAC has failed to provide a definitive diagnosis. In extended parotid tumors, often the situation will occur that ultrasound does not allow visualizing the parotid tumor completely, due to its location in the deep lobe. In such a situation, or if FNAC or a biopsy argue for a malignant disease, further imaging with computed tomography (CT) or magnetic resonance imaging (MRI) are indicated. MRI is the first choice. If a malignant parotid tumor is suspected, MRI and CT scanning are important for the tumor staging of the primary tumor and the neck.

10.1 Introduction

The clinical diagnosis of an extended parotid tumors starts with a history and examination of the complete head and neck region including all salivary glands and not only the affected parotid gland [1, 2]. Concerning the differential diagnosis, the duration of the history and the clinical features of the tumor are relevant. Any history of systemic disease should also be carefully assessed as the parotid tumor can be the expression of a systemic disease. Nevertheless, the symptoms of a parotid mass are often nonspecific. Several investigative methods might be necessary to confirm the final diagnosis. Sonography is the easiest, a cheap, noninvasive, and fast method for

O. Guntinas-Lichius, MD
Department of Otorhinolaryngology, University Hospital Jena, Jena, Germany
e-mail: orlando.guntinas@med.uni-jena.de

© Springer International Publishing Switzerland 2016

V.-V. Costan (ed.), *Management of Extended Parotid Tumors*, DOI 10.1007/978-3-319-26545-2_10

completing the initial clinical examination. Sonography is appropriate to get an overview about the dimension of the tumor and its relation to the neighboring structures. Sonography can be immediately combined with fine-needle examination of the tumor itself but also neighboring structures if there is any suspicion that the mass has expanded outside the parotid space.

10.2 Medical History and Important Clinical Signs

A careful history will often already confirm a probable diagnosis of a parotid tumor and rule out other diseases, respectively [1]. The duration of the disease, the description of the symptoms, and the patient's age in particular are important: Developing an extended parotid tumor takes time. It is not an acute disease occurring within a few days, although the patient might have detected the disease as a painless swelling only a few days before the consultation. Especially malignant tumors are more frequent in older age (>60 years of age). Older age may contribute to a delayed notice of the parotid tumor. Normally, a parotid tumor does not disturb the salivary function of the affected gland. Due to his larger size, an extended parotid tumor could lead to an obstruction of the main excretory duct (Stenson's duct). A blockage of the saliva flow usually does not affect the moistening of the mouth and throat because the other major salivary glands work normal. But such a blockage could produce symptoms similar to a blockage by sialolithiasis, i.e., acute painful swelling of the affected gland related to eating, which gradually subside after eating, and rising of the pain again with the next meal.

Ultrasonography or other imaging (see below) excludes this differential diagnosis of sialolithiasis.

If the obstruction exists over a longer period, the accumulation of saliva could lead to a retrograde bacterial infection. Untreated, the parotid gland even can become abscessed. Both infection and abscess can obscure the parotid mass as primary disease. Therefore, persistent swelling after antibiotic treatment of a local infection or abscess drainage has to be inspected for a persistent parotid mass.

Primary and secondary, benign and malignant parotid tumors usually present as painless enlargement [2]. Both benign and malignant tumors typically manifest as a slowly growing tumor. If the patient presents case of an extended parotid tumor, this fact alone, unless proven otherwise, argues for an aggressive and malignant tumor. A primary tumor typically involves only the affected parotid and surrounding structures but not the other salivary glands. Lymphomas and metastases are the only malignant parotid tumors that might occur bilaterally. There are at present no specific clinical signs, tests, or tumor markers available to definitively predict malignancy of the discovered parotid tumor. Smoking is the only known risk factor, but only for a Warthin tumor. Warthin tumors normally do not present as parotid tumor with extension beyond the parotid space. Fast growth but also a sudden growth spurt of the mass, local pain, immobility of the mass, skin infiltration, and concurrent facial palsy are indicators for a malignant disease. Pain may be an expression of the tumor infiltration into the surrounding structures. Facial palsy typically occurs due to a facial nerve infiltration by the tumor. The incidence of facial nerve infiltration by parotid cancer with consecutive facial palsy on presentation has been reported to be <20 %.

A direct sign of the extension of the tumor into the neighborhood beyond the parotid space is an immobility resulting from a fixation to adjacent tissue. Thereby, by proceeding infiltration, the overlying skin or mucosa or the adjacent tissues may become swollen, inflamed, or even ulcerated. Complaints indicating an extension of the parotid tumor beyond the parotid space are:

- Muscle weakness on one side of the face
- Numbness in part of the face
- Persistent local pain in the parotid
- Dysphagia
- Difficulty in opening the mouth

Nevertheless, it has to be emphasized that most patients with parotid cancer present with a slowly enlarging, painless mass. A discrete mass in an otherwise normal-appearing gland is the usual finding. Even the local extension into the surrounding tissue might be discrete and symptomless.

10.3 Clinical Examination

Examination of the patient comes first and is the basis of any diagnostic workup for patients with parotid masses. Further investigations are directed on the results of the clinical examination. The clinical examination comprises a complete head and neck examination including an investigation of all major salivary glands (Fig. 10.1). Otoscopy or ear microscopy, for instance, is important to detect or rule out an extension of the parotid tumor in posterior direction through infiltration of the outer ear canal. Inspection of the mouth is mandatory to detect an extension of the tumor into the parapharyngeal space. This is indicated by a swelling or displacement of the tonsillar region. The salivary gland examination includes bimanual palpation of the upper neck tissues located under the mandible for the submandibular and sublingual glands and anterior to the ear for the parotid gland. In order to detect a lump, all major salivary glands, not only the suspicious gland, are palpated for masses and asymmetry of the soft tissues around the mandible and anterior and inferior to the ear. Especially for extend tumors, it is necessary to perform bimanual palpation of the salivary gland in order to detect dumbbell-shaped tumors that grow into the deep lobe of the parotid gland and to evaluate lateral pharyngeal wall extension. It is to check if the parotid tumor is mobile or fixed, as fixation is a sign of malignant tumor infiltration, especially when also the skin is involved into the fixation. Involvement of the masseter muscle or of the deeper lying pterygoid muscles is indicated by painful or painless trouble or blockage to open the mouth. Asking the patient to clench on his teeth also helps to demarcate the masseter muscle from the parotid gland and the tumor mass. Movement of the tumor mass during contraction of the masseter muscle is a hint for an extension of the tumor into the masseter muscle. A secondarily acute inflamed parotid gland is tender, while the gland is usually non-tender beyond the tumor mass. Fever and swelling, pain, or erythema over the affected parotid gland can go along with the acute sialadenitis. Erythema combined with fluctuating swelling in the region of the mass is a signal for a secondary abscess formation. Abscess formation can be confirmed by ultrasound examination (see below) and/or puncture and aspiration of pus. Of course, the neck is also examined for lymphadenopathy, in case of the malignant parotid tumor to clinically stage the neck.

Intraoral inspection and bimanual palpation and massage of the submandibular gland duct orifices anterior to the base of the tongue in the floor of the mouth and parotid gland duct punctum opposite to the upper second molar are necessary in order to assess the salivary flow out of the related salivary duct punctum. In a healthy patient, massaging the parotid gland from posterior to anterior expresses clear saliva from the parotid duct. Purulent saliva is expressed when there is bacterial parotitis, and clear saliva with small yellow curds may be expressed in chronic sialadenitis. Both parotitis and chronic sialadenitis accompany and thereby camouflage a parotid tumor. If no saliva appears, a blockage of the salivary duct or severe chronic sialadenitis might be the underlying reason.

It is mandatory to evaluate the facial nerve (VII) function (Fig. 10.2): Both facial symmetries at rest and during movement have to be examined in all facial regions in order to detect even minor and partial facial nerve palsy [3]. In case of a facial palsy, electrodiagnostics is recommended. Electromyography can reveal signs of a degenerative lesion of the facial, indicating a malignant etiology in case of a parotid tumor [4, 5]. Sensation of the facial skin has to be tested to check the function of the trigeminal nerve (V). Of utmost importance is the testing of the maxillary nerve (V2) as this branch is passing the skull through the foramen rotundum to cross the pterygopalatine fossa. Numbness in the dermatome V2 is indicating a parotid tumor with infiltration of the pterygopalatine fossa. The cranial nerve

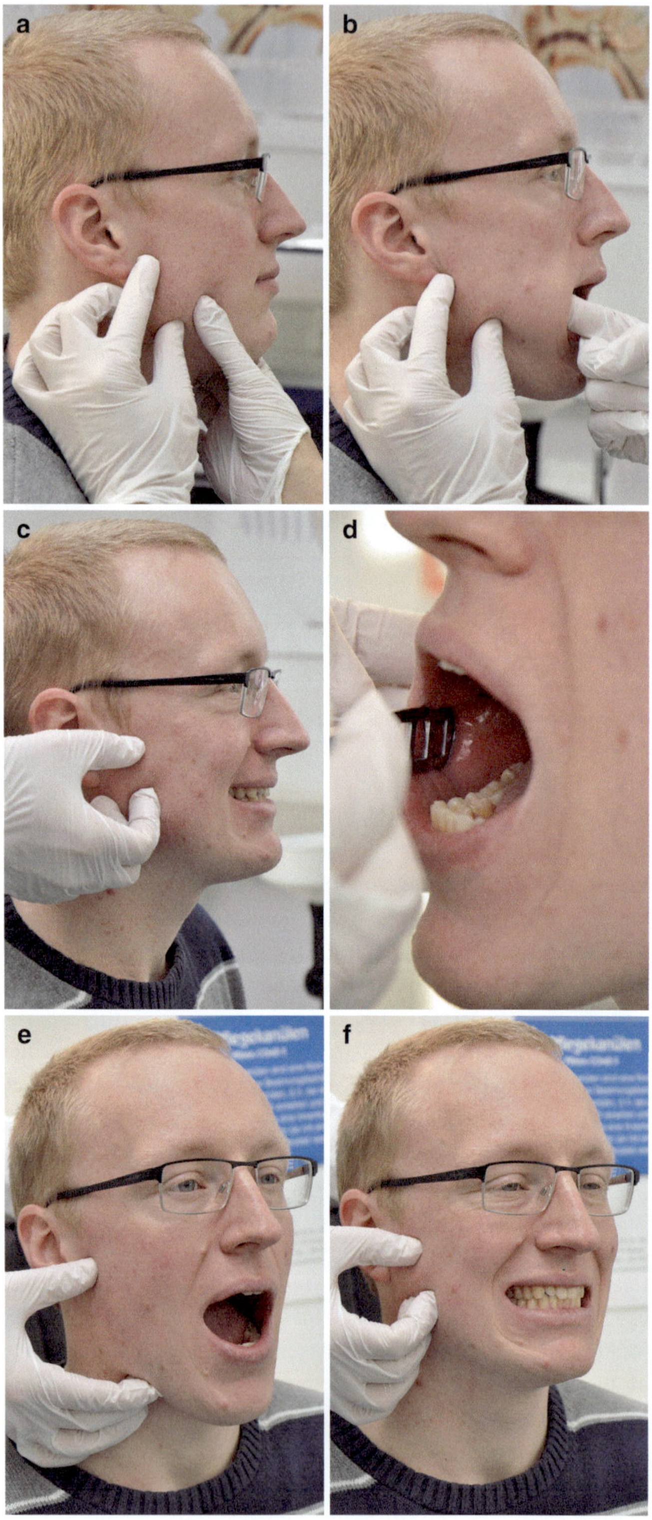

Fig. 10.1 Additional examinations in patients with extended parotid tumors. (**a**, **b**) Bimanual palpation of the parotid tumor in the right parotid gland. (**c**) Clenching the teeth helps to determine an infiltration of the masseter muscle. (**d**) Inspection of the orifice of the Stenon's duct. (**e**, **f**) Opening the mouth and clenching teeth are tests to discover functional deficits of the chewing muscles because of a tumor infiltration

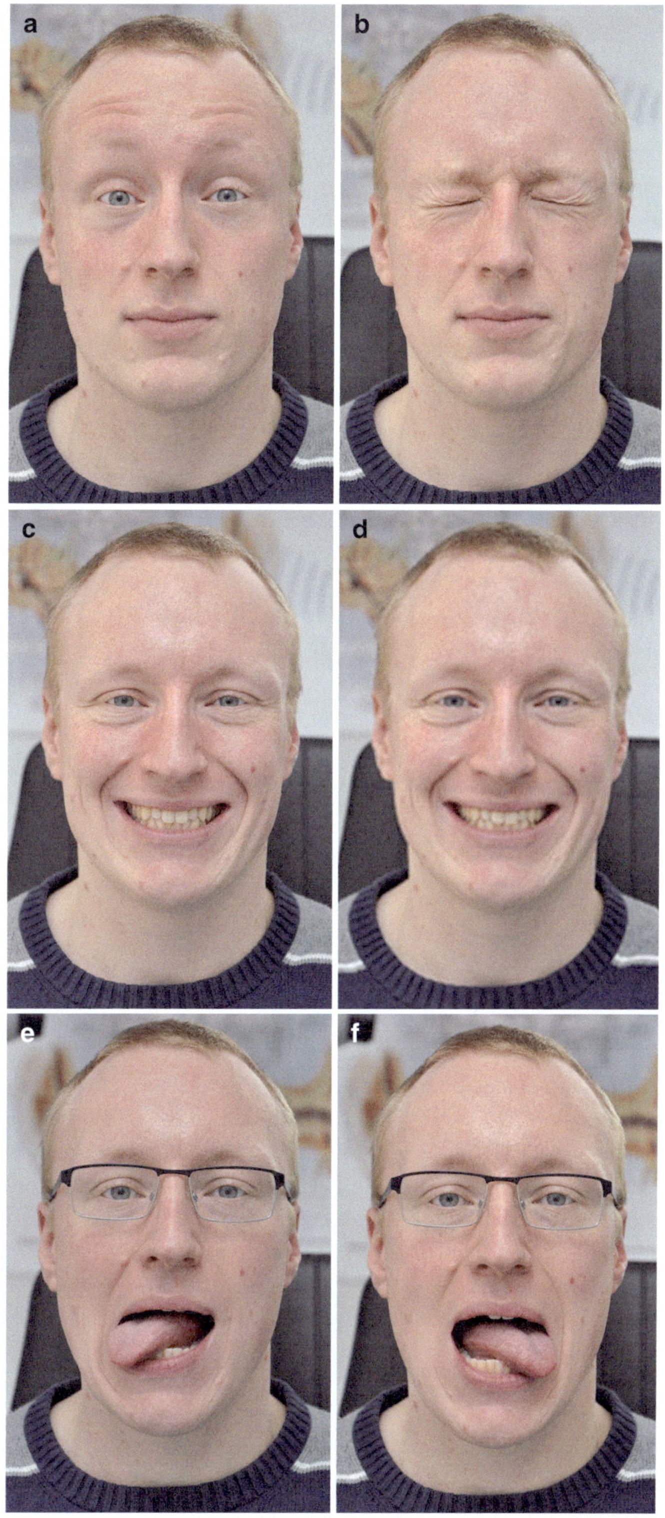

Fig. 10.2 (**a**–**f**) Examination of facial nerve function

examination should be completed. Of particular attention are also the glossopharyngeal nerve (IX), vagal nerve (X), and the accessory nerve (XI) because they are all exiting the skull through the jugular foramen. Functional deficits of these cranial nerves are signifying a tumor extension along the skull base up to the jugular foramen. Nearby is the hypoglossal canal for the hypoglossal nerve (XII). Therefore, tongue function has to be tested, too. Besides, normal hypoglossal function is a prerequisite to use this nerve for facial reanimation in case of severe facial nerve lesion (see Chap. 21).

10.4 Serologic and Saliva Examinations

The indication for serology tests is limited to differential diagnosis [6]. There are so far no specific serology tests for parotid tumors specific enough to be incorporated into clinical practice. In case of severe secondary acute bacterial sialadenitis, it might be necessary to analyze saliva samples to identify pathogens and their antibiotic resistance profile in some special or refractory situations or when a salivary abscess develops [7].

10.5 Ultrasound

Ultrasound is a quick, noninvasive, and inexpensive method to assess parotid tumors and their extension without any radiation exposure [8, 9]. If it is available, ultrasound is the first-choice imaging technique for assessing the salivary glands and a parotid tumor. The method is presented together with the clinical examination as both go hand in hand, at best by the same examiner, and can even be combined with fine-needle aspiration cytology (FNAC; see below and Fig. 10.3) [10]. In many European countries in Europe, ultrasound examination of the head and neck is part of routine training for head and neck surgeons. Ultrasonography usually is performed using linear-array transducers with a frequency of 7–12 MHz. The entire salivary glands and all

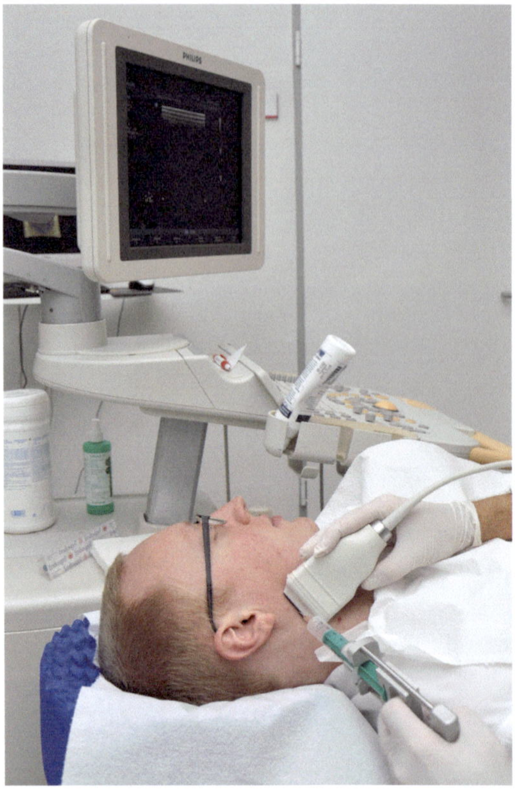

Fig. 10.3 Ultrasonographic examination of parotid tumor of the right side including fine-needle aspiration cytology

pathologies have to be evaluated and documented in frozen images on at least two perpendicular planes during ultrasonography [11]. The whole neck and both thyroid lobes are also be scanned to assess any potential lymph node enlargement and to search for concomitant or related disease. In large lesions as it is often the case in parotid tumors with considerable extension, additional transducers with a lower frequency are advisable in order to delineate the lesion completely. Using the color Doppler and the power Doppler imaging mode, the method is helpful for assessing the vascularity of the tumor and in deciding whether a mass lesion is solid or cystic. It is important to notice the limitations of the method: Ultrasonography is operator dependent and does not allow complete cross-sectional imaging of the parotid gland like with computed tomography or magnetic resonance imaging. The deep lobe of the parotid gland may be difficult to visualize or even impossible due to the adjacent mandible.

Parotid tumors with extension often affect the deep lobe. Therefore, ultrasound might underestimate the tumor size in the depth. In addition, ultrasound does not show the extratemporal facial nerve and its branches. Ultrasound is not suited to evaluate a tumor infiltration of the skull base or of the mandible.

From the point of view of the ultrasound examiner, it is important to know that the parotid gland is located in the retromandibular fossa, anterior to the ear and sternocleidomastoid muscle. Extended parotid tumors can infiltrate or displace the sternocleidomastoid muscle. Parts of the superficial lobe cover the mandible and the posterior part of the masseter muscle. Extended parotid tumors can also infiltrate or displace the masseter muscle. The intraparotid facial plexus of the facial nerve is normally not visible with standard sonography. The retromandibular vein is the landmark to separate approximately superficial and deep lobe of the gland. The deep parotid lobe can only partially be visualized. Parts are hidden behind the mandible. Therefore, parts of an extended parotid tumor reaching the deep lobe can also be hidden behind the mandible. Stenson's duct, lying on the masseter muscle, is seldom visible with standard ultrasonography unless dilated by obstruction. Normal parotid lymph nodes have a hyperechoic hilum, a short axis of <5 to 6 mm, and central vessels may be seen with Doppler ultrasound.

The parotid gland has high acoustic impedance and a homogeneous echotexture. Therefore a parotid tumor is easily detected within a normal echogenic parotid gland [12]. Ultrasound is not able to differentiate a benign from a malignant tumor. It only can give indirect hints for a malignant disease: Malignant tumors generally have a hypoechoic texture and irregular shape and have poorly defined borders. The presence of metastatic-appearing lymph nodes accompanying the tumor in the parotid gland is another hint for a malignant disease. However, malignant tumors may look just the same as benign tumors on ultrasound. Skull base involvement in malignant tumors cannot be proven. In case of secondary inflammation, the demarcation of the tumor from the surrounding inflamed parotid tissue might be impaired.

10.6 Fine-Needle Aspiration Cytology

FNAC is an important and reliable tool in the diagnostic workup of parotid tumors [13, 14]. However FNAC continues to be a matter of debate among some head and neck surgeons. It is not available in all centers dealing with salivary gland diseases. One major problem is that the accuracy of FNAC stands or falls with the availability of adequately trained cytopathologists with the requisite skills and experience. The aim of FNAC and the subsequent cytological examination is to determine whether the parotid tumor process is inflammatory and/or reactive, benign, or malignant and if possible to give a specific diagnosis. Knowing beforehand whether the parotid tumor is malignant might aid in surgical planning, may expedite or delay the decision in favor of surgery, and is important for patient counseling. If the lesion is small or is localized deep in the parotid tissue, it can be helpful to perform FNAC under sonographic control. If initial FNAC did not reveal a clear diagnosis, it might be necessary to repeat the procedure.

10.7 Parotid Biopsy

A parotid biopsy allowing a histological examination of the tissue is possible by core-needle biopsy or by open biopsy [15]. Core-needle biopsy may offer an additional effective diagnostic tool in cases in which FNAC has failed to provide a definitive diagnosis and the aim is to avoid open biopsy. In order to avoid accidental puncture of large blood vessels, core-needle biopsy should always be carried out under ultrasound control. Local anesthesia is needed. In the hands of an experienced pathologist, the accuracy of ultrasound-guided core-needle biopsies is comparably high as final histological findings. An open parotid biopsy is only indicated when the likely diagnosis of a pleomorphic adenoma has been excluded to avoid cell spreading of the pleomorphic adenoma. In cases of extended parotid tumors, especially with skin infiltration, an open tissue biopsy is a fast way to assure a malignant disease.

10.8 Magnetic Resonance Imaging and Computed Tomography

In extended parotid tumors, often the situation will occur that ultrasound does not allow visualizing the parotid tumor completely, due to its location in the deep lobe. In such a situation, or if FNAC or a biopsy argues for a malignant disease, further imaging with computed tomography (CT) or magnetic resonance imaging (MRI) is indicated [16, 17]. These methods are presented in detail in Chap. 11. If ultrasound is not available or does not demonstrate a clear tumor margin or capsule, MRI is the first choice [18]. If a malignant parotid tumor is suspected, MRI and CT scanning are important for the tumor staging of the primary tumor and the neck.

References

1. Chen S, Paul BC, Myssiorek D. An algorithm approach to diagnosing bilateral parotid enlargement. Otolaryngol Head Neck Surg. 2013;148(5):732–9. PubMed.
2. Carlson ER, Webb DE. The diagnosis and management of parotid disease. Oral Maxillofac Surg Clin North Am. 2013;25(1):31–48. v. PubMed.
3. Guntinas-Lichius O. The facial nerve in the presence of a head and neck neoplasm: assessment and outcome after surgical management. Curr Opin Otolaryngol Head Neck Surg. 2004;12(2):133–41. PubMed.
4. Grosheva M, Wittekindt C, Guntinas-Lichius O. Prognostic value of electroneurography and electromyography in facial palsy. Laryngoscope. 2008;118(3):394–7. PubMed Epub 2007/12/20. eng.
5. Volk GF, Klingner C, Finkensieper M, Witte OW, Guntinas-Lichius O. Prognostication of recovery time after acute peripheral facial palsy: a prospective cohort study. BMJ Open. 2013;3(6):e003007. PubMed Pubmed Central PMCID: 3669721.
6. Nieuw Amerongen AV, Ligtenberg AJ, Veerman EC. Implications for diagnostics in the biochemistry and physiology of saliva. Ann N Y Acad Sci. 2007;1098:1–6. PubMed.
7. Isa AY, Hilmi OJ. An evidence based approach to the management of salivary masses. Clin Otolaryngol. 2009;34(5):470–3. PubMed.
8. Gritzmann N, Rettenbacher T, Hollerweger A, Macheiner P, Hubner E. Sonography of the salivary glands. Eur Radiol. 2003;13(5):964–75. PubMed.
9. Katz P, Hartl DM, Guerre A. Clinical ultrasound of the salivary glands. Otolaryngol Clin N Am. 2009;42(6):973–1000. Table of Contents. PubMed.
10. Kraft M, Lang F, Mihaescu A, Wolfensberger M. Evaluation of clinician-operated sonography and fine-needle aspiration in the assessment of salivary gland tumours. Clin Otolaryngol. 2008;33(1):18–24. PubMed.
11. Bialek EJ, Jakubowski W, Zajkowski P, Szopinski KT, Osmolski A. US of the major salivary glands: anatomy and spatial relationships, pathologic conditions, and pitfalls. Radiographics. 2006;26(3):745–63. PubMed.
12. Shimizu M, Ussmuller J, Hartwein J, Donath K, Kinukawa N. Statistical study for sonographic differential diagnosis of tumorous lesions in the parotid gland. Oral Surg Oral Med Oral Pathol Oral Radiol Endod. 1999;88(2):226–33. PubMed.
13. Verma K, Kapila K. Role of fine needle aspiration cytology in diagnosis of pleomorphic adenomas. Cytopathology. 2002;13(2):121–7. PubMed.
14. Zbaren P, Nuyens M, Loosli H, Stauffer E. Diagnostic accuracy of fine-needle aspiration cytology and frozen section in primary parotid carcinoma. Cancer. 2004;100(9):1876–83. PubMed.
15. Pijpe J, Kalk WW, van der Wal JE, Vissink A, Kluin PM, Roodenburg JL, et al. Parotid gland biopsy compared with labial biopsy in the diagnosis of patients with primary Sjogren's syndrome. Rheumatology. 2007;46(2):335–41. PubMed eng.
16. Howlett DC, Kesse KW, Hughes DV, Sallomi DF. The role of imaging in the evaluation of parotid disease. Clin Radiol. 2002;57(8):692–701. PubMed.
17. Lee YY, Wong KT, King AD, Ahuja AT. Imaging of salivary gland tumours. Eur J Radiol. 2008;66(3):419–36. PubMed eng.
18. Yerli H, Aydin E, Haberal N, Harman A, Kaskati T, Alibek S. Diagnosing common parotid tumours with magnetic resonance imaging including diffusion-weighted imaging vs fine-needle aspiration cytology: a comparative study. Dentomaxillofac Radiol. 2010;39(6):349–55. PubMed Pubmed Central PMCID: 3520240.

11 The Diagnostic Imaging of Extended Parotid Tumors

Orlando Guntinas-Lichius
and Hartmut Peter Burmeister

Abstract

Extended parotid tumors require a precise preoperative assessment. Imaging is an indispensable part of the diagnostic work-up. The algorithm for the imaging of extended or suspected extended parotid tumors is basically easy to describe: If available, ultrasonography gives a first overview about the tumor. It can be combined with fine-needle aspiration cytology to get first information if the tumor is benign or malignant. The exact extent of an extended parotid tumor is most often not to be determined by ultrasonography, especially when the tumor is located in the deep parotid lobe. High-resolution magnetic resonance imaging (MRI) is mandatory to delineate the exact borders of the tumor and its extent into surrounding structures. If MRI is not available or contraindicated, computed tomography (CT) is an alternative. Furthermore, CT allows a good evaluation of the relation of the parotid tumor to the bony skull base. The chapter presents in detail the advantages and disadvantages of ultrasonography, MRI, and CT. Furthermore, the role of other imaging technique like of contrast-enhanced positron emission tomography (PET) together with CT (PET-CT) is discussed.

11.1 Introduction

In case of an extended parotid tumor, imaging should of course show the complete extent and the exact localization and borders of the primary tumor. Furthermore, it is equally important that imaging is exactly depicting the extension or infiltration of the parotid tumor into neighboring structures. Finally, in case of neoplasms, imaging should allow at best a staging of the primary tumor and of neck status concerning lymph node metastasis. In case of a multinodular recurrence

O. Guntinas-Lichius, MD (✉)
Department of Otorhinolaryngology, University Hospital Jena, Jena, Germany
e-mail: orlando.guntinas@med.uni-jena.de

H.P. Burmeister, MD, Priv.-Doz. Dr. med. habil.
Institute of Diagnostic and Interventional Radiology, Neuroradiology, and Nuclear Medicine, Klinikum Bremerhaven Reinkenheide,
Bremerhaven, Bremen, Germany

© Springer International Publishing Switzerland 2016

V.-V. Costan (ed.), *Management of Extended Parotid Tumors*, DOI 10.1007/978-3-319-26545-2_11

of a pleomorphic adenoma, multiple nodules are typically found beyond the prior scar line. Here, imaging should be able to detect as much of the sometimes very small recurrent nodules. In general, imaging of parotid tumors, not only of extended tumors, is difficult, because of the huge number of histological subtypes. Imaging can give some information about the characteristics of the tumor and can give hints that the tumor might be malignant. Up to now, imaging cannot substitute a histological examination, i.e., imaging alone cannot confirm the diagnosis of a malignant tumor when faced with an extended parotid tumor. This chapter presents the imaging work-up before and after treatment of an extended parotid tumor. Especially, the role of ultrasonography, computed tomography (CT), magnetic resonance imaging (MRI), and positron emission tomography/CT (PET/CT) are presented.

11.2 Selecting the Appropriate Imaging Technique and Imaging Work Flow

If available, especially when available and performed in the same department in which also the surgery is performed, ultrasonography is the first, fast, and easiest imaging method to get an overview about the tumor and the neck status [1, 2]. Even if the primary tumor cannot be depicted completely, ultrasonography might help to differentiate between a benign and malignant lesion because ultrasonography-guided fine-needle aspiration cytology (FNAC) might reveal a malignant tumor [3]. In that case, or if cytology is inconclusive, deep tumor spread is suspected, or if facial palsy is present, the next and mandatory step is an MRI examination. MRI for lesions of the deep lobe is mandatory, because deep lobe parotid gland lesions are partially not seen by ultrasonography (Fig. 11.1). It is also important that often the extension of a parotid tumor into the pterygoid muscles cannot be seen by ultrasonography. Even to differentiate an extension from an infiltration into the masseter or sternocleidomastoid muscle might be difficult by ultrasonography. If MRI is not available, or when MRI is contraindicated because of other reasons, CT is the best alternative. However, MRI is superior to CT for soft tissue differentiation and detection of perineural tumor spread. During the follow-up of the patient after surgery or radiotherapy, ultrasonography still is the first choice, but to differentiate posttherapeutic fibrosis and edema from a recurrence might be not possible. Or it might be impossible to differentiate a new muscle infiltration from fibrosis from a prior muscle infiltration treated earlier. Nevertheless, ultrasonography might assist FNAC to increase the probability to hit a small recurrent tumor in the fibrotic parotid region. MRI, CT, and PET/CT are better choices in the recurrent situation. CT is inferior to MRI and PET/CT for such an assessment during follow-up. It is still a matter of debate if PET/CT is superior to MRI to detect a recurrent parotid tumor.

11.3 Ultrasonography

Basic technical aspects and advantages of ultrasonography were presented in detail in Chap. 10. Ultrasonography is able in most cases of a circumscribed inexplicit mass to differentiate if a tumor is located in the parotid gland, outside or both [1, 2]. This is true also for most cases if the tumor is located in the superficial lobe. If the disease is accompanied by an inflammatory reaction, it might even be difficult to detect a small tumor. This is much more difficult in large lesion and lesion of the deep parotid lobe as it is frequently the case for tumors extending from the gland to the surrounding tissue medial and deep to the parotid gland (Figs. 11.2c and 11.3b). Ultrasonography nicely can describe if a lesion is cystic or solid but that does not help to validly differentiate benign from malignant tumors. Nevertheless, there are some features that are suspicious for a malignant lesion: irregular border, heterogeneous echotexture, necrosis, and cystic changes. Local invasions into the subcutaneous tissues and skin are other signs but often such features become obvious already during the clinical examination and palpation. If such features are detected, it is indicated to perform MRI

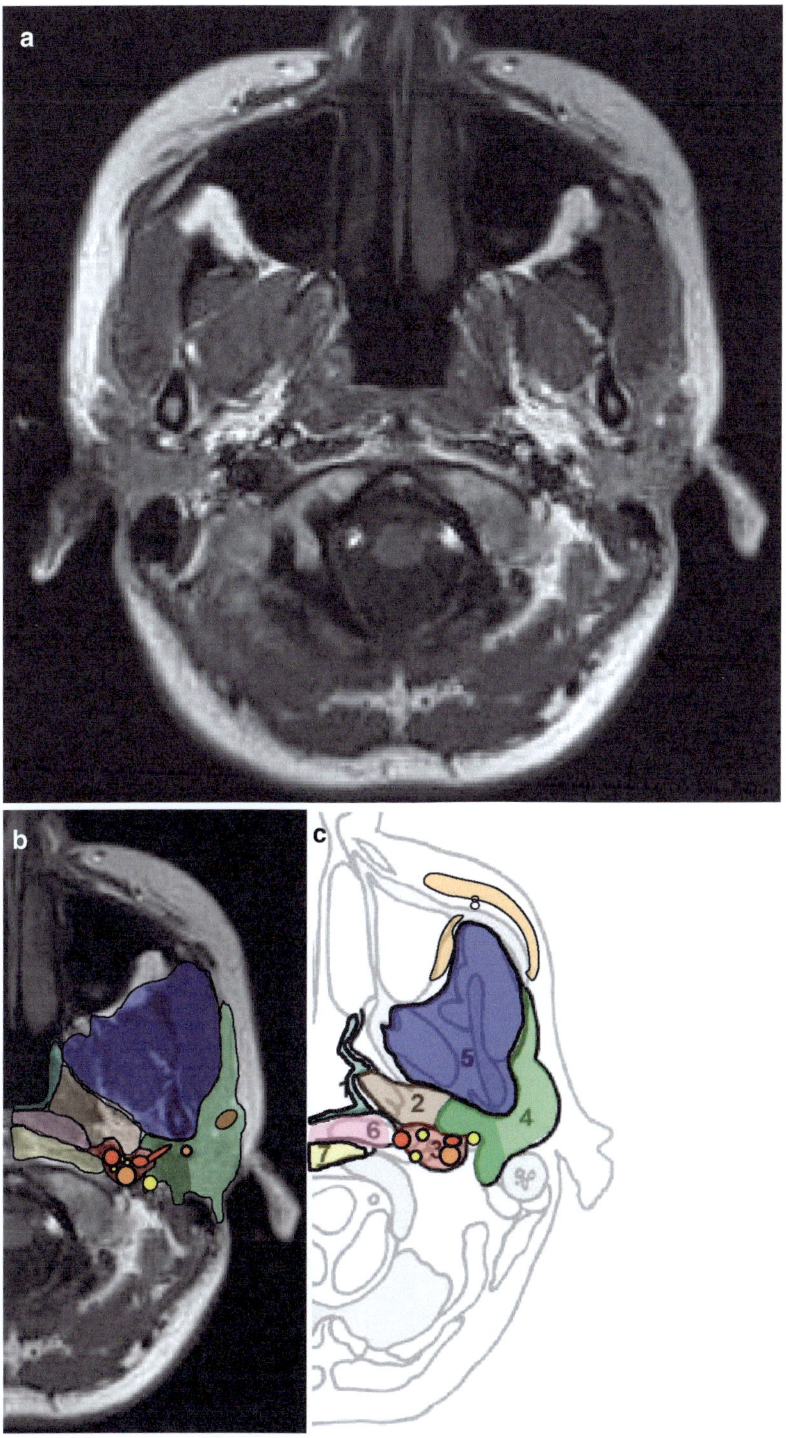

Fig. 11.1 (**a–c**) MRI clearly depicts the neighboring soft tissue compartments of the parotideal region and therefore could precisely detect the infiltration of an extended parotid tumor into the surrounding structures. *1* uperficial compartment, mucosa, *2* parapharyngeal compartment, *3* carotid compartment, *4* parotid compartment, *5* masticator compartment, *6* retropharyngeal compartment, *7* prevertebral compartment, and *8* buccal compartment

St 11.,Sono 1, CT 001-0, MR 006-0

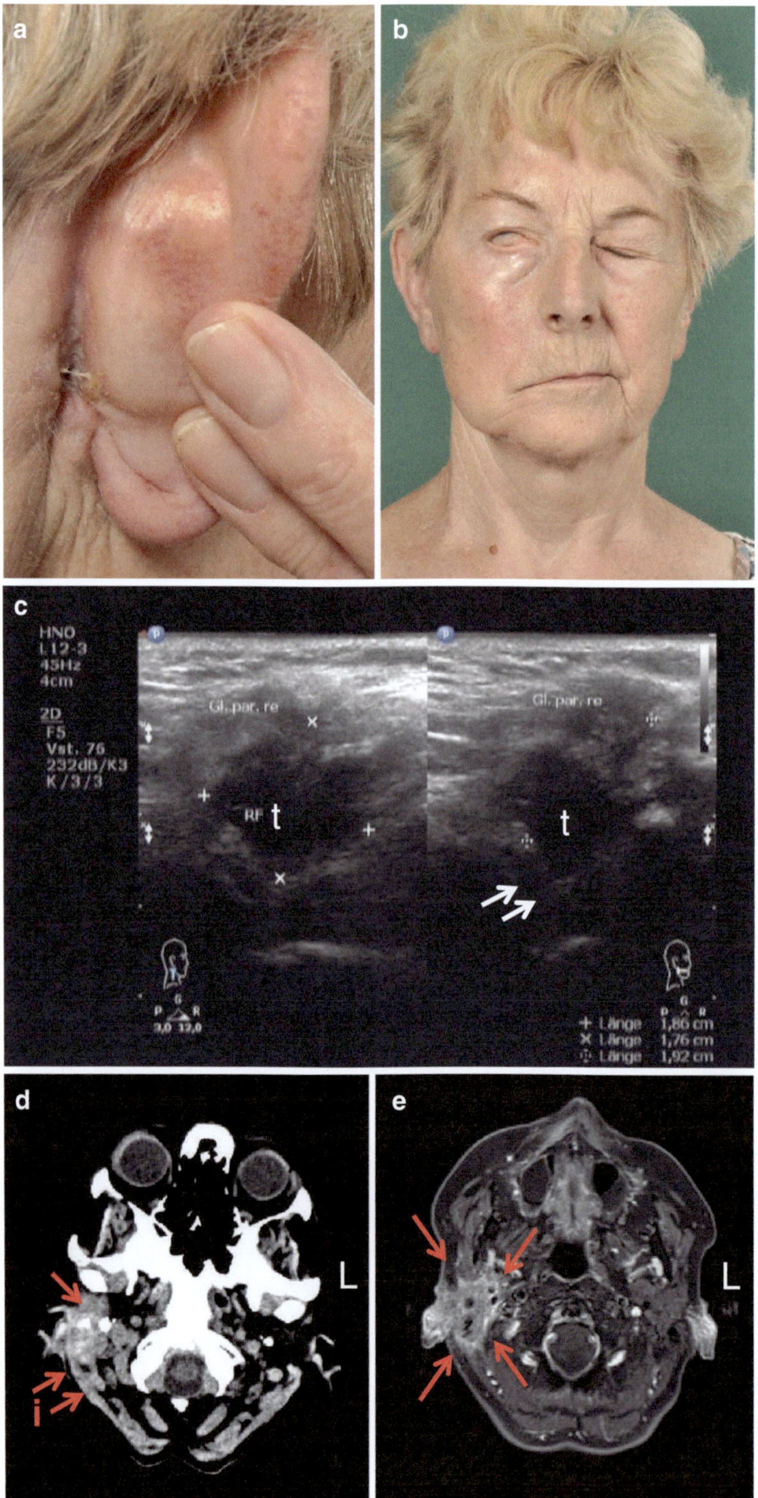

Fig. 11.2 Parotid carcinoma of the right side with facial palsy. (**a**) Skin infiltration of the tumor behind the right ear. (**b**) Complete facial palsy on the affected right side. (**c**) Ultrasonography of the right parotid and of the tumor (*t*) cannot show the infiltration of the surrounding tissue (*white arrows* and *i* = infiltration). (**d**) Axial CT shows the retroauricular extension but the delineation of the tumor's borders (*red arrows*) is difficult (*I* = cutaneous infiltration?). (**e**) Axial MRI most suitable depicts the tumor and its extension (*red arrows*)

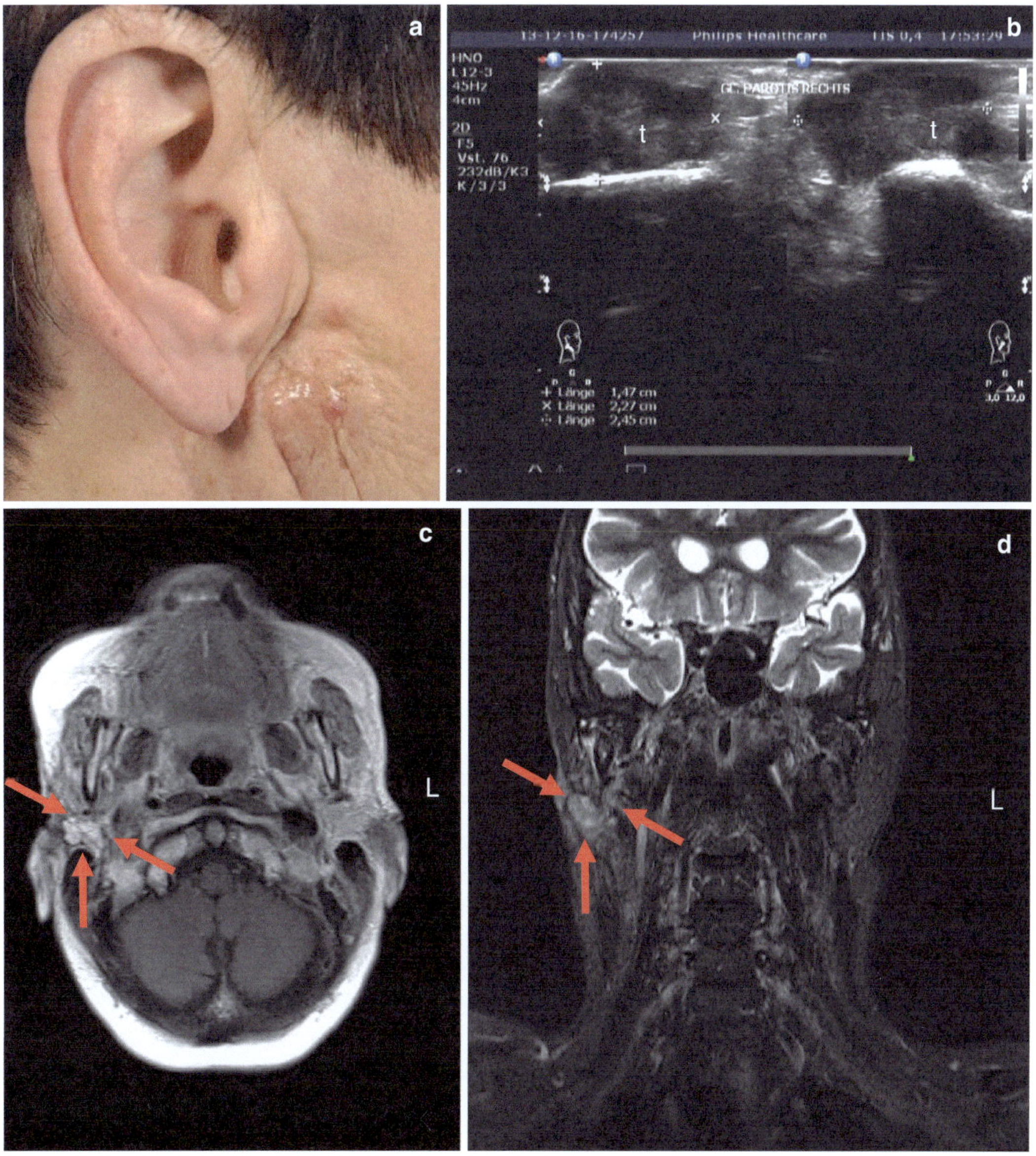

Fig. 11.3 Recurrent adenocarcinoma of the right parotid gland with normal facial function. Primary treatment 2 years ago was parotidectomy and postoperative radiotherapy. (**a**) The tumor became obvious by the skin infiltration (*arrows*). (**b**) Ultrasonography showing the recurrent tumor (*t*). (**c**) Axial MRI showing in contrast to the ultrasonography the tumor infiltration into the former deep lobe area and the pterygoid fossa (*red arrows*). The infiltration of the masseter that was revealed later during surgery is not clearly seen. (**d**) Coronal MRI of the tumor extension (*red arrows*)

or if not available a CT as the next diagnostic step. If ultrasonography shows an extension of the tumor into the deep lobe, or extension into the surrounding muscles, MRI or CT is also mandatory. Be aware that ultrasonography cannot show or rule out bony invasion at the skull base.

One special situation for a benign tumor has to be addressed: In case of current pleomorphic adenoma, the number of recurrent nodules that are detected by palpation is often lower than the number of nodules seen by ultrasonography. Further, the number of nodules seen by ultrasonography still is often much lower than the actual number of nodules. At best, MRI is necessary to detect as much of a multinodular recurrence as possible.

11.4 Magnetic Resonance Imaging

If ultrasonography is not available or does not demonstrate a clear tumor margin or capsule, MRI is the first choice [4, 5]. If a malignant parotid tumor is suspected by ultrasonography, MRI is also the next step in the imaging work-up (see Figs. 11.2e and 11.3c, d). MRI shows a much better tissue contrast and therefore anatomical details than CT or ultrasonography. MRI can also show the involvement of cranial nerves and perineural spreading. If the patient has an allergy to contrast media, it is better to perform MRI than CT without contrast media. Because MRI does not include the exposure to X-rays, it is preferred to CT in children. Dental artifacts are normally less disturbing than with CT. Not all patients tolerate MRI, e.g., due to claustrophobia. Related to this, it is also disadvantageous that MRI needs a much longer scanning time than CT. MRI also might be contraindicated in some patients with medical implants. Finally, it is more expensive than CT.

Field strength of 1.5 T is nowadays a standard for MRI of the parotid gland. If available, 3.0 T delivers even better images. The parotid gland is depicted with head and neck coils and surface coils. Standard are thin section (3–4 mm, 0–1 mm intersection gap, $\geq 20 \times 20$ cm field of view, $\geq 512 \times 257$ acquisition matrix), T1-weighted, gadolinium contrast-enhanced T1-weighted MR images with and without fat saturation, and short tau inversion recovery (STIR) sequences. In case of an extended parotid tumor, especially the fat suppression technique together with the application of contrast medium is very helpful. This fat suppression technique makes it much easier to follow the borders of the tumor and its extension into surrounding structures. If available, 3D techniques with T1-weighted gradient echo (GRE), volumetric interpolated breath-hold examination (VIBE), or the sampling perfection with application-optimized contrast using different flip angle evolutions (SPACE) sequence help to precisely describe deep tumor expansion and invasion.

In general, in MRI parotid neoplasms can show irregular tumor margins without or with infiltration into surrounding tissues, intermediate to low signal intensity on T2-weighted images, and a general heterogeneity in signal intensity. But be careful, these characteristics have to be interpreted together with other clinical findings. Benign tumors like pleomorphic adenoma also can show heterogeneity of the tissue signal. A definitive differentiation between benign and malignant disease is not possible with MRI. The future must show if newer techniques like diffusion-weighted MRI (DW-MRI) can help for better differentiating between benign and malignant parotid tumors [6, 7]. So far, the number of tumors examined is too low to draw final conclusions. Perineural tumor spread can be suspected if gadolinium enhancement is seen for involved cranial nerve or by a widening of the related bony foramen at the skull base on MRI. CT only shows the late aspect of perineural spread – it is the changes of the bony foramens at the skull base. Loss of perineural fat is another MRI sign for perineural tumor spread. This is of course also important for a tumor infiltration of the extratemporal facial nerve. Loss of fat is also an important sign for other fat-bearing areas: If the parotid tumor extends via the palatine nerves to the pterygopalatine fossa, the fat within the fossa typically is obliterated. When the parotid tumor invades the base of the skull or the mandible, MRI can show the cortical erosions (but less precise than using CT) and detects marrow infiltration (low signal intensity on T2-weighted images and moderate enhancement with contrast medium). Finally, MRI is also used to stage the neck of the patient.

11.5 Computed Tomography

CT has a wide availability. It normally has a faster acquisition time than MRI. If an MRI is not available, a contrast-enhanced CT is the method of choice [8, 9]. Additionally, CT allows evaluation of the bony skull base. Artifacts due to dental implants may be a problem in extended parotid tumors as this can impede an evaluation of deep muscle infiltration in the pterygoid fossa [10]. Contrast-enhanced CT is, of course, contraindicated in patients with known allergy to iodinated contrast media. Using contrast-enhanced CT provides the advantage that the majority of malignant processes show a contrast enhancement (see Fig. 11.2d). Nevertheless, mucoepidermoid carcinoma, adenoid cystic carcinoma, and acinic cell carcinoma sometime do not show any contrast enhancement. CT helps to detect tumor irregularities, necrosis, and extension beyond the parotid gland, muscle infiltration, and infiltration of the subcutaneous tissue and of the skin. Moreover, invasion of the base of the skull, of the mandible, and of large vessels can be seen. Concerning bony invasion, high-resolution CT – including the acquisition of very thin slices – should be performed. High-resolution CT can detect cortical erosions with greater accuracy than MRI. Compared to MRI, computed tomography is also advantageous to differentiate between reactive bone marrow edema and tumor invasion. In such situations, MRI might overestimate the bony invasion. Like for the primary disease, CT is helpful to stage the neck: Metastases of lymph nodes in the neck can be classified.

11.6 Other Imaging Techniques

Meanwhile, positron emission tomography (PET) with fluorine 18 fluorodeoxyglucose (FDG) and especially the combination of PET with CT (PET/CT) are widely used for oncologic imaging [11]. The idea behind is to receive information about the metabolic state of the parotid tumor that cannot be provided by ultrasonography, MRI, or CT. Combining PET and CT in one scanner can localize the metabolically abnormal parotid tumor and metastasis precisely. Nevertheless, only few studies have compared the value of PET/CT in comparison to MRI and CT in parotid gland imaging. PET/CT can definitively help, when histologic work-up cannot differentiate metastasis of the parotid gland from a primary parotid tumor. One should know that there is a physiological bilateral tracer uptake. In case of a malignant, and/or extended parotid tumor, an asymmetric tracer uptake is suspicious for a malignant parotid tumor. But be careful interpreting the result: Overall, the accuracy to differentiate between benign and malignant disease in the parotid gland is poor. Finally, the role of PET/CT during follow-up after treatment for an extended malignant parotid tumor has not been defined yet.

Besides PET/CT, other imaging techniques like conventional X-ray, or scintigraphy, applied for some other salivary diseases, do not play any role for diagnostics in extended parotid tumors.

References

1. Gritzmann N, Rettenbacher T, Hollerweger A, Macheiner P, Hubner E. Sonography of the salivary glands. Eur Radiol. 2003;13(5):964–75. PubMed.
2. Katz P, Hartl DM, Guerre A. Clinical ultrasound of the salivary glands. Otolaryngol Clin N Am. 2009;42(6):973–1000. Table of Contents. PubMed.
3. Kraft M, Lang F, Mihaescu A, Wolfensberger M. Evaluation of clinician-operated sonography and fine-needle aspiration in the assessment of salivary gland tumours. Clin Otolaryngol. 2008;33(1):18–24. PubMed.
4. Howlett DC, Kesse KW, Hughes DV, Sallomi DF. The role of imaging in the evaluation of parotid disease. Clin Radiol. 2002;57(8):692–701. PubMed.
5. Lee YY, Wong KT, King AD, Ahuja AT. Imaging of salivary gland tumours. Eur J Radiol. 2008;66(3):419–36. PubMed eng.
6. Yabuuchi H, Matsuo Y, Kamitani T, Setoguchi T, Okafuji T, Soeda H, et al. Parotid gland tumors: can addition of diffusion-weighted MR imaging to dynamic contrast-enhanced MR imaging improve diagnostic accuracy in characterization? Radiology. 2008;249(3):909–16. PubMed.

7. Yerli H, Aydin E, Haberal N, Harman A, Kaskati T, Alibek S. Diagnosing common parotid tumours with magnetic resonance imaging including diffusion-weighted imaging vs fine-needle aspiration cytology: a comparative study. Dentomaxillofac Radiol. 2010;39(6):349–55. PubMed Pubmed Central PMCID: 3520240.
8. Yousem DM, Kraut MA, Chalian AA. Major salivary gland imaging. Radiology. 2000;216(1):19–29. PubMed.
9. Thoeny HC. Imaging of salivary gland tumours. Cancer Imaging. 2007;7:52–62. PubMed Pubmed Central PMCID: 1866314.
10. Yerli H, Aydin E, Coskun M, Geyik E, Ozluoglu LN, Haberal N, et al. Dynamic multislice computed tomography findings for parotid gland tumors. J Comput Assist Tomogr. 2007;31(2):309–16. PubMed.
11. Antoch G, Vogt FM, Freudenberg LS, Nazaradeh F, Goehde SC, Barkhausen J, et al. Whole-body dual-modality PET/CT and whole-body MRI for tumor staging in oncology. JAMA. 2003;290(24):3199–206. PubMed.

12 Extended Parotidectomy

Julio Acero and Belen Guerra

Abstract

The type of surgical treatment of parotid tumors is based on the tumor histology and stage, ranging in the majority of cases from superficial parotidectomy with preservation of the facial nerve to radical parotidectomy including resection of the facial nerve. A detailed work-up including a fine-needle aspiration cytology (FNAC) and imaging techniques such as computed tomography (CT) or magnetic resonance imaging (MRI) are required in order to select the surgical strategy. In case of extension of the lesion to the adjacent structures, such as the skin, the external ear, and the bone including the temporal bone or the mandible, etc, an extended parotidectomy including the parotid gland and the involved structures is indicated. Adequate repair of the defect will contribute to the recovery of the patient.

12.1 Introduction

Treatment of the tumors affecting the parotid gland is based currently on surgery. Histological type and tumor stage determine the extent of the surgical procedures [1]. Parotid gland tumors constitute a heterogeneous group being the preoperative diagnosis frequently a challenge. Imaging techniques such as computed tomography (CT) and magnetic resonance imaging (MRI) are indicated in order to identify infiltration of adjacent structures (muscle, vessels, bone, skin, etc.) and extension of the tumor into neighboring anatomical regions (Fig. 12.1). Positron emission tomography (PET) imaging has recently being introduced and still requires evaluation. Potential involvement of the prestyloid compartment of the parapharyngeal space should be excluded, especially in case of tumors originated in the deep portion of the gland or relapsing tumors such as recurrent pleomorphic adenoma as it was discussed in the previous chapters. Surgical treatment can range from enucleation to extended parotidectomy being the treatment goal to remove the tumor while preserving or restoring function and aesthetics, if possible (Table 12.1).

J. Acero, MD, DMD, PhD (✉)
Department of Maxillofacial Surgery, Ramón y Cajal University Hospital, University of Alcala, Madrid, Spain
e-mail: J-acero@telefonica.net

B. Guerra, MD, DMD
Department of Oral and Maxillofacial Surgery, Quiron Madrid University Hospital, European University Madrid, Madrid, Spain

Department of Maxillofacial Surgery, Quiron Madrid University Hospital, Madrid, Spain

© Springer International Publishing Switzerland 2016
V.-V. Costan (ed.), *Management of Extended Parotid Tumors*, DOI 10.1007/978-3-319-26545-2_12

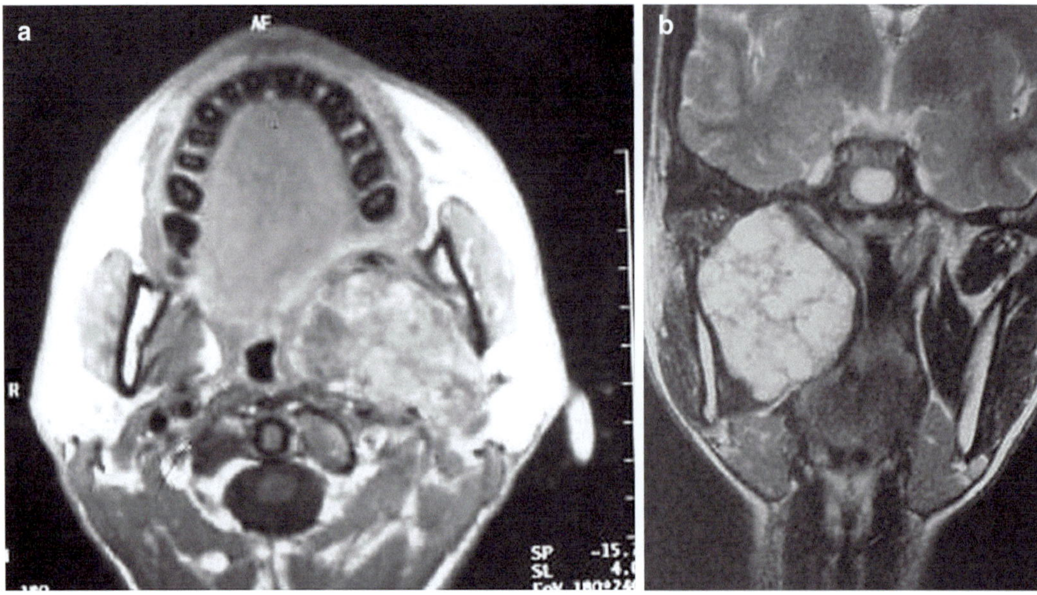

Fig. 12.1 (**a**, **b**) Pleomorphic adenoma. Magnetic resonance imaging (MRI) showing extension to the parapharyngeal region of the tumor

Table 12.1 Parotidectomy: surgical options

Enucleation
Superficial parotidectomy
Partial parotidectomy
Total parotidectomy
Extended parotidectomy

Enucleation is associated with a high recurrence rate and is indicated only in selected cases of tumors showing a low recurrence rate, such as lipoma. Currently, the standard surgical technique for the majority of benign tumors is conservative parotidectomy [2]. Superficial parotidectomy is performed in the case of benign neoplasms of the superficial lobe, while conservative total parotidectomy is performed in the case of benign neoplasms affecting the deep portion of the gland or malignant neoplasms with absence of facial nerve infiltration. Modified techniques such as partial parotidectomy and extracapsular dissection have been introduced in the treatment of selected benign tumors. Radical parotidectomy, with sacrifice of the facial nerve, is indicated in case of neoplastic involvement of the facial nerve. Reconstruction of the facial nerve through anastomosis or nerve graft is carried out usually in case of nerve resection.

Extended radical parotidectomy is reserved for parotid neoplasms in an advanced stage affecting several structures. This therapeutic approach can be also necessary in case of secondary involvement of the gland by primary tumors located in other structures (secondary infiltration of the parotid gland by skin tumors or metastatic tumors to the parotid gland). Extended parotidectomy includes the removal of the parotid gland with sacrifice of the facial nerve in case of malignant tumors as mentioned and the resection en bloc of the adjacent structures affected by neoplastic extension, such as the mandibular ramus and condyle, the overlying skin, the temporal bone, the parapharyngeal spaces, the auditory canal, or the external ear. Radical or functional neck dissection can be indicated depending on the tumor histology and stage. Resection of these structures can cause significant alteration of facial symmetry and contour, which can lead to a devastating situation both functionally and aesthetically for the patient. Therefore, an adequate reconstruction is an important component of the treatment. Reconstructive methods after extended parotidectomy can be non-vascularized skin or fat grafts, cervicofacial skin flaps, pedicled myocutaneous flaps, or microvascular free flaps.

In addition to the surgical treatment, postoperative radiotherapy can be used in case of close margins or residual disease. According to De Vicentiis et al. (2005), total extended radical parotidectomy combined with postoperative radiotherapy shows the best results in terms of quality of life and life expectancy in patients with an advanced stage of malignant neoplasms of the parotid gland [3].

12.2 Types of Extended Parotidectomy

The selection of the technique to be used should be based on the site, size, and type of the primary lesion and on the extension and type of infiltration to the adjacent structures (Table 12.2). Different types can be defined depending on the structures involved in the resection. In case of a massive tumor, a combination of techniques approaching the different areas involved needs to be used:

Table 12.2 Types of extended parotidectomy based on the affected tissues

Skin	Includes a portion of the cheek, temporal or cervical skin
Mandibular bone	Partial mandibulectomy
Temporal bone	Partial mastoidectomy
	Dissection of the temporal bone
	Total mastoidectomy or temporal bone resection
Auditory canal	Resection of the auditory canal in selected cases
	Temporal bone resection if bone destruction is manifested
External ear	Amputation of the external ear and the overlying skin
Parapharyngeal space	Dissection of the prestyloid parapharyngeal space
	Mandibulotomy with paralingual extension

12.2.1 Parotidectomy Extended to the Skin

Surgical resection of the tumor will include the parotid gland in monoblock with a portion of the skin adjacent to the tumor, including the cheek and temporal or cervical skin depending on the tumor extension.

12.2.2 Parotidectomy Extended to the Mandibular Bone

The radical treatment of parotid malignant tumors, especially those located in the deep lobe, may require a partial mandibulectomy thus including in the resection a part of the mandible which can be directly infiltrated by the tumor or be considered as a safety margin. In the case of a segmental resection, the postoperative situation potentially can result in facial asymmetry characterized not only by the absence of the part of the mandible but also by the deviation of the remaining mandible toward the affected side, loss of occlusion, and impaired chewing. Surgical resection can involve the temporomandibular joint in case of infiltration of the articular and periarticular structures.

12.2.3 Parotidectomy Extended to the Temporal Bone

In case of tumors that reach but not invade the mastoid and the lower portion of the tympanic annulus or tumors confined to the parotid gland needing a wide resection in order to achieve safe margins, a limited resection of the temporal bone can be done (partial mastoidectomy) in conjunction with total parotidectomy, while the external auditory canal and the middle ear are preserved (Fig. 12.2) [4]. For lesions located in the preauricular area over the stylomastoid foramen or in case of involvement of the external ear canal, limited dissection of the temporal bone can aid to localize the facial nerve through a posterior approach thus giving access to the dissection plane that lies medial to the nerve [5]. When the tumor has invaded the middle ear and the mastoid process or has infiltrated the temporal bone in depth, a radical parotidectomy with total mastoidectomy or temporal bone resection is required [6].

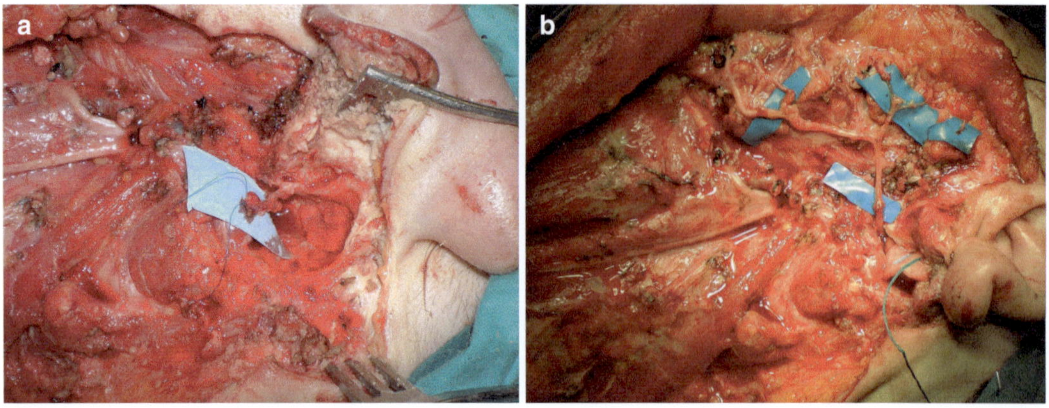

Fig. 12.2 (**a**, **b**) Radical parotidectomy with partial mastoidectomy. Reconstruction of the facial nerve with sural nerve graft

12.2.4 Parotidectomy Extended to the Auditory Canal

If the tumor is adherent to or invades the auditory canal, a locally aggressive resection with excision of the cartilaginous auditory canal is required. If the tumor does not involve the external ear, the pinna can be safely preserved with resection limited to the auditory canal which is reconstructed with a skin graft. If bone destruction is evident, a temporal bone resection should be considered.

12.2.5 Parotidectomy Extended to the External Ear

When the tumor involves the external ear, the treatment requires resection of this anatomical structure and of the overlying skin and the repair of the surgical defect (Fig. 12.3). Reconstruction techniques after extended parotidectomy will be discussed later in this chapter.

12.2.6 Parotidectomy Extended to the Parapharyngeal Space

The parapharyngeal space is described as an inverted pyramid-like space whose base is at the sphenoid bone and its ápex is at the greater cornu of the hyoid bone. It can be divided into two compartments on the basis of its relationships to the styloid process or to the tensor-vascular-styloid fascia: prestyloid or poststyloid compartments [7]. The tumors arising from the deep lobe of the parotid gland are the most common extrinsic tumors involving the prestyloid parapharyngeal space, being frequently benign lesions although also malignant tumors can affect this region. Several surgical approaches have been described for the management of lesions affecting this anatomical region: transcervical, transoral, transparotid-transcervical, and transmandibular approaches. In case of extended parotidectomy, usually a transparotid-transcervical approach is performed. In some patients, removal of the tumor through this approach is not possible due to the size of the tumor, the presence of multiple recurrent tumors affecting the parapharyngeal region, or in cases where lesions are located in a high situation in the parapharyngeal region internally to the mandible, which makes it not possible to access the tumor without performing an osteotomy in the ascending ramus of the mandible as an approach to this space. After the excision of the tumor, the mandible fragments are repositioned and fixed with miniplates previously preshaped before the osteotomy was performed (Fig. 12.4). In large benign tumor of the parapharyngeal region as an alternative or in case of malignant tumors affecting the parotid gland with extension to the parapharyngeal region, a lip-split approach with paramedian mandibulotomy should be considered to access the parapharyngeal region. This approach combined with a neck dissection allows to control the carotid artery at the neck. Finally, in extensive malignant tumors affecting both the mandible and the parapharyngeal space, an en bloc resection including the mandibular ramus, the parotid gland, and the parapharyngeal extension of the tumor has to be performed.

12.3 Reconstruction after Extended Parotidectomy

Extended parotidectomy may result in extensive compound defects with devastating aesthetic and functional sequelae, such as facial palsy, loss of facial symmetry, and a visible defect in the

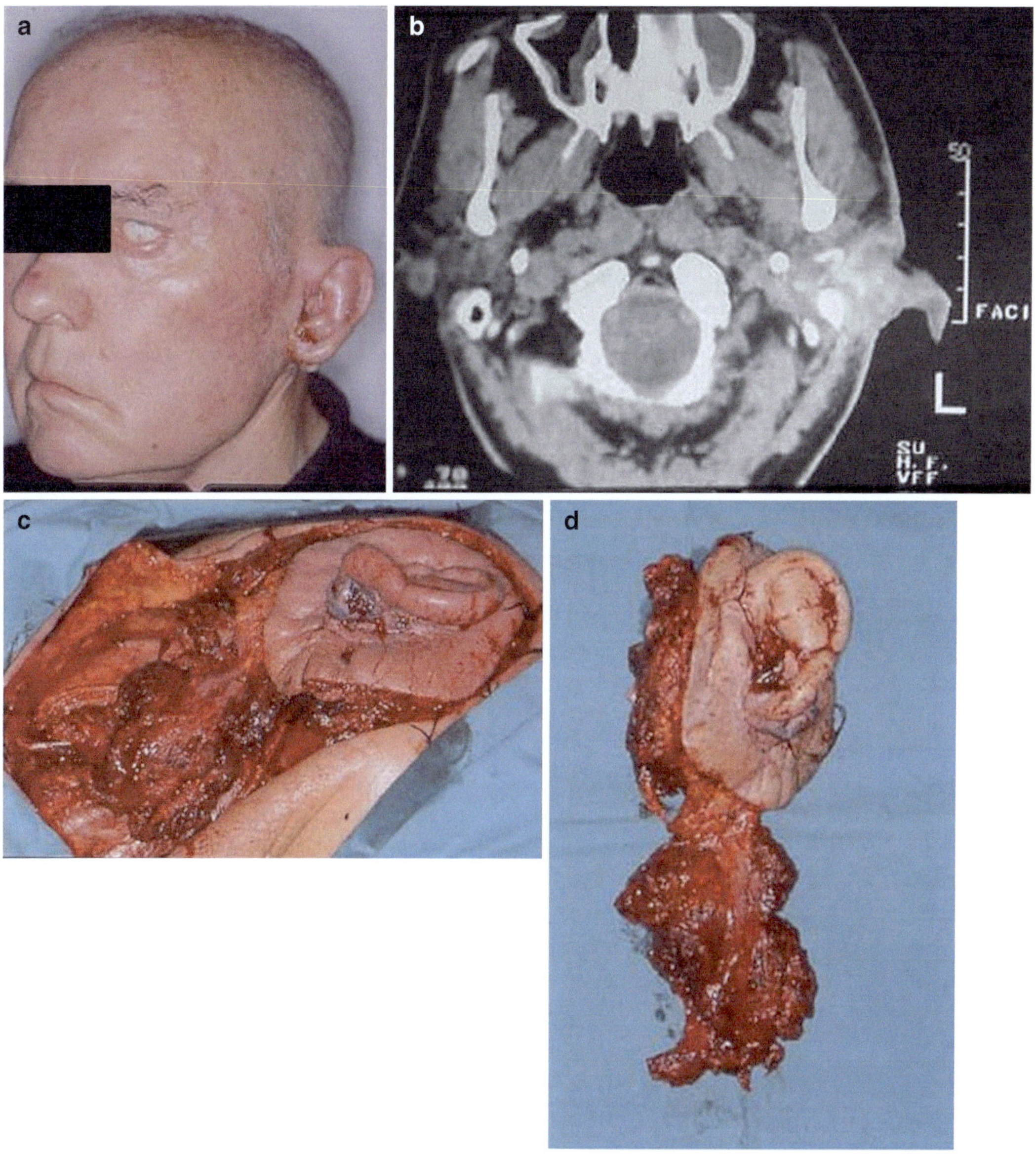

Fig. 12.3 (**a**, **b**) Squamous cell carcinoma affecting the parotid gland with extension to the skin and the temporal bone. (**c**, **d**) Neck dissection and extended parotidectomy including the overlying skin, external ear, pinna, and temporalis bone. Surgical specimen. (**e**) Reconstruction with a pectoralis major myocutaneous pedicled flap

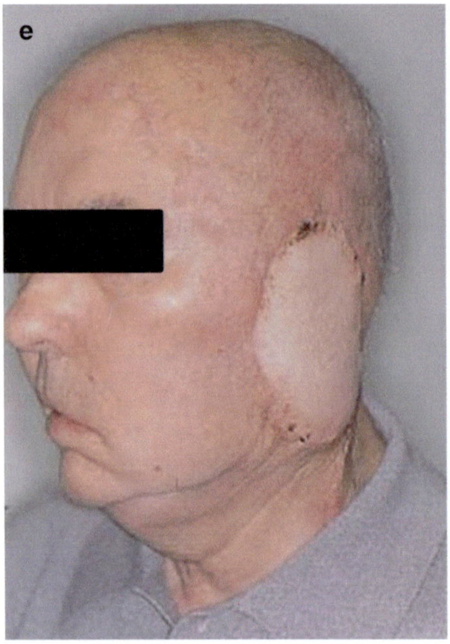

Fig. 12.3 (continue)

parotid region. In case of facial nerve excision, nerve reconstruction must be considered in order to recover its function. Immediate nerve grafting should be carried out if possible. Donor sites are the contralateral greater auricular or the sural nerve [8]. Mandibular resection associated with radical parotidectomy leads also to important postoperative sequelae including chin deviation toward the defect's side with loss of dental occlusion and chewing impairment. In order to avoid these sequelae and to achieve an adequate result with a positive impact in the quality of life of the patient, immediate reconstruction of the defect is mandatory after extended parotidectomy (Table 12.3).

Several reconstructive options have been described to repair the defects after extended parotidectomy, including non-vascularized derma-fat grafts, local skin or muscle pedicled flaps, regional mucocutaneous flaps, and microvascular free tissue transfer. Repair of the defect follows a reconstructive ladder:

- Contour defects without skin loss can be repaired with local flaps like the superficial musculocutaneous aponeurotic system flap (SMAS flap), which is not indicated in case of malignancy or after recurrent pleomorphic adenoma excision, or the temporal-parietal fascia flap. Derma-fat grafting has been used for filling postsurgical subcutaneous defects after parotidectomy. LipoStructure seems to be more predictable for soft tissue augmentation [9], although its role in the repair of major defects after extended parotidectomy is not well established.
- Moderate skin resection with small contour defects after extended parotidectomy can be restored with different *local and regional pedicled flaps* (local skin rotation flaps, temporalis muscle flaps, sternocleidomastoid muscle flap, cervicofacial rotation-advancement flap, submental island flap, Fig. 12.5). The cervicofacial rotation/advancement flap is very useful for the repair of large skin defects. Elevation of the flap is simple and, as other local or regional flaps, provides a good aesthetic result due to an excellent skin color and texture match although this type of flaps is limited for the reconstruction of major defects, not being able to restore the loss of volume after major resection in the parotid region [10, 11].
- *Distant pedicled myocutaneous flaps* are used to cover large skin defects which require a bulky flap to restore the postoperative defect. The pectoralis major myocutaneous flap is a reliable flap based on the pectoral branch of the thoracoacromial artery which has many advantages, including a long pedicle and an easy and quick dissection providing a bulky tissue able to fill big contour defects and to protect deep structures like the dura (see Fig. 12.3). This type of flap, however, provides a poor color match in cases where a skin paddle is required. Other drawbacks, common to other pedicled flaps, are the limited arch of rotation, the donor-site morbidity, and a less precise contour reconstruction in comparison with free flaps repair. As a primary reconstructive procedure is especially indicated in elderly and medically compromised patients. Other pedicled distant flaps such as the posterior or vertical trapezius flap, using the trapezius muscle based on the transverse cervical

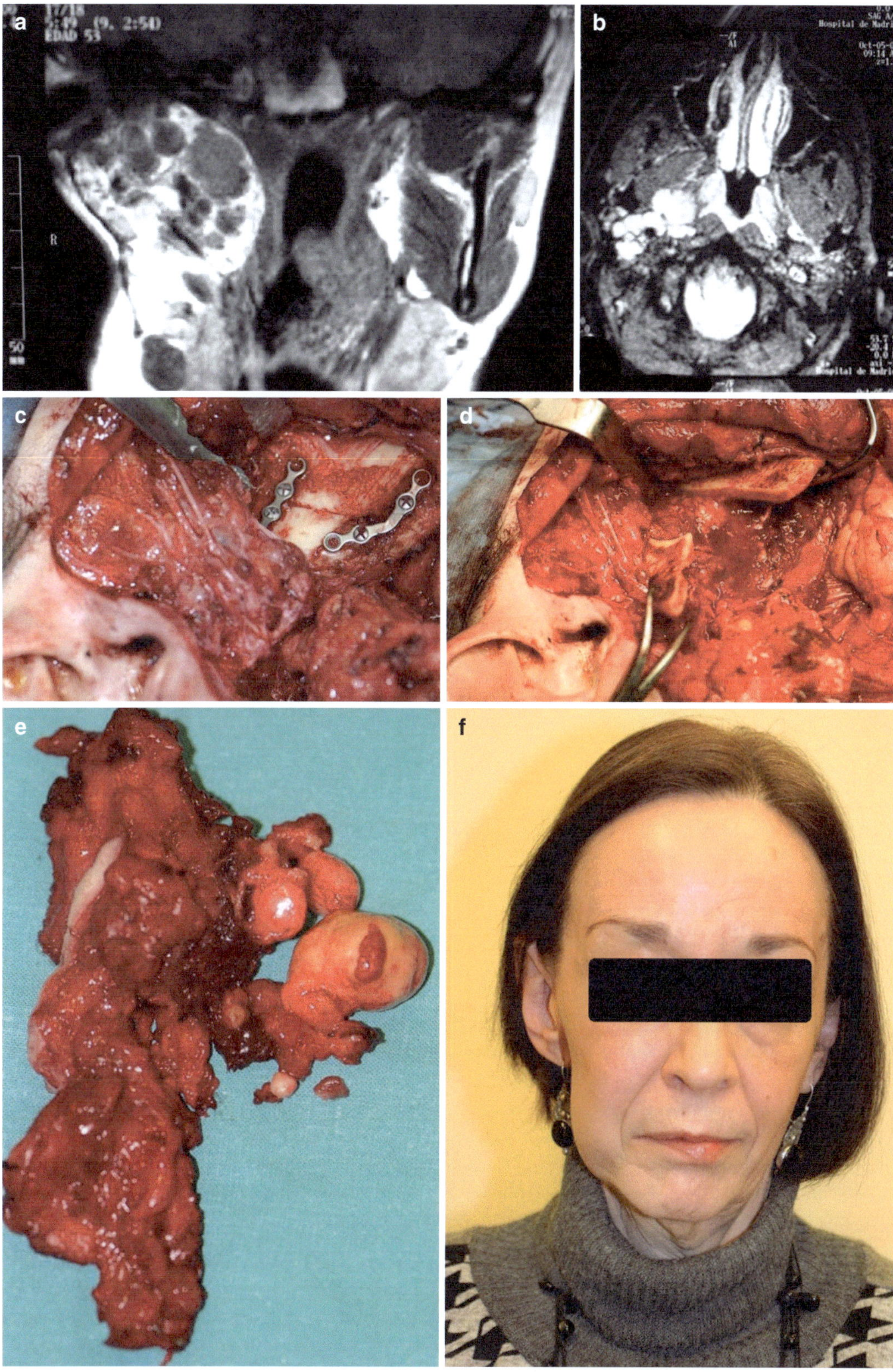

Fig. 12.4 (**a**, **b**) Multinodular relapsing pleomorphic adenoma extended to the parapharyngeal space. (**c–e**) Total parotidectomy and dissection of the parapharyngeal region. Approach to the parapharyngeal space through ramus osteotomy. Surgical specimen. (**f**) Postoperative aspect of the patient. Good function of the facial nerve

Table 12.3 Algorithm of reconstruction in extended parotidectomy

Soft tissue loss	Lateral arm, ALT, rectus abdominis free flap
Soft tissue loss with facial nerve extension	Lateral arm free flap and posterior cutaneous nerve of the forearm
	ALT free flap with fascia lata and nerve graft of vastus lateralis
	Latissimus dorsi and thoracodorsal nerve
	Rectus abdominis flap with intercostal nerve anastomosis
Soft tissue and mandibular bone loss	Scapular/parascapular system free flap
	Latissimus dorsi flap with rib fibula
	No bone reconstruction can be considered in lateral defects
Soft tissue-mandibular bone loss and facial nerve extension	Latissimus dorsi free flap with thoracodorsal nerve and rib
	Osteofasciocutaneous scapular/parascapular system flap and nerve graft
Elderly and medically compromised patients	Regional myocutaneous flaps
	Sural nerve graft if nerve excision with recipient bed preparation with muscle flap

artery with its overlying skin, the sternocleidomastoid, and the platysma myocutaneous flap, provide an alternative for the repair of major surgical defects in extended parotidectomy with or without temporal bone resection. These flaps can be harvested easily, showing minimal donor-site morbidity and a predictable outcome [12, 13].

- Reconstruction of large and complex defects after extended parotidectomy requires the use of free flaps [14]. Advantages of these flaps are the versatility in orientation concerning tissue (skin, muscle, bone, nerves), the reduction of irradiation-induced complications, and the ability to perform facial nerve repair allowing for the restoration of shape and function in one single operation for complex defects. Disadvantages of free microvascular transfer are the technical difficulty requiring an additional training, longer operation times, and the donor-site morbidity. A variety of donor sites available allows for the simultaneous resection and flap harvest. Selection of the flap will depend on the type of tissue requirements (skin, muscle, bone) and the size of the defect. The most frequently used free flaps for reconstruction of the parotid region are described in the following sections.

12.3.1 Rectus Abdominis Free Flap

The rectus abdominis has a reliable vascular supply with a pedicle relatively large in caliber and length based on the deep inferior epigastric vessels, providing a bulky soft tissue which can be indicated for skull base coverage [15]. Rectus abdominis flap is segmentally innervated from the lower intercostal nerves which can be anastomosed to the contralateral facial nerve if necessary. Disadvantages of this flap are poor skin color match and flap ptosis.

12.3.2 Latissimus Dorsi Free Flap

Latissimus dorsi free flap is a muscle flap which may be harvested with a wide skin paddle (Fig. 12.6). This flap may be ideal for the reconstruction of extensive defects involving the skin and the underlying soft tissues including coverage of the skull basis. Vascular supply depends on the thoracodorsal artery of the subscapular system with a single comitans vein. The length of the pedicle is up to 15 cm, which is an advantage in case of difficult recipient vessels. Innervation through the thoracodorsal nerve can be used for functional repair after facial nerve resection [16]. This flap offers the possibility of harvesting a rib together with the flap allowing for mandibular reconstruction (condyle and ramus) if necessary.

Fig. 12.5 (**a–d**) Dermatofibrosarcoma protuberans affecting the parotid gland. Superficial parotidectomy and wide skin resection. Submental island pedicled flap design. (**e**) Postoperative aspect of the patient. Good aesthetic and functional result

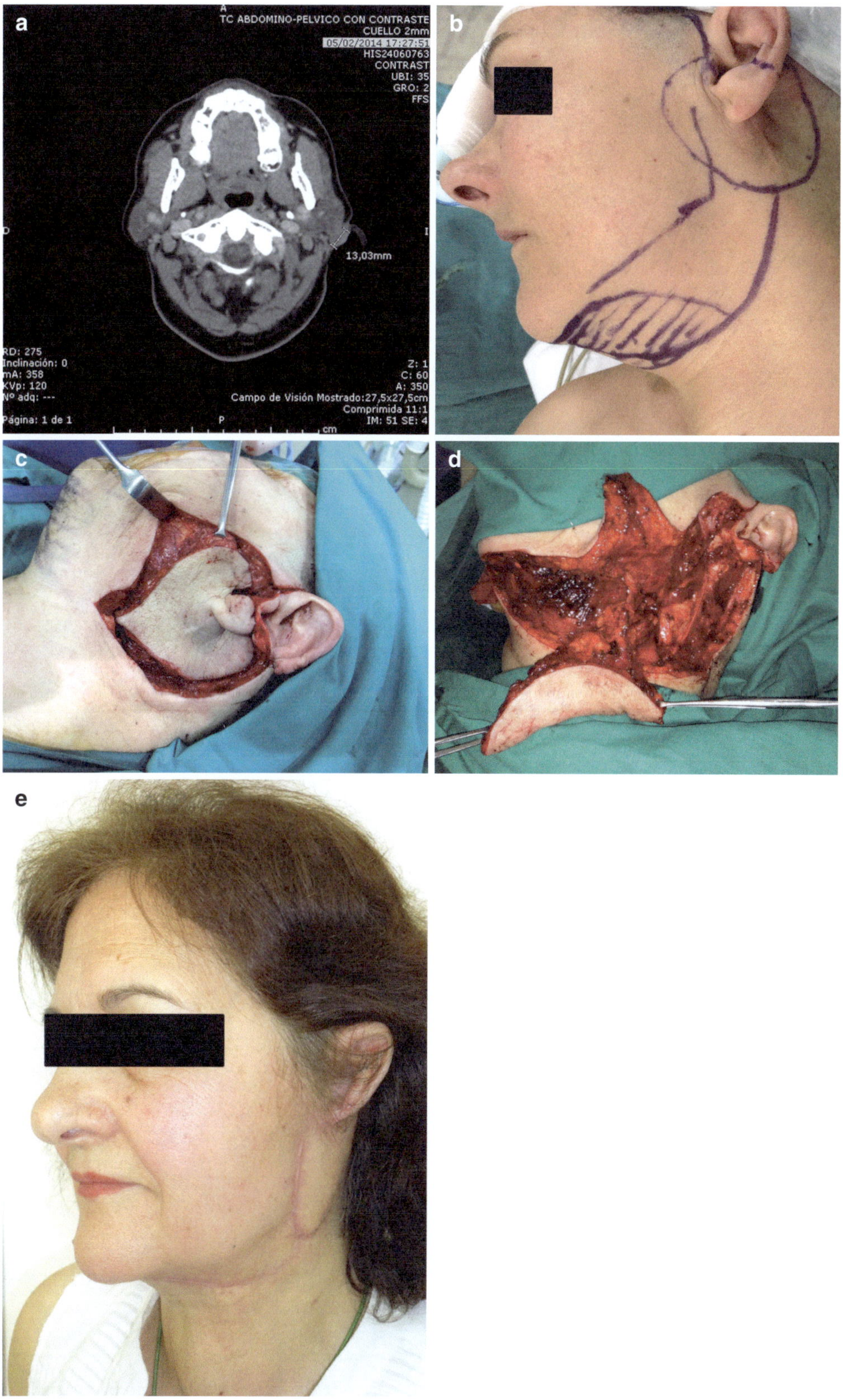
a
b
c
d
e
TC ABDOMINO-PELVICO CON CONTRASTE
CUELLO 2mm
05/02/2014 17:27:51
HIS24060763
CONTRAST
UBI: 35
GRO: 2
FFS
13,03mm
RD: 275
Inclinación: 0
mA: 358
KVp: 120
Nº adq: ---
Página: 1 de 1
Z: 1
C: 60
A: 350
Campo de Visión Mostrado:27,5x27,5cm
Comprimida 11:1
IM: 51 SE: 4
cm

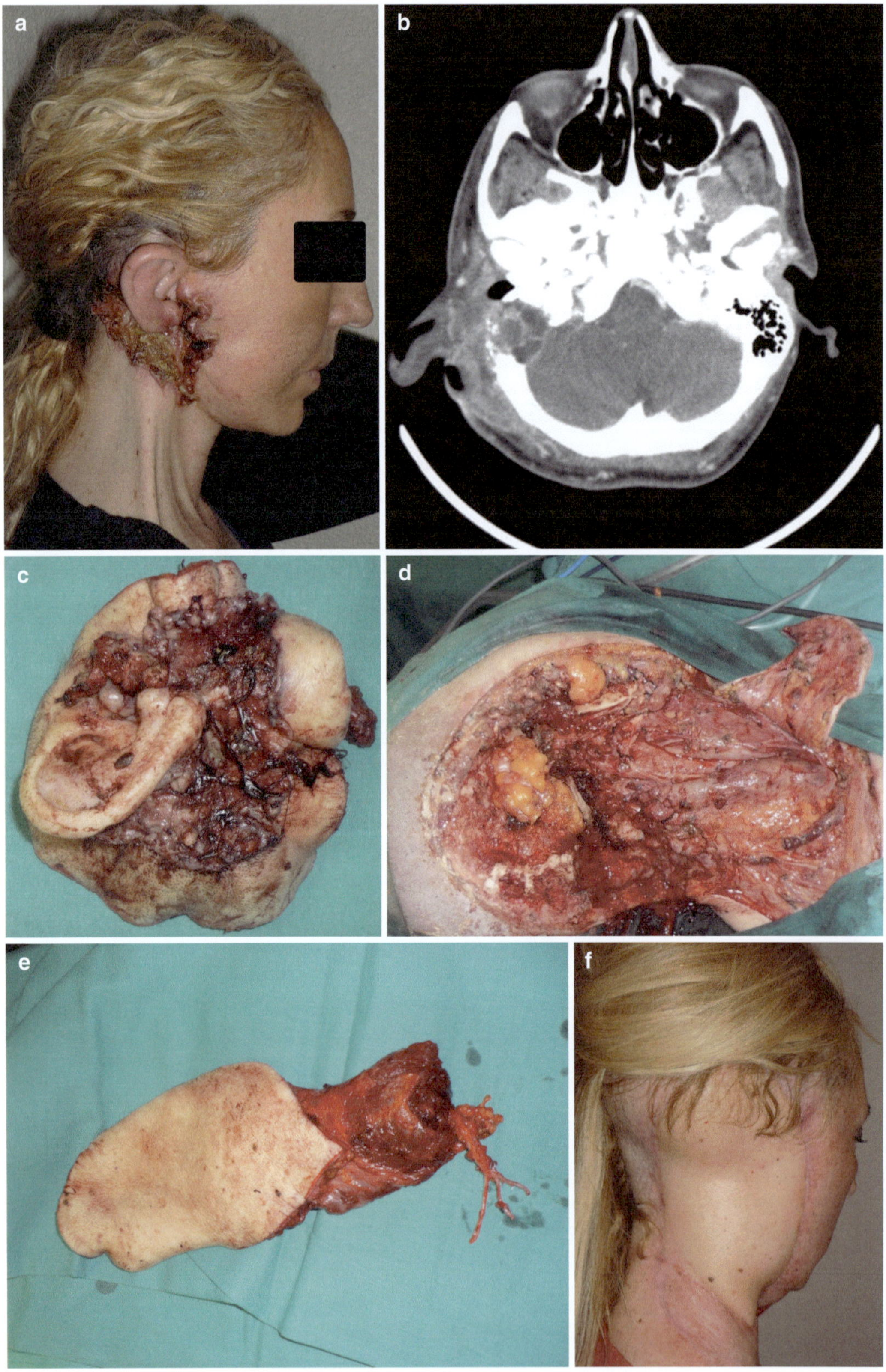
a
b
c
d
e
f

A major problem in raising this flap concerns the necessity of changing the patient's position thus increasing the operation time.

12.3.3 Lateral Arm Free Flap

The reconstruction of complex parotidectomy defects using the lateral arm free flap was described by Teknos [17]. The lateral arm flap is a fasciocutaneous flap based on the posterior collateral artery. A portion of the humerus can be used to repair composite defects but this use is not frequent. The main disadvantage of this flap is the short length and caliber of the vascular pedicle, often less than 1.5 mm in diameter, which makes the anastomosis technically difficult.

The posterior cutaneous nerve of the forearm can be simultaneously harvested for facial nerve reconstruction. This flap has the advantages of being easily harvested in a two-team approach showing ideal color match and minimal donor-site morbidity. However, due to the small bulk of the lateral arm, this free flap may not provide complete an adequate coverage of the defect.

12.3.4 Scapular/Parascapular Flap System

This flap is optimal for reconstruction of extensive soft tissue defects providing a well-vascularized large skin paddle with the possibility of including an osseous component from the scapula with an independent pedicle. One of the advantages of the parascapular flap is the length and caliber of the vascular pedicle (circumflex scapular artery). The main disadvantages are that harvesting cannot be possible in a two-team approach needing change of the position of the patient and a poor color match [18].

12.3.5 Anterolateral Thigh Free Flap (ALT)

ALT flap offers a potentially large skin paddle which can be as large as 8 by 25 cm with minimal patient morbidity and can be raised in a two-team approach. In the right patient, the skin and subcutaneous fat of the anterolateral thigh can be thin, making this flap a versatile tool for the reconstruction of large defects especially those affecting the skull base coverage. Large defects of the lateral temporal bone associated with parotidectomy are adequately reconstructed using the ALT free flap. The approach to ALT harvest also exposes the tensor fascia lata, which can be harvested as a vascularized sling for facial reanimation procedures [19]. The flap has a large caliber pedicle based on the descending branch of the lateral femoral circumflex artery, but the anatomy of the perforator vessels can be variable, requiring most of them dissection of musculocutaneous perforators, and is infrequently supplied solely by septocutaneous perforators. Perforator dissection can be difficult to the inexperienced microsurgeon.

12.3.6 Fibula Flap

The fibular osteocutaneous free flap is based upon the peroneal artery and associated veins. This flap can be considered currently as the workhorse for mandibular reconstruction [20, 21] with potential advantages like a good pedicle and the great length of available bone (up to 27 cm), but the limited extension of the associated soft tissues and the high incidence of skin paddle failure make this flap rarely indicated in reconstruction after extended parotidectomy.

12.3.7 Iliac Crest Free Flap

This flap, based upon the deep circumflex iliac artery (DCIA) and vein, is considered anatomi-

Fig. 12.6 (**a**, **b**) Basal cell carcinoma infiltrating the parotid gland, external ear, and skull base. (**c**–**f**) Extensive resection including skin, ear, total parotidectomy, mandibular condyle, and skull base. Safe reconstruction of the defect by means of a latissimus dorsi free flap cally ideal for reconstruction of mandibular defects [22], although the skin paddle is very poor and its use is limited in the reconstruction of post-parotidectomy defects.

References

1. Shah JP, Ihde JK. Salivary gland tumors. Curr Probl Surg. 1990;27(12):775–883.
2. Bianchi B, Ferri A, Ferrari S, Copelli C, Sesenna E. Improving aesthetic results in benign parotid surgery: statistical evaluation of facelift approach, sternocleidomastoid flap, and superficial musculoaponeurotic system flap application. J Oral Maxillofac Surg. 2011;69(4):1235–41.
3. De Vincentiis M, Magliulo G, Soldo P, Manciocco V, Pagliuca G, Del Gaizo R, et al. Extended parotidectomy. Acta Otorhinolaryngol Ital. 2005;25(3):169–73.
4. Mehra S, Morris LG, Shah J, Bilsky M, Selesnick S, Kraus DH. Outcomes of temporal bone resection for locally advanced parotid cancer. Skull Base. 2011;21(6):389–96.
5. Munir N, Tandon S, Brown JS, Lesser THJ. Transmastoid facial nerve localisation for malignant neoplasms confined to the parotid gland. Br J Oral Maxillofac Surg. 2012;50(8):736–8.
6. Ho B, Solares CA, Panizza B. Temporal bone resection. Oper Tech Otolaryngol Head Neck Surg. 2013;24(3):179–83.
7. Friedman ER, Saindane AM. Pitfalls in the staging of cancer of the major salivary gland neoplasms. Neuroimaging Clin N Am. 2013;23(1):107–22.
8. Biglioli F, Colombo V, Pedrazzoli M, Frigerio A, Tarabbia F, Autelitano L, et al. Thoracodorsal nerve graft for reconstruction of facial nerve branching. J Craniomaxillofac Surg. 2014;42(1):e8–14.
9. Clauser L, Polito J, Mandrioli S, Tieghi R, Denes SA, Galiè M. Structural fat grafting in complex reconstructive surgery. J Craniofac Surg. 2008;19(1):187–91.
10. Fa-yu L, Zhong-fei X, Peng L, Chang-fu S, Rui-wu L, Shu-fen G, Jun-lin L, Shao-hui H, Xuexin T. The versatile application of cervicofacial and cervicothoracic rotation flaps in head and neck surgery. World J Surg Oncol. 2011;9(135):1–7. doi:10.1186/1477-7819-9-135.
11. Soler-Presas F, Cuesta-Gil M, Borja-Morant A, Concejo-Cútoli C, Acero-Sanz J, Navarro-Vila C. Midface soft tissue reconstruction with the faciocervico-pectoral flap. J Craniomaxillofac Surg. 1997;25(1):39–45.
12. Kumar V, Gaud U, Shukla M, Pandey M. Sternocleidomastoid island flap preserving the branch from superior thyroid artery for the reconstruction following resection of oral cancer. Eur J Surg Oncol (EJSO). 2009;35(9):1011–5.
13. Liu H, Li Y, Dai X. Modified face-lift approach combined with a superficially anterior and superior-based sternocleidomastoid muscle flap in total parotidectomy. Oral Surg Oral Med Oral Pathol Oral Radiol. 2012;113(5):593–9.
14. Cannady SB, Seth R, Fritz MA, Alam DS, Wax MK. Total parotidectomy defect reconstruction using the buried free flap. Otolaryngol Head Neck Surg. 2010;143(5):637–43.
15. Cappiello J, Piazza C, Taglietti V, Nicolai P. Deep inferior epigastric artery perforated rectus abdominis free flap for head and neck reconstruction. Eur Arch Otorhinolaryngol. 2012;269(4):1219–24.
16. Biglioli F, Pedrazzoli M, Rabbiosi D, Colletti G, Colombo V, Frigerio A, et al. Reconstruction of complex defects of the parotid region using a lateral thoracic wall donor site. J Craniomaxillofac Surg. 2013;41(3):265–9.
17. Teknos TN, Nussenbaum B, Bradford CR, Prince ME, El-Kashlan H, Chepeha DB. Reconstruction of complex parotidectomy defects using the lateral arm free tissue transfer. Otolaryngol Head Neck Surg. 2003;129(3):183–91.
18. Mitsimponas KT, Iliopoulos C, Stockmann P, Bumiller L, Nkenke E, Neukam FW, et al. The free scapular/parascapular flap as a reliable method of reconstruction in the head and neck region: a retrospective analysis of 130 reconstructions performed over a period of 5 years in a single department. J Craniomaxillofac Surg. 2014;42(5):536–43.
19. Elliott RM, Weinstein GS, Low DW, Wu LC. Reconstruction of complex total parotidectomy defects using the free anterolateral thigh flap: a classification system and algorithm. Ann Plast Surg. 2011;66(5):429–37.
20. Hidalgo DA, Cordeiro P, Disa J. Refinements in mandible reconstruction. Oper Tech Plast Surg. 1996;3:257–62.
21. Disa JJ, Cordeiro PG. Mandible reconstruction with microvascular surgery. Semin Surg Oncol. 2000;19:226–34.
22. Urken ML. Iliac Crest osteocutaneous and osteomusculocutaneous. In: Urken ML, Cheney ML, Sullivan MJ, Biller HF, editors. Atlas of regional and free flaps for head and neck reconstruction. New York: Raven Press; 1995. p. 261–90.

Part III

Treatment Planning for Extended Parotidectomy

13 Issues in General Anesthesia

Otilia Boisteanu

Abstract

The preoperative management of patients with extensive parotid tumors poses a real challenge for the anesthesiologist. Generally, the patients are elderly, cachectic, and immunodeficient and often associate other multiple comorbidities. The anesthetic management requires a correct preoperative diagnosis and treatment of the general coexisting diseases in order to reduce the risks of surgery. The adequate preanesthetic preparation reduces preoperative morbidity and mortality. When the extensive parotid tumors reach the deep structures of the neck, they can create a difficult airway. The fiber-optic tracheal intubation (flexible fiberscope) must be considered as the first option in predicted difficult intubation. Intubation is performed by oral or nasal route, while the patient is awake, in spontaneous breathing, or while the patient is under general anesthesia. The monitoring of muscle relaxation in parotid surgery is very important, the neuromuscular blockade being interrupted or reversed and the function of the facial nerve evaluated before the surgical intervention reaches its proximity. Extubation is performed when there is no major risk of airway obstruction by hemorrhage, hematoma formation, or edema. In case of reconstruction of loss of substance with free transferred microvascular flaps due to the scale of the intervention, both in terms of duration and complexity, extubation is possible in the first or second day after surgery. The patient's surgical wound and general condition is monitored postoperatively to prevent complications, some of which with a vital prognosis.

13.1 Introduction

Anesthesia in the oral and maxillofacial surgery presents a range of features. The surgeon and the anesthesiologist have a common working "front"; they "share" the same territory more than in any other surgical branch, so the chosen anesthetic

O. Boisteanu, MD, PhD
Department of Anesthesiology, Faculty of Dental Medicine, "Grigore T. Popa" University of Medicine and Pharmacy, Iasi, Romania
e-mail: otilia.boisteanu@yahoo.com

© Springer International Publishing Switzerland 2016

V.-V. Costan (ed.), *Management of Extended Parotid Tumors*, DOI 10.1007/978-3-319-26545-2_13

technique shall be strongly influenced by the type of intervention practiced.

In the intraoperative oral and maxillofacial surgery, the head of the patient being covered with surgical drapes, the safety of the respiratory tract is compulsory. A free, clean, unobstructed respiratory tract is the main concern of the anesthesiologist. The tracheal intubation allows the protection of the respiratory tract against contamination with blood, gastric content secretions, controlled or assisted ventilation, the possibility of obstruction of the upper respiratory tract, and the easy access to the respiratory-digestive tract.

The intubation probe is fitted and secured, so as not to be displaced and not to produce facial or tissue distortions. Usually, during the surgical interventions performed at the level of the lateral part of the head and of the neck, the patient is subject to an oral tracheal intubation, and the probe is fitted on the opposite part of the oral cavity. As a general rule, they use metal armored tracheal probes or tracheal probes which present preformed curving, as they have a minimum curving potential or compression potential through the rotation of the head. The anesthetic circuit is connected to the patient, so as not to be intraoperatively disconnected and to ensure a good surgical access. Moreover, the oral and maxillofacial surgery performs in a strongly reflexogenic area which concentrates in a restricted area several formations belonging to different systems (respiratory, digestive, vascular, nervous) [1–4].

The surgical and/or anesthetic manipulation can determine a range of serious accidents and incidents, so it is compulsory to perform an adequate monitoring of the physiological parameters and a very good intraoperative vegetative protection. In the oral maxillofacial surgery, the head of the patient being covered with surgical drapes, there are difficulties in the clinical follow-up of the anesthesia stage by supervising the movements of the eyeballs, of the palpebral reflexes.

Surgical interventions in the cervical territory involve a range of risks: activation of the carotid sinus depressor reflexes with the occurrence of arterial hypotension and sinus bradycardia up to asystolia; injury of the cervical vegetative nervous system, mainly of the right stellar ganglion, which determines the decrease of the activation threshold of ventricular fibrillation via the prolongation of the QT interval; the occurrence of gas embolisms; and also, during the radical neck dissection, the apical pleura can be injured, with the occurrence of pneumothorax and subcutaneous emphysema.

Lesions present at the level of the neck can produce modifications of the regional anatomy and local distortions which predispose to a difficult tracheal intubation [5–7].

13.2 Management of the Difficult Respiratory Tract

In case of the extended parotid gland tumors, when the development of the tumor formation extends toward the deep structures of the throat, we can confront with a difficult air pathway

The difficult tracheal intubation represents a balance moment for the anesthesiologist and for the patient, to the same extent.

Before an abnormal respiratory tract, any anesthesiologist must be prepared for three emergency situations: the possibility of a difficult intubation, the impossibility of performing the intubation, and the "can't intubate," "can't ventilate."

The American Society for Anesthesiologists (ASA) defines the difficult intubation as the inability of placing the endotracheal tube in 10 min or from three attempts at direct laryngoscopy.

The American Society for Anesthesiologists (ASA) defines the difficult mask ventilation as the inability of an anesthesiologist (having an appropriate training level) in maintaining the oxygen saturation of a patient above 90 %, by using a ventilation facial mask, when we start from a normal basal saturation [8–10].

The tracheal intubation supposes a complete and correct clinical assessment, command of diverse techniques of approaching the respiratory tract, endowment with multiple and diverse devices for the achievement of the maneuver, use of a specific medication which facilitates the maneuver, and last but not least the personal experience. The intubation equipment must also contain adjuvant devices of the intubation: optic probe, bougie, fiber-optic bronchoscope, rigid fiberscope, and video-laryngoscope. The role of the bougie is still under assessed in the management of the difficult respiratory tract. Before a difficult tracheal intubation, the anesthesiologist may raise certain problems: whether the patient must remain awake or he can be sedated, whether he maintains or not the spontaneous ventilation, whether he needs or not muscular relaxation, and whether the patency of the respiratory tract shall be maintained surgically or nonsurgically [9, 11–13].

When an intubation is assessed to be difficult, the first intubation option must be the use of the flexible fiberscope (fiber-optic tracheal intubation), which should be at hand to each specialist. The decision is whether the patient shall be orally or nasally intubated and whether the intubation shall be performed in the patient awake, with spontaneous breathing, or in the patient under general anesthesia. If one assesses that the mask ventilation is not possible, if there are antecedents of difficult intubation or great aspiration risk, it is compulsory that the fiber-optic tracheal intubation be performed on the patient awake, conscious, and sedated, in spontaneous breath. The patients who can be adequately ventilated on mask shall be subject to a fiber-optic intubation under general anesthesia [14]. In the absence of the flexible fiberscope, when there is a suspicion or history of difficult intubation, one shall practice: the "blind" vigil intubation, the tracheotomy, the use of the esophageal-tracheal combitube, and the use of LMA, ILMA, or other new means of supraglottic ventilation [8–13].

The performance of the vigil ("blind" or fiberscope) intubation needs a good collaboration with the patient and a good intranasal and intraoral local anesthesia. The lidocaine spray 5–10 %, applied on the vocal chords (135 mg/75 kg), does not alter the pressor response to the tracheal intubation; in exchange, in the postoperative period, there is the risk of incompetence of the vocal chords and of difficulties in deglutition [15]. An alternative for the intubation of the patient awake is remifentanil in dose of 0.5–2 μg/kg. The good conditions which allow the tracheal intubation in safety conditions are offered by associating the propofol (1–2 mg/kg) with remifentanil, using the inhalator induction with sevoflurane, or using the succinylcholine (depolarized curare), but we cannot talk anymore of the patient awake, vigil [16–18].

Even if the use of curare for the tracheal intubation is the first recommendation, the French Society of Anesthesia and Reanimation (SFAR) recommends the selection of the non-depolarizing curare according to the type of surgery (is it necessary to administer curare?) and the intervention duration. When the surgical intervention does not require muscular relaxation but only to secure the respiratory tract and maintain the ventilation and the oxygenation, satisfactory intubation conditions are offered by the association of hypnotic-opioid or by the inhalatory anesthesia, the main advantage being the fast reversibility of drugs in case of a possible difficult intubation. Rocuronium is the only non-depolarizing relaxant which offers optimal conditions for the tracheal intubation in almost 1 min (similar to succinylcholine) and whose complete neuromuscular block can be reversed by sugammadex in almost 90 s. Sugammadex extended the use of rocuronium for the tracheal intubation, even in emergencies. Vecuronium was less studied in terms of the fast reversion of the profound block – by sugammadex. With regard to the difficult respiratory tract, the essential objective is to maintain the oxygenation of the patient. The use of sugammadex for the fast antagonization of the neuromuscular block, given by rocuronium or vecuronium, is an alternative which must be taken into consideration before resorting to the invasive maneuvers of access and security of the respiratory tract [19–21].

13.3 Preanesthetic Assessment and Premedication

The anesthesiologist must be highly prepared for the multiple and complex anesthesia variants, for the purpose of ensuring security and a particular comfort to the patient and to the surgical team.

According to the ASA guides (American Society of Anesthesiologist), the preanesthetic assessment is the responsibility of the anesthesiologist and consists in the clinical and paraclinical assessment of the patient, for the purpose of performing an anesthesia for a surgical or non-surgical intervention. The preanesthetic consult compulsorily includes the analysis of the medical documents of the patient, the anamnesis, and the evaluation of the data included in the general examination and in the complementary examinations. As for the preanesthetic assessment process, the anesthesiologist can require the consult of other medical branches, so as to obtain information or services relevant for the perioperative anesthetic care. The documentation of an anterior anesthesia can show diverse important difficulties or complications, such as the difficult intubation, history of malign hyperthermia, and the individual response to the surgical stress or to drugs.

Moreover, during the preanesthetic consultation, the patient shall be informed with regard to the anesthesia, the perioperative management, and pain treatment, the purpose being that of reducing the anxiety and facilitating the collaboration in the postoperative period. After the preanesthetic assessment, the anesthesiologist shall frame the patient into an anesthetic risk class and shall choose an anesthetic protocol, taking into account the data obtained and the opinion of the patient. The global purpose of the preoperative assessment is to reduce the perioperative morbidity and death rate and to diminish the anxiety of the patient. The most important guides and protocols regarding the preanesthetic assessment were drafted by the American Society of Anesthesiologists (ASA), the American College of Cardiology (ACC), and the American Heart Association (AHA), with regard to the assessment of the patients with cardiovascular pathology programmed for the noncardiac surgery.

The main score used for the assessment of the anesthetic risk is the ASA score (American Society of Anesthesiologists), which reflects the physical status of the patient regardless of the nature of the planned surgical intervention [22–25].

ASA Classification:

ASA 1: normal, healthy patient
ASA 2: patient with mild or moderate systemic disease, with no functional limit (mild form of diabetes, high blood pressure stage 1–2, anemia, obesity, aged patient)
ASA 3: patient with severe systemic disease that borders the activity (angina, BPOC, heart failure in antecedents, ICC NyHA 1–2)
ASA 4: patient with severe systemic disease that constantly endangers the life of the patient (ICC NyHA 3–4, instable angina, acute respiratory, hepatic renal failure)
ASA 5: dying patient who will not survive 24 h without surgical intervention

After the preanesthetic examination, one shall fill in the "preanesthetic examination file" which contains the main information regarding the health condition of the patient and the informed consent.

Generally speaking, the patients who are subject to certain surgical interventions for parotid gland extended tumors are aged patients. Elderly patients normally present structural and functional modifications at the level of the cells and tissues, but additionally they often associate a range of chronic compensated or decompensated diseases, cachexia, immunodeficiency and addictions, therefore the anesthetic management compulsorily requires diagnostic and treatment of the coexisting pathology and a stringent preanesthetic preparation with the balance and correction of all the preexisting dysfunctions/ insufficiencies [26, 27].

The aged patients have a higher risk of perioperative morbidity and death rate as compared to young persons, because of the high incidence of the concomitant pathology. Although they present risks, the age and the associated diseases must not be deemed as an anesthetic contraindication if the surgery is required.

As the discussions with the patient during the preanesthetic visit cannot totally remove the anxiety and cannot offer sedation, analgesia, and amnesia, it is often necessary to resort to the preanesthetic medication. Nowadays, there is a wide range of drugs used in preanesthesia in the non-codified and confuse protocols. The premedication choice shall be performed according to age, weight, clinical condition of the patient, anxiety degree, allergic antecedents, and tolerance to drugs.

The objectives which have to be achieved through the preoperative medication are: fighting against anxiety, amnesia, and sedation, fighting against the preoperative pain, shortening the induction and reducing the necessary of intraoperative analgesic, using drugs which reduce the incidence of postoperative nausea and vomit, using the vagolytic agents when one anticipates an important dejection of the cardiovascular reflexes in induction, and using antihistamine drugs in allergic persons and in the patients with asthma [28].

13.4 The Anesthetic Monitoring

The anesthetic monitoring is an essential aspect of the anesthetic act. It has allowed the significant increase of the intra-anesthetic safety and also the increase of the complexity of the surgical interventions. The effective monitoring reduces the potential of the postoperative complications and detects the abnormalities, before the injury becomes irreversible.

The standard for the intra-anesthetic monitoring established by the American Society of the Anesthesiologists (ASA), initially in 1986 and subsequently modified, the most recent in 2011, comprises human, technical, or technological means compulsorily present, regardless of the surgical intervention or the health conditions of the patient [29].

In the parotid surgery, it is essential to monitor the muscular relaxation (neuromuscular blockade).

Besides the minimum compulsory standard, one shall also use all the monitoring means necessary for maintaining the safety of the patient and for guiding the therapeutic intervention (of the intraoperative intensive care). The presence of a blood gas analyzer in the operative block is very useful.

It is compulsory to protect the eyes and prevent the peripheral nerve elongations, preventing bedsores [30–33].

13.5 General Anesthesia

Regardless of the anesthetic technique used, all the surgical interventions at the parotid level impose the tracheal intubation, ensuring comfort and safety to the patient, over the entire duration of the surgical intervention. The choice of the anesthesia technique for the surgical intervention depends on a range of objective and subjective factors regarding the patient, surgeon, anesthesiologist, and the material conditions. The surgeon and the anesthesiologist must collaborate very well; the careful planning, preoperative assessment, and close cooperation are essential.

13.5.1 Arrangement of the Anesthesiologist in the Operating Room

In the OMF surgery, anesthesiologist's position is dictated by the surgical or anesthetic access, by the respiratory tract, and by the isolation of the head with sterile drapes. So as to ensure the space necessary to the surgeon and to the instruments, the anesthesiologist and the anesthetic equipment shall be placed in the lateral position of the patient or at the feet of the patient. That is why a good collaboration with the surgeon is required, together with a careful monitoring of the impermeability and pressure in the anesthetic circuit. The surgeon is obliged to inform the anesthesiologist with regard to any modification which appears in the operative field or if he performs maneuvers at carotid level. In emergency situations, when there are concerns regarding the respiratory tract, it is necessary to allow the fast access to the respiratory tract, even by removing the sterile drapes. Anesthesia induction is always performed with the anesthesiologist located at the head of the patient. The presence of the surgeon during the induction is compulsory. The advantage of the anesthesiologist who works in the OMF surgery is that he becomes specialized in difficult intubations and he receives the support of the surgeon, who is an expert in the emergency tracheotomy. In the case of the patients where a difficult intubation is anticipated, the neck of the patient must be prepared for tracheotomy, before starting any attempt of intubation. It is preferable to perform the induction on inhaler path, so that the patient can be easily awakened if there are ventilation difficulties. The surgeon, washed and clothed with the sterile equipment, must be prepared to interfere during the intubation maneuvers and to carry out the emergency tracheotomy when the situation imposes it. If the tracheotomy is carried out, the anesthesiologist remains at the head of the patient, from where he monitors and controls the tracheal tube. Because of the long distance between the respiratory tract of the patient and the anesthesia device, one must use an anesthetic circuit having a length higher than the one used regularly. In case of the use of the circuits with a higher length, there may appear ventilation problems, mainly in the patients with low pulmonary compliance [1–4].

13.5.2 Position of the Head and of the Body

Most of the interventions in the OMF surgery impose the rotation of the head and the extension of the neck, so one has to take into consideration measures for preventing the significant compression of the internal and external jugular veins and of the carotid artery in the vulnerable patients. A lateral inclination of the operative table can improve the surgical access without the need for the excessive rotation of the head and of the neck.

13.5.3 Monitoring of the Facial Nerve

In the parotid surgery, in the direction of the facial nerve, so as to decrease the incidence of its iatrogenic lesions, the surgeon needs to test the integrity of the facial nerve and of its branches, and this is why the neuromuscular blockade is contraindicated.

The complete or partial neuromuscular block produced by the muscular relaxants used in anesthesia induction reduces or abolishes the activity of this nerve, and its accidental section does not generate signal. It is very important that the neuromuscular blockade be interrupted or reversed and the function of the facial nerve assessed before the surgical intervention reaches in the neighborhood of the facial nerve. The monitoring of the parotid surgery is important for the muscular relaxation.

For the monitoring of the facial nerve, we use the nerve stimulator. One places electrodes at the level of the face, which shall detect the nervous activity when the nerve is stimulated. An auditory or visual signal shall be generated [2, 3].

13.5.4 Controlled Hypotension

Because of the rich vascularization of the territory, the intraoperative bleeding is important, that is why controlled hypotension is required (the systolic blood pressure between 85 and 90 mmHg). The induced hypotension requires a careful assessment of the risks and benefits and is not to be performed in patients with preexisting heart troubles. The controlled hypotension and the elevation of the head with 10–15°, reduce the bleeding and ensure a "clean" operative field which facilitates the dissection of the facial nerve, allowing at the same time a good central vascularization. The drugs used for this purpose include beta-blockers (metoprolol, labetalol), α-2-agonist (clonidine), and opioid (remifentanil) drugs [34].

As for the expansive parotid tumors in which we practice the substance loss reconstruction with free transferred microvascular flap, the intraoperative blood loss can be high, the controlled hypotension being a solution for reducing this loss. This technique is contraindicated in those with cardiac pathology, diseases of the central nervous system, anemia, and intercranial high blood pressure. When we anticipate high intraoperative blood loss and the general condition of the patient allows it, we can perform the preoperative hemodilution (conservation of the autologous blood, autologous blood transfusion). Moreover, blood loss reduction can be determined by the local infiltration with a local anesthetic solution with vasoconstrictor (adrenalin or noradrenalin 1/100,000) [1–7].

13.5.5 Additional Attitudes Depending on the Extent of the Surgical Procedure

The prophylaxis of the profound venous thrombosis must be established for all the interventions that do not have a very short duration. It is recommended to avoid hypoxemia and hypercapnia, sampling arterial gas (ASTRUP) for the long surgical interventions. One shall monitor the temperature, avoid hypothermia and hyperthermia, and maintain the normal temperature of the patient (37 °C peripheral). The central venous catheterization (CVC) is indicated when high blood losses are anticipated or when the patient is hemodynamically unstable. The urinary catheterization shall be taken into consideration for the long surgical interventions [1–6]. In parotid surgery, it is indicated to perform the maintenance of the anesthesia at least until the dissection of the facial nerve, by using only hypnotics and analgesics without muscular relaxation [1–7].

13.6 Awakening from Anesthesia

Like the induction, it represents a key moment for the anesthesiologist, sometimes being marked by the occurrence of certain specific complications. After a general anesthesia, the patient has to be permanently monitored until the complete awakening. The patient shall be detubated only when there is not a major risk of obstruction of the respiratory tract through hemorrhage, hematomas, or edema formation. The optimal choice is to detubate the patient after the complete awakening and not in profound anesthesia, when the protection reflexes of the respiratory tract are present. According to the ampleness of the anesthesia, the detubation is usually possible within the first 24 h following the surgery [1–10].

In case of a difficult intubation, the patient is detubated when he is completely awake. If the patient is agitated because of the probe and he is in the second stage of anesthesia, he will be sedated, supported by the ventilator, and as soon as the patient is awake, he is oriented, and there is efficient ventilation, one shall enforce the standard detubation protocol regarding the detubation of a patient with difficult intubation. The use of the "probe exchanger" is a common practice in the case of a difficult intubation. It is a metallic guide, made of rayon or elastic caoutchouc, it is passed through the probe in the trachea, and then the probe is extracted, letting the guide in the trachea. The patient shall tolerate the guide, and he will even be able to talk. If within almost 30 min there are no objective signs of obstruction, the guide shall be extracted. If there appears an obstruction or a deterioration of the respiratory tract, another intubation shall be performed, by using the guide and a probe having a smaller number than the former. The difficult intubation has to be notified in the medical record, and the staff that will continue supervising the patient must be informed with regard to this situation. When the reconstruction of the substance losses with free transferred microvascular flaps is performed, because of the intervention ampleness, in terms of duration and complexity, the patient is detubated in the first day following the surgery [35, 36].

13.7 Postoperative Care Management

Although most patients wake up fine from anesthesia, any patient operated under general anesthesia must be treated and monitored after surgery, as complications may occur, some with a vital prognostic. The first 24 h after surgery are critical, mostly in patients who underwent difficult and lengthy surgery and in patients with associated disorders. When managing postoperative patients, the complexity of the surgery and the associated general pathology are considered, and they are placed either in the recovery unit of the oral and maxillofacial surgery clinics or in the intensive care unit of the hospital.

All patients that undergo free flap reconstruction are admitted in the intensive care unit. The anesthesiologist provides the postoperative care. Each patient is made a postoperative/postanesthesia monitoring record in which the monitored parametric values at preset intervals (every 5 min in the first 15 min and after that, every

15 min), patient's condition at admission and at discharge, and medication are recorded [35–40, 43–47].

Postoperatively, the general condition and the surgical lesion (hemorrhage, drainage) of the patient are monitored and assessed in order to identify early and treat quickly any complication before it gets worse.

The postoperative care plan includes the following procedures: monitoring the respiratory function (pattern, effort, and rate of breathing, peripheral blood oxygen saturation – SpO2, viable airway), the cardiovascular function (noninvasive systemic blood pressure, electrocardiogram, pulse rate, and rhythm), and the neuromuscular function (clinically), monitoring consciousness (clinically), diuresis, temperature, pain, nausea, and drainage/bleeding. Patients that underwent complex surgery and patients with associated complex general pathology are kept under diversified complex monitoring depending on the specific traits of their particular cases [30, 31, 36–45] (Table 13.1).

If the flap is highly vascularized, well-perfused, and no complication occurs within 12 h (which in clinical practice means next morning), sedation may be reduced to restore patient's spontaneous breathing. The patient is kept under low sedation to enable communication and to provide optimal condition for extubation, which are no noticeable rise in blood pressure and excessive coughing. Standard criteria for extubation must be observed, because reintubation is risky for the flap [7, 35, 46–53] (Table 13.2).

Fluid administration is a regular practice, depending on patient's volume status. The amount and rhythm of administration depend on the chemical and hemodynamic recordings of the patient. Balanced electrolytic solutions and coloidal solutions are administered. Hemodynamic parameters are maintained at patients' specific values (not at theoretically normal values), to make efficient the tissue perfusion (ensuring the appropriate oxygen intake). Besides fluid administration (optimization of the circulating blood volume), it is necessary sometimes to optimize cardiac output/contractility by correcting heart rate and by inotropes, vascular resistance by means of vasoactive drugs, and oxygen transport capacity by correcting hypoxia (oxygen therapy) and to optimize (not to normalize) hemoglobin levels. In free flap reconstruction, vasoconstrictive therapy should be administered for short periods of time until other therapies reestablish an efficient hemodynamics, as they aggravate tissue hypoperfusion despite the maintenance of vital organ perfusion [31, 35, 40–45].

The decision to administer a transfusion should be made individually. The total amount of lost blood, the hemoglobin level or red blood cells, the systemic blood pressure, the cardiac output, the oxygen saturation in arterial (SaO2) and peripheral blood (SpO2), and the temperature are monitored.

Severe anemia should be corrected by transfusion as it lowers oxygen transport capacity. The target hemoglobin of 7–9 g/dl is recommended. Hemoglobin shall not be normalized as it increases

Table 13.1 Routine and selective monitoring of patients

	Routine	Selective
Respiratory function	Respiratory function, viable airway, oxygen saturation	Capnography, sanguine gas
Cardiovascular function	Noninvasive blood pressure, pulse frequency	Invasive blood pressure, electrocardiograph, volume status assessment
Neuromuscular function	Clinically	
State of consciousness	Clinically	
Pain	Pain scale	
Nausea	Clinically	
Drainage and bleeding	Clinically	
Temperature		
Diuresis		Urinary volume, hourly dieresis

Table 13.2 Criteria for extubation following free flap reconstruction

Examination of the flap
Warm, perfused, good venous drainage, swelling within acceptable limits
Examination of the patient
Warm peripherally with normal blood pressure indicating good cardiac output
Good peripheral arterial oxygen saturation and blood gases
Good urine output (0.5–1 ml/kg body weight/h)
Drains working and accumulation of blood in drainage bottles acceptably low
Swelling in the neck or airway minimal and not worsening

blood viscosity and stresses microcirculation disorders. The administration of the packed red blood cells is recommended when hemoglobin level is low (Hb<7 g/dl in a healthy young patient), mostly in conditions of acute anemia. When hemoglobin is 7–9 g/dl, the decision to administer packed red blood cells depends on patient's risk factors, bleeding potential, rate and size of bleeding, intravascular volume, and presence of organ ischemia. When blood loss is quick and large, over 1500 ml or>30 % of blood volume and bleeding is not controlled quickly, blood transfusion is indicated. Acute normovolemic hemodilution and intraoperative red cell recovery are options, although they are rarely used, with the purpose of reducing the usage of transfused blood units [36–40, 54–60].

An essential objective in the postoperative period is pain management. The presence of the sensation of pain produces psychomotor agitation, peripheral vasoconstriction, pallor, sweat, arterial hypertension, and tachycardia. Pain is assessed using a pain scale, initially every 10 min, and then it is tailored to the patient. Surprisingly in oral maxillofacial surgery, major interventions do not produce intense pain. In practice, small doses of opiates (morphine) associated with anti-inflammatory nonsteroidal painkillers and paracetamol provide a good analgesia and hemodynamic stability (good blood pressure, warm extremities, and efficient urinary flow). It is preferable to have multimodal analgesia by associating drugs of different classes administered by different methods, avoiding in this way the adverse effects of medication. Local anesthesia techniques are many times extremely useful [36–40, 58–63, 70].

Nausea control is another concern of the anesthesiologist. It is a minor postoperative side effect, but it is unpleasant to the patient and may generate side effects in other systems and apparatuses (in the cardiovascular system, intracranial pressure). Like in pain, multimodal prophylaxis is used, substances from different classes being administered. Superior effects are obtained when doses of each individual substance are gradually reduced. Patients are administered receptor antagonists 5-HT3 (ondansetron), dexamethasone, antihistamine, metoclopramide, and propofol. An adequate volemic status contributes to nausea decrease. Colloidal solutions are much more efficient compared to crystalloid solutions [36–40, 64–70].

Prophylaxis of deep venous thrombosis and pulmonary embolism is applied in patients under risk. Mechanic measures to prevent venous stasis in lower limbs (compressive bandages, pneumatic dressing of foreleg musculature) are combined with medication (heparin or low molecular weight heparin).

Hypothermia and shivering are frequently met complications in the postoperative period. They occur in hypothermic patients after prolonged general anesthesia. The treatment involves warming the patient, oxygen, and myalgin administration.

Additional oxygen administration is made when there is a risk of hypoxemia [31, 40–46].

Any postoperative complications of the central nervous system, of the cardiovascular system, and of the respiratory system and renal, hepatic, laryngeal, ocular, and neuromuscular complications are treated.

Hematological and biochemical investigations are conducted in patients to ascertain and to correct early any hydro-electrolytic and acido-basic imbalance (although in oral and maxillofacial surgery, significant imbalances rarely occur) [40–46].

Surgical complications may occur: hemorrhage, drainage blocking, and infection. In case of flap reconstruction, good vascularization is essential; this is why the anesthesiologist should inspect regularly and see the aspect of the flap. He always informs and talks to the surgical team before planning extubation, being aware that any failure is his responsibility [36–40, 48, 50–53].

Enteral nutrition (EN) or parenteral nutrition (PN) should start early (in the first 24 h, no more than 48 h). In hemodynamically stable patients with functional digestive tract, the administration of the nutritional support (NS) is made by early enteral nutrition (EEN), which is superior to parenteral nutrition, as it is associated with lower infectious complications and hospitalization period. Enteral nutrition decreases gastrointestinal permeability and prevents bacterial translocation. Enteral nutrition is administered per os through a nasojejunal tube or orojejunal tube. If 2 days after starting early enteral nutrition (EEN), the caloric needs are not met (25 Kcal/kg body/day), parenteral nutrition (PN) is added to meet the caloric needs [71–75].

To all patients in which substance loss was replaced by microvascular flap reconstruction, pentoxifylline is administered for 5 days. Pentoxifylline is an anti-ischemic vasodilator with musculotropic action that facilitates microcirculation and improves red blood cell deformability.

The patient will be transferred to the surgical section when he meets the discharge criteria: perfectly normal state of consciousness, cardiovascular stability, adequate peripheral perfusion, viable airway, present pharyngeal reflex, satisfactory ventilator parameters, pain and nausea under control, thermally normal, and normal vascularized flap [36–40, 43–45].

References

1. Aitkenhead AR, Rowbotham DJ, Smith G. Textbook of anaesthesia. 4th ed. Philadelphia: Elsevier; 2002.
2. Morgan GE, Maged SM, Murray MJ. Clinical anesthesiology. 4th ed. New York: McGraw-Hill; 2006.
3. Miller RD. Miller's anesthesia. 7th ed. Philadelphia: Elsevier; 2010.
4. Acalovschi I. Anestezie clinică. 2nd ed. Cluj-Napoca: Clusium; 2005.
5. Hargrave SA. Anesthesia for dental and faciomaxilarry surgery. In: Healy TE, Cohen PJ, editors. A practice of anesthesia. 6th ed. London: Edward Arnold; 1996. p. 1205–22.
6. Gotta AW, Ferrari LR, Sullivan CA. Anesthesia for ENT surgery. In: Barash PG, Cullen BT, Stoelting RK, editors. Clinical anesthesia. Philadelphia: Lippincott–Raven; 1996. p. 929–43.
7. Patel H, editor. Anaesthesia for burns, maxillo-facial and plastic surgery. London: Edward Arnold; 1993.
8. American Society of Anesthesiologists. Practice guidelines for the management of the difficult airway. Anesthesiology. 1993;78:597–600.
9. American Society of Anesthesiologists Task Force on Management of the Difficult Airway. Practice guidelines for management of the difficult airway. Anesthesiology. 2003;98:1269–77.
10. Slater R, Bharia K. Cannot ventilate, difficult to intubate. Eur J Anaesthesiol. 2007;24:377–8.
11. Benumof JL. Management of the difficult adult airway. With special emphasis on awake tracheal intubation. Anesthesiology. 1991;75:1087–110.
12. Mort TC, Gabrielli A, Coans TJ, Behringer EC, Layon AJ. Airway management. In: Gabrielli A, Layon AJ, Yu M, editors. Civetta, Taylor and Kirby's critical care. 4th ed. Philadelphia: Lippincott Williams & Wilkins; 2009. p. 519–55.
13. Henderson JJ, Popat MT, Latto IP, Pearce AC. Difficult airway society. Difficult airway society guidelines for management of the unanticipated difficult intubation. Anaesthesia. 2004;59:675.
14. Robin AS. Fiberoptic airway management. Anesthesiol Clin N Am. 2002;20:933–51.
15. Koirala S, Tripathi M, Subani A, Bhattarai B. Topical anaesthesia of the vocal cords by nebulized lidocaine inhalation to facilitate fiberoptic nasotracheal intubation in a head – size parotid tumour patient. J Nepal Med Assoc. 2011;51:34–6.
16. Puchner W, Egger P, Puhringer F, Löckinger A, Obwegeser J, Gombotz H. Evaluation of remifentanil as single drug for awake fiberoptic intubation. Acta Anaesthesiol Scand. 2002;46:350–4.
17. Machata AM, Gonano C, Holzer A, Andel D, Spiss CK, Zimpfer M, et al. Awake nasotracheal fiberoptic intubation: patient comfort, intubating conditions, and hemodynamic stability during conscious sedation with remifentanil. Anesth Analg. 2003;97:904–8.
18. Lallo A, Billard V, Bourgain J. A comparison of propofol and remifentanil target – controlled infusions to facilitate fiberoptic intubation. Anesth Analg. 2009;108:852–7.
19. Woods AW, Allam S. Traheal intubation without the use of neuromuscular blocking agents. Br J Anaesth. 2005;94(2):150–8.
20. Lee C, Jahr JS, Candiotti KA, Warriner B, Zornow MH, Naquib M. Reversal of profound neuromuscular block by sugammadex administered three minutes after rocuronium. A comparison with spontaneous recovery from succinylcholine. Anesthesiology. 2009;110:1020–5.
21. McTernan CN, Rapeport DA, Ledowski T. Successful use of rocuronium and sugammandex in an anticipated defficult airway scenario. Anaesth Intensive Care. 2010;38(2):390–2.

22. Committee on Standards and Practice Parameters, Apfelbaum JL, Connis RT, Nickinovich DG; American Society of Anesthesiologists Task Force on Preanesthesia Evaluation, Pasternak LR, Arens JF, Caplan RA, Connis RT, Fleisher LA, Flowerdew R, Gold BS, Mayhew JF, Nickinovich DG, Rice LJ, Roizen MF, Twersky RS. Practice advisory for preanesthesia evaluation: an updated report by the American Society of Anesthesiologists Task Force on Preanesthesia Evaluation. Anesthesiology. 2012; 116(3):522–38.
23. Roizen MF. Preoperative assessment: What is necessary to do? 45th Annual Refresher Course Lectures and Clinical Update Program. American Society of Anesthesiologists, San Francisco, 1994;132:1–7.
24. Barash PG, Cullen B, Stoelting RK, Cahalan MK, Stock MC. Handbook of clinical anesthesia. 6th ed. Philadelphia: Lippincott Williams & Wilkins; 2009. p. 333–45.
25. Pasternak LR. Preoperative laboratory testing: general issues and considerations. Anesthesiol Clin N Am. 2004;22(1):13–25.
26. Copotoiu M, Azamfirei L. Anestezia la varstnic, in vol actualitati in anestezie. Targu Mures: University Press; 2011.
27. Jancovic R, Bogicevic A, Storsic B, Panlovic A, Petrovic A, Marcovic D, Vuceva C. Preoperative preparation of geriatric patients. Acta Chir Iugos. 2011;52(2):169–75.
28. Evers AS, Maze M. Anesthetic pharmacology physiologic principles and clinical practice. A companion to Miller's anesthesia. Philadelphia: Churchill Livingstone; 2004.
29. American Society of Anesthesiologists. Standards for basic anesthetic monitoring. Committee of origin: Standards and Practice Parameters (Approved by the ASA House of Delegates on October 21, 1986, and last amended on October 25, 2005), American Society of Anesthesiologists. Standards, Guidelines and Statements. 2009.
30. http://www.asahq.org/quality-and-practice-management/standards-and-guidelines.
31. Grigoraş I. Anestezie şi terapie intensivă. Principii de bază. Iasi: Editura Institutul European; 2007.
32. Miller RD, Eriksson LI, Fleisher LI, Weiner-Kronish JP, Young WL. Miller's anesthesia. 7th ed. Philadelphia: Churchill Livingstone Elsevier; 2010.
33. Morgan GE, Mikhail MS, Murray M, editors. Clinical anesthesiology. 4th ed. New York: McGraw–Hill; 2005.
34. Van Acken H, Miller Jr E. Deliberate hypotension. In: Miller RD, editor. Anesthesia. 4th ed. New York: Churchill Livingstone; 1994. p. 1441–503.
35. Marsh M, Elliot S, Anand R, Brennan PA. Early postoperative care for free flap head and neck reconstructive surgery – a national survey of practice. Br J Oral Maxillofac Surg. 2009;47:182–5.
36. Vimlati I, Gilsanz F, Goldik Z. Quality and safety guidelines of postanesthesia care. Eur J Anaesthesiol. 2009;26:715–21.
37. Practice Guidelines for Postanesthetic Care – A report by the American Society of Anesthesiologists Task Force on Postanesthetic Care. Anesthesiology. 2002;96:742–52.
38. Barone CP, Pablo CS, Barone GW. Postanesthetic care in the critical care unit. Crit Care Nurse. 2004;24:38–45.
39. Prien T, Van Aken H. The perioperative phase as a part of anesthesia. Tasks of the recovery room. Anaesthesist. 1997;46 Suppl 2:S109–13.
40. American Society of Anesthesiologists Task Force on Postanesthesic Care. Practice guidelines for postanesthetic care. Anesthesiology. 2002;96:742.
41. Fu ES, Downs JB, Schweiger JW. Supplemental oxygen impair detection of hypoventilation by pulse oximetry. Chest. 2004;126:1552–8.
42. Dibenedetto RJ, Graves SA, Gravenstein N, Konk C. Pulse oximetry monitoring can change routine oxygen supplementation practices in the postanesthesia care unit. Anesth Analg. 1994;78(2):365–8.
43. Aitkenhead AR. Postoperative care. In: Rowbotham DJ, Smith G, editors. Textbook of anaesthesia. 4th ed. New York: Churchill Livingstone; 2001. p. 524–44.
44. Zelcer J, Wells DG. Anesthetic – related recovery room – complications. Anaesth Intensive Care. 1996;15:168.
45. Mecca RS. Postoperative recovery. In: Barash PG, Cullen BF, Stoelting RK, editors. Clinical anesthesia. 5th ed. Philadelphia: Lippincott Williams & Wilkins; 2006. p. 1397–405.
46. Aps C. Surgical critical care: the overnight intensive recovery (OIR) concept. Br J Anaesth. 2004;92:164–6.
47. Sabir N, Martin S, Vaughan D. Clinical and cost effectiveness of an overnight intensive recovery (OIR) for patients undergoing complex airway and head and neck surgery in a regional unit. Anaesthesia. 2008;63:1388.
48. Cobbett JR. Free digital transfer. J Bone Joint Surg. 1969;51B:677.
49. Haljame H. Anesthetic risk factors. Acta Chir Scand Suppl. 1989;550:11–9.
50. Farwell DG, Reilly DF, Weymuller EA, Greenberg DL, Staiger TO, Futran NA. Predictors of perioperative complications in head and neck patients. Arch Otolaryngol Head Neck Surg. 2002;128:505–11.
51. Baker SR. Microsurgical reconstruction of the head and neck. New York: Churchill Livingstone; 1989.
52. Head C, Sercarz JA, Abemayor E, Calcatterra T, Rawnsley I, Blackwell K. Microvascular reconstruction after previous neck dissection. Arch Otolaryngol Head Neck Surg. 2002;128(3):328–31.
53. Mc Carthy JG. Plastic surgery. In: Tumors of the head and neck and skin, vol. 5. Philadelphia: WB Saunders; 1990.
54. Vincent JL, Piagnerelli M. Transfusion in the intensive care unit. Crit Care Med. 2006;34:S96–101.

55. Vincent JL, Baron JF, Reinhart K, Gattinoni L, Thijs L, Webb A, et al. Anemia and blood transfusion in critically ill patients. JAMA. 2002;288(12): 1499–507.
56. Kemming IG. Anemia in the ICU. Tolerance or therapy? Refresher course. Euroanesthesia. 2003.
57. Fung MK, Moore K, Ridenour M, Mook W, Triulzi DJ. Clinical effects of reverting from leukoreduced to nonleukoreduced blood in cardiac surgery. Transfusion. 2006;46:386–91.
58. American Society of Anesthesiologists Task Force on Perioperative Blood Transfusion and Adjuvant Therapies. Practice guidelines for perioperative blood transfusion and adjuvant therapies: an updated report by the American Society of Anesthesiologists Task Force on perioperative blood transfusion and adjuvant therapies. Anesthesiology. 2006;105(1):198–208.
59. Vincent JL, Werl MH. Fluid challenge revisited. Crit Care. 2006;34:1333–7.
60. Crawford JH, Isabel TS, Huang Z, Shiva S, Chacko BK, Schechter AN, et al. Hypoxia, red blood cells, and nitrite regulate NO-dependent hypoxic vasodilation. Blood. 2006;107:566–74.
61. Gan TJ, Lubarsky DA, Flood EM. Patient preferences for acute pain treatment. Br J Anaesth. 2004;92(5): 681–8.
62. Strassels SA, Mcnicol E, Suleman R. Postoperative pain management: a practical review. Am J Health Syst Pharm. 2005;62(19):2019–25.
63. White PF. The changing role of non-opioid analgesic techniques in the management of postoperative pain. Anesth Analg. 2005;101(5 Suppl):S5–22.
64. Scuderi PE, James RL, Harris L, Mims GR. Multimodal antiemetic management prevents early postoperative vomiting after outpatient laparoscopy. Anesth Analg. 2000;91:1408–14.
65. Tramer MR, Reynolds DJM, Moore RA, McQuay HJ. Efficacy, dose-response, and safety of ondansetron in prevention of postoperative nausea and vomiting: a qualitative systemic review of randomised placebo-controlled trials. Anesthesiology. 1997;87:1277–89.
66. Henzi I, Walder B, Tramer MR. Dexamethasone for the prevention of postoperative nausea and vomiting: a quantitative systemic review. Anesth Analg. 2000;90:186–94.
67. Khalil S, Philbrook L, Rabb M, Wells L, Aves T, Villanueva G, et al. Ondasetron/prometazine combination or prometazine alone reduces nausea and vomiting after middle ear surgery. J Clin Anesth. 1999;11:596–600.
68. Sinclair DR, Chung F, Mezei G. Can postoperative nausea and vomiting be predicted? Anesthesiology. 1999;91:109–18.
69. Morette EW, Robertson KM, El-Moalem H, Gan TJ. Intraoperative colloid administration reduces postoperative nausea and vomiting and improves outcomes compared with crystalloid administration. Anesth Analg. 2003;96:611–7.
70. Maharaj CH, Kallam SR, Malik A, Hassett P, Grady D, Laffey JG. Preoperative intravenous fluid therapy decreases postoperative nausea and pain in high risk patient. Anesth Analg. 2004;99:1630–7.
71. Kreymann KG, Berger MM, Deutz NEP, Hiesmayr M, Jolliet P, Kazandjiev G, et al. ESPEN guidelines on enteral nutrition: intensive care. Clin Nutr. 2006;25:210–23.
72. Singer P, Berger MM, Van den Berghe G, Biolo G, Calder P, Forbes A, et al. ESPEN guidelines on parenteral nutrition: intensive care. Clin Nutr. 2009;28: 387–400.
73. Sandstrom R, Drott C, Hyltander A, Arfvidsson B, Scherstén T, Wickström I, et al. The effect of postoperative intravenous feeding (TPN) on outcome following major surgery evaluated in a randomised study. Ann Surg. 1993;217:185–95.
74. Peter JV, Moran JL, Philips-Hughes J. A metaanalysis of treatment outcomes of early enteral versus early parenteral nutrition in hospitalized patients. Crit Care Med. 2005;33:213–20.
75. Braunschweig CL, Levy P, Sheean PM, Wang X. Enteral compared with parenteral nutrition: a metaanalysis. Am J Clin Nutr. 2001;74:534–42.

14 Arising Problems in Extended Parotidectomy

Victor-Vlad Costan, Daniela A. Trandafir, and Eugenia I. Popescu

Abstract

The extended parotidectomy is a complex surgery reserved, generally, for the advanced parotid malignant lesions that interest several anatomical structures, with the objective of eradicating malignancy by en bloc resection of all tumor involved tissue. Besides the problem of the extent of tissues that will be removed in order to ensure oncological safety limits (with radical neck dissection usually performed at the same time), the reconstructive surgery techniques addressed to these cases are of particular interest, because they must correct both the aesthetic deficit (depression of the parotid and superior laterocervical regions due to the missing tissues surgically removed) and the functional one (the facial nerve palsy and Frey's syndrome), for optimal results of the postoperative survival. In large defects following extended parotidectomy, the use of the thicker free transferred soft tissue flaps or, better, the radial forearm fasciocutaneous flaps (but usually followed by lipostructure in the latter cases, from our experience) is recommended, allowing a proper restoration of the facial contours and skin coverage and also avoid Frey's syndrome. The paralytic lagophthalmos consecutive to total or extended parotidectomy for malignancy requires a special attention, due to the risk of developing a keratopathy, corneal abrasions or ulcers, or even blindness, due to the absence of the long-term protection provided by the ocular conjunctiva.

V.-V. Costan, MD, DMD, PhD (✉)
Department of Oral and Maxillo-Facial Surgery, Faculty of Dental Medicine, "Grigore T. Popa" University of Medicine and Pharmacy, "St. Spiridon" University Hospital, Iasi, Romania
e-mail: victorcostan@gmail.com

D.A. Trandafir, MD, PhD • E.I. Popescu, DMD, PhD
Department of Surgery (Dentoalveolar Surgery, Oral and Maxillofacial Surgery), Faculty of Dental Medicine, "Grigore T. Popa" University of Medicine and Pharmacy, Iasi, Romania

14.1 Introduction

Extensive surgery such as total parotidectomy and extended parotidectomy is generally followed by aesthetic and functional sequelae. The functional sequelae refer to Frey's syndrome, locally loss of the skin sensitivity in the parotid region and earlobe and the facial paralysis, which is the most important of them. The striking aesthetic consequence is

© Springer International Publishing Switzerland 2016

V.-V. Costan (ed.), *Management of Extended Parotid Tumors*, DOI 10.1007/978-3-319-26545-2_14

the preauricular, retromandibular and upper laterocervical depression but also the depression due to malar bone resection. To diminish these problems, several techniques were proposed, especially to restore the normal facial contour by filling the depression of the parotid region and the upper laterocervical region but also to avoid Frey's syndrome or sequelae of the facial nerve palsy at the same time. Total and extensive parotidectomies create major defects that often cannot be restored only by local soft tissue flaps.

We present in this chapter a summary of issues raised during the extended parotidectomy, while the details of these problems are separately discussed in the following chapters addressed to the different types of reconstructive surgery.

14.2 Issues Related to the Extent of the Surgical Resection That Removes the Parotid Extended Malignancy

Extended parotidectomy is a surgical procedure that aims to eradicate the malignant tumors that interest the parotid gland and neighboring anatomical structures, such as the overlying skin, the masseter muscle (most commonly), the temporal bone, the mandible, or the malar bone. This complex surgery is usually reserved for malignant parotid lesions in advanced stages, which involve several anatomical structures. The surgical resection refers to en bloc resection of the malignant tumor extended from the parotid to neighboring tissues, namely: the parotid gland, the covering skin, the adjacent muscles and vessels, the tumor infiltrated temporal, mandibular and malar bones, and, where is required, the ear (Fig. 14.1a–c). If necessary, the radical or functional neck dissection is performed and, possibly, the facial nerve reconstruction by anastomosis. The reconstruction of the substance loss is usually made by use of a myocutaneous flap from the major pectoralis (it is probably the simplest method for the bulky defects) or with adjacent flaps.

The surgical technique is chosen depending on the location of the primary tumor and the malignant tumor infiltration of the adjacent anatomical structures [1]. The parotidectomy extended to the skin includes surgical resection of a portion of the cheek and temporal or cervical region of the skin. In parotidectomy extended to the mandible, the surgical resection includes osteo-myo-articular structures and the temporomandibular joint infiltrated by tumor. Bony resection is also necessary

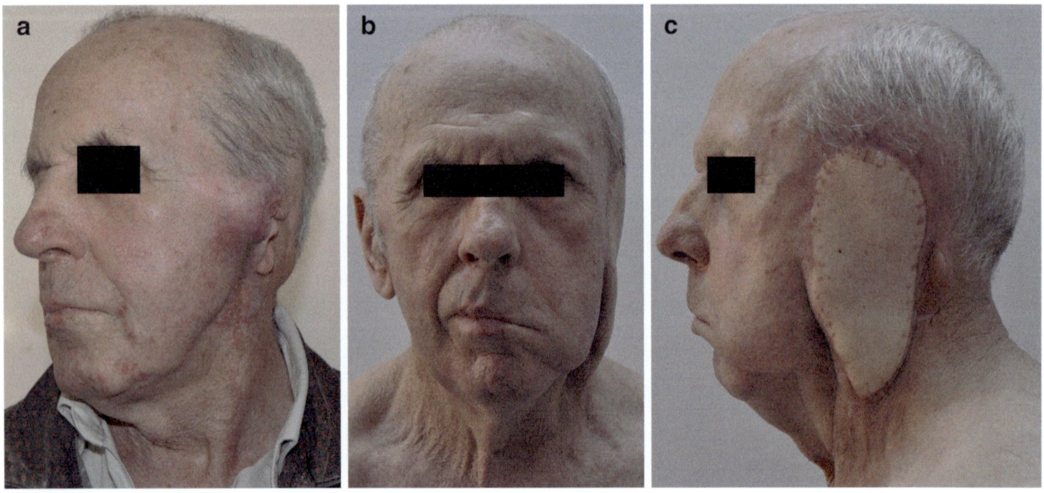

Fig. 14.1 (**a**) Squamous cell carcinoma in the left parotid region, multiple operated and relapsed in left parotid gland and external ear. (**b**, **c**) Treatment consisted of extended parotidectomy with partially sacrificing the facial nerve, external ear resection and partial temporal bone resection. Defect plasty was performed using a musculocutaneous free flap transfer of the latissimus dorsi. Besides the paralysis of the facial nerve, the main damage was the esthetic one, with facial asymmetry in which contributed left external ear disappearance

in the case of temporal bone invasion, including the middle ear. In this aspect, a vertiginous syndrome can develop postoperatively following the unilateral impairment of the middle ear. In our experience, the symptoms spontaneously disappear within the first two weeks after surgery. When the tumor reaches but does not invade the mastoid and the lower portion of the tympanic ring, partial mastoidectomy is performed. In such cases, total parotidectomy, radical or modified neck dissection, and partial mastoidectomy are performed, with preservation of the external ear canal and middle ear and sacrifice of the upper and lower peripheral branches of the facial nerve. When the tumor invades the lower portion of the tympanic ring, complete mastoidectomy is performed. When tumor invades the glenoid fossa, the petrous portion of the temporal bone is also removed. In such advanced tumors, the soft tissues from the parapharyngeal space, the ninth cranial nerve, the pterygoid apophysis, and the internal pterygoid muscle are also removed.

Note that sometimes advanced malignant parotid tumors will also require the surgical excision of the squamous part of the temporal bone or the wings of the sphenoid bone, reaching up to the meningeal level. In such situations of extensive resections, a special attention will be given to the reconstruction techniques, which should provide a good "sealing" (closing) at this level, avoiding the leakage of the cerebrospinal fluid and thus, the meningitis or meningoencephalitis. The musculocutaneous flaps – free transferred (which are preferred) or pedicled (such as, for instance, the pectoralis major flap) – have elective indication. The great pectoral musculocutaneous pedicled flap, for example, is located at the end of the vascular pedicle and often has small marginal necrosis. On the contrary, the situation is exactly the reverse for the latissimus dorsi free flap, since the latter free flap provides adequate sealing of the receiving area.

The tumor size, the histopathological type, the involvement of the facial nerve, and the neighboring tissues are important prognostic markers for patients with primary parotid carcinoma [2]. The long-term survival depends mainly on histopathological characteristics and tumoral stage. For enlarged parotid malignant tumors, the radical extended parotidectomy associated with postoperative radiotherapy is the treatment of choice that improves the life expectancy of these patients.

A special attention is given to the resection of the mandible. It may cause functional disorders (disorders of mastication, swallowing, and, phonation) and aesthetic disorders (lateral deviation of the chin, depression of the masseter and cheek regions). The mandibular condyle resection is also included here (but more commonly encountered than other resections in such situations) and it has minimal functional and aesthetic implications.

Due to the position of the parotid tumors around the vertical mandibular ramus, the mandibular resection (which is required in cases of extensive bone tumors) does not involve the mandibular arch, and, therefore, there is no need to perform a reconstruction of the mandible; the aesthetic and functional consequences are relatively less obvious. This is important because, as already mentioned, the extended parotidectomies are often needed in patients with a poor general condition, in which any extension of the surgery duration may result in a significant increase of the postoperative morbidity.

The proximity of the malar bone sometimes makes it necessary to remove (usually partially) this bone together with the specimen, in order to ensure tumor free margins of the wound (Fig. 14.2a–c). Fortunately, in most of the cases, this kind of resection has only esthetical consequences.

14.3 The Problem of Facial Nerve Palsy following the Total and Extended Parotidectomy

Interruption of the facial nerve is a consequence of radical parotidectomy (to note that the facial nerve sacrifice can also be partial depending on tumor extension). The decision to interrupt the facial nerve can be simple if the tumoral invasion of the nerve is present form the beginning (Fig. 14.3a, b). Loss of the facial nerve leads to loss of eye protection, nasal inspiration, and oral competence. Besides the serious problem of

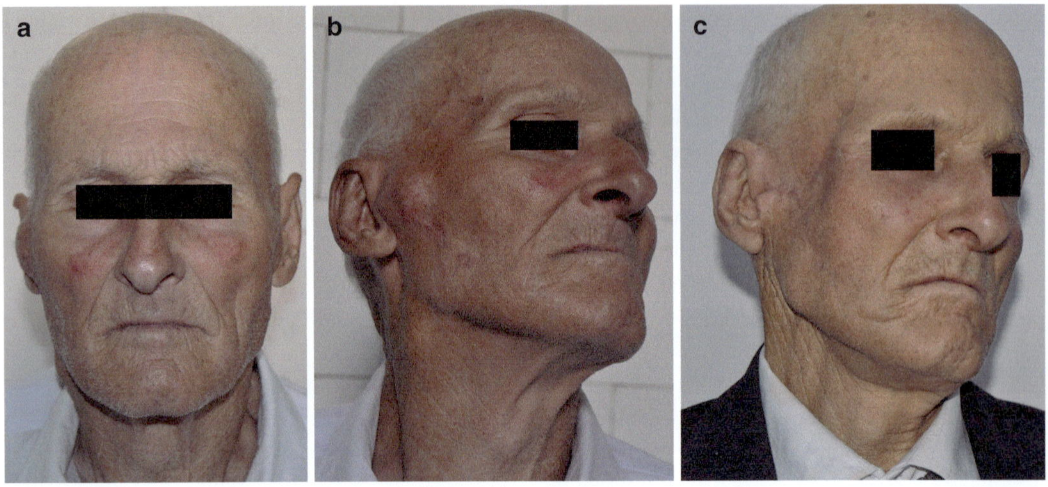

Fig. 14.2 (**a**, **b**) The patient presented a squamous cell carcinoma in the right masseteric region, operated, locally cured, with metastatic lymphadenopathy of the right parotid gland extended to right malar bone. (**c**) Removal of lymph node metastasis made necessary an extended parotidectomy to right malar bone, with sacrificing of the superior branch of the facial nerve and closure of the defect by direct suture. There was a depression in the malar bone region, postoperatively. This depression can be corrected with minimal trauma using lipostructure

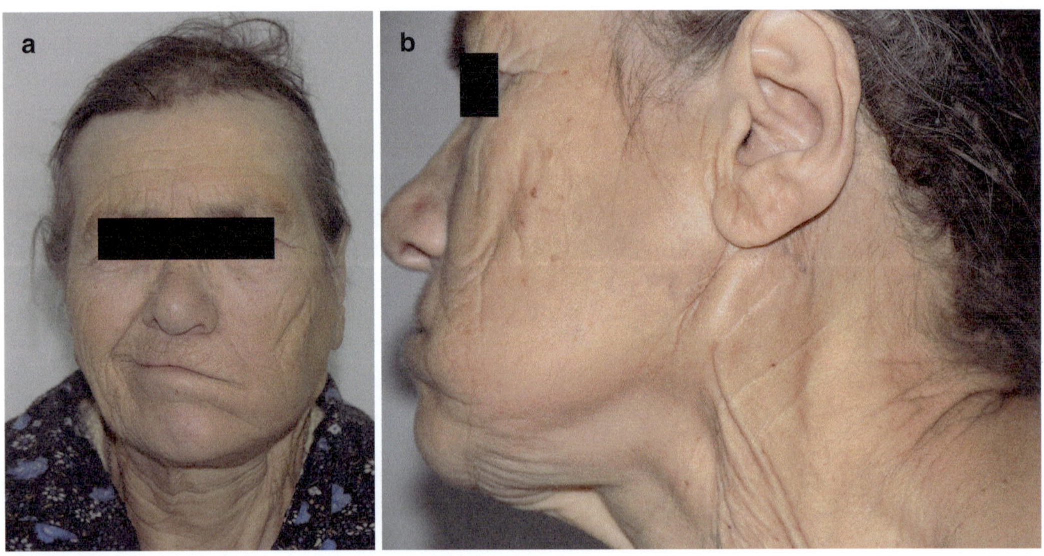

Fig. 14.3 (**a**, **b**) Facial nerve paralysis in left parotid gland adenoid cystic carcinoma, extended to skin

lagophthalmos, we should not minimize the problem of perioral muscle denervation; the incontinence of the oral cavity with the decreasing of the cheek muscle tone and diminishing of the sensitivity at this level has the unpleasant consequence of food retention (Fig. 14.4a, b). The aesthetic defect and the disrupted communication of these patients may also have a negative psychological effect, especially in young patients and female sex. Effective restoration of the affected territory with respect to the interrelations of mimic muscles cannot be guaranteed. Therefore, the main objectives of these interventions for nervous restoration are the protection of

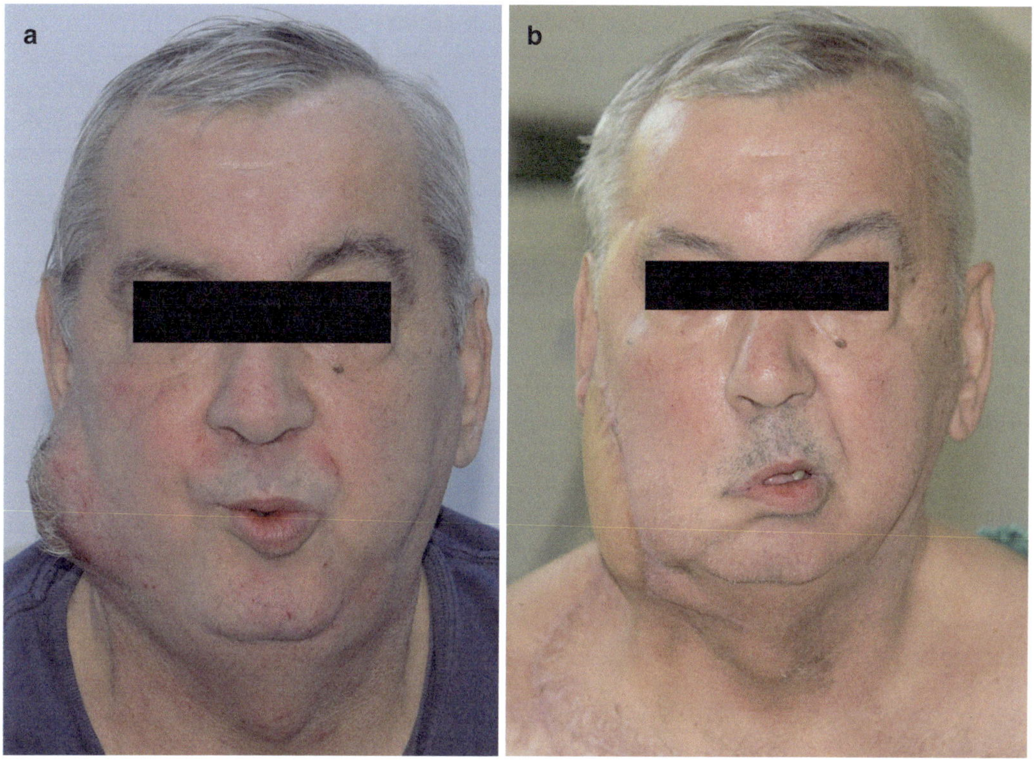

Fig. 14.4 (**a**) Carcinoma ex pleomorphic adenoma, extended to skin. (**b**) Treatment consisted of extended parotidectomy, defect plasty being performed with a musculocutaneous latissimus dorsi free flap. It was necessary to sacrifice the facial nerve, with classical aesthetic and functional consequences

vision function, nasal air passage and oral cavity continence, the restoring of facial symmetry, and trying to achieve facial symmetry during facial muscle movements [3].

In cases of radical parotidectomy, direct reconstruction of the facial nerve is not always possible due to the defect size. If the trunk of the facial nerve is preserved, then grafting the branches is considered. In some cases, nerve elongation through tumor bulkiness provides enough length for direct suture of the nerve stumps after resection of the intratumoral nerve path. The great auricular nerve which is highlighted during extirpation of the tumor and neck dissection can be used as a donor graft due to its caliber, lower donor site morbidity, and its length. Other options of nerve graft include the dorsal cutaneous nerve of the foot and the sural nerve. Other nerve transfers use the hypoglossal nerve for end-to-end or end-to-side neurorrhaphy. Masseter innervation is another alternative for nervous transferring, which proved to be effective in producing a spontaneous and dynamic response, consequence of activation [4]. Static reconstruction refers to the use of tendon "straps" that can support the external nasal wing, maintain the mouth continence, and provide the facial symmetry. The wires (barbed or not) suspended in the temporal region can also be used, according to our experience. But, dynamic reconstruction is certainly superior and can be obtained by free transfered or regional muscle flaps. The masseter and temporal muscles are two models of regional transfers, particularly useful to improve the oral function and facial communication. The loss of the marginal mandibular branch of the facial nerve will lead to paralysis of the lower lip and angle mouth descending muscle, producing an asymmetric smile and a flaccid lower lip, rotated on the affected side. A local muscle transfer that corrects this imbalance is one that uses the anterior belly of the digastric muscle, with the central tendon inserted into the lower lip vermillion edge, 1–2 cm medial to the mouth corner [5].

14.4 Problems in the Restoration of the Normal Facial Contour and Avoiding Frey's Syndrome

Additional issues of radical parotidectomy include the depression of the parotid region contour and the loss of skin coverage [3]. The local options that correct these problems are cervicofacial or submental flaps. But fasciocutaneous free flaps represent "the gold standard" for skin coverage and facial contours restoration. Frey's syndrome is a potential complication following the radical parotidectomy [1].

Extended parotidectomy is a complex intervention both in terms of anatomical structures to be excised and facial contour reconstruction problems. Removal of the whole parotid gland with cervical neck dissection leads to changes in the contour of the head and neck characterized by retromandibular and upper cervical depression [6]. The exceeding parotid gland tumors that infiltrate the covering skin require excision of the invaded skin, and those that infiltrate the facial nerve can reach up to the mastoid and temporal bone, imposing the removal of the affected bone structures and facial nerve decompression at the exit from the stylomastoid foramen. The loss of the facial nerve or its branches leads to different degrees of functional and aesthetic subsequent deficits. Any motor denervation is followed by the atrophy of the structures, in this case of the innervated muscle structures, which accentuates the facial asymmetry. For this reason, the dynamic recovery of the facial nerve function should be performed as early as possible, with decreasing atrophy but getting the best functional results. We should not omit the fact that many of these patients will be further treated by postoperative radiotherapy. In case of facial nerve paralysis, the radiotherapy will further contribute to the interested tissue atrophy.

The post-extensive parotidectomy defects that require reconstructive surgery vary from loss of subcutaneous soft tissue defects to extensive defects that involve the skin, soft tissue, and bone tissue, with facial paralysis. Therefore, the reconstructive surgery should be adapted in such cases to the peculiarities of the defect. The preauricular, retromandibular, and upper cervical soft tissue loss, as a result of performing a total parotidectomy, require a flap reconstruction of an adequate thickness to restore the normal facial contour and any lack of skin [7]. The anterolateral thigh flap has shown an increasing popularity in reconstructive surgery of the head and neck, because it can be designed as fasciocutaneous or myocutaneous flap or in many other configurations. The advantages that recommend it are the long pedicle, the large palette of skin and soft tissue and the anatomical location which allows its harvesting during the tumor resection. Additionally, the donor site can be extended to access the lateral femoral cutaneous nerve (which can be used to reconstruct the facial nerve and for the commissuroplasty). Another advantage is the minimum morbidity at the donor site [8, 9]. Our experience showed a good result in the reconstructions following extensive parotidectomy by using the radial forearm free transferred flap and performing the autologous fat transfer in one or more postoperative sessions (see Chapters. 20 and 23 for more details). For bulky or large-area defects, the musculocutaneous free flaps from latissimus dorsi are a good indication. An additional benefit of the soft tissue reconstruction is the decreased incidence of postoperative Frey's syndrome [10]. The mastoidectomy and the lateral temporal bone resection require the use of musculocutaneous and thick fasciocutaneous flaps for reconstructive purposes. The functional deficits resulting from injury of the facial nerve branches should be restored (when possible) with nerve grafts. The reconstructive plan must always take into account the effect of the adjuvant radiotherapy on the surrounding soft tissue, nerves, and bones.

The preauricular and retroauricular defects following total parotidectomy are often a source of dissatisfaction, particularly in young patients.

Frey's syndrome is another common result of these operations, caused by aberrant regeneration of parasympathetic fibers of auriculotemporal nerve. This nerve ensures the parotid parenchyma innervation, but after parotidectomy, the nerve fibers innervate the sweat glands causing the gustatory sweating. Frey's syndrome is quoted in 10–50 % of cases of parotidectomy [11, 12]. If Frey's syndrome (Fig. 14.5a–c) can be satisfactorily treated by injecting botulinum toxin A, the area of the tissue defect is a problem that remains after parotid tumor excision surgery [13]. Both sequelae (aesthetic and functional) can be minimized by interposing a tissue flap filling the resulting post-parotidectomy cavity. For this purpose, various procedures have been proposed: fascia lata grafts and dermal-fat grafts (resorption and infection risk) [14], local flaps from parotid fascia and superficial muscular aponeurotic system (ineffective when extended tissues are removed) [15], the temporal fascia flap with superficial temporal artery pedicle (Frey's syndrome may be prevented but it only partially replaces the tissue lack) [16], and the platysma muscle – cervical fascia – and the sternocleidomastoid flap (inconclusive results) [17]. However, in an extended parotidectomy, the volume of tissue to be transpositioned is much higher. The technique that has been used for a long time was the sternocleidomastoid muscle flap (it is effective in preventing Frey's syndrome but inadequate to restore the aesthetic defect) [6]. The reconstructive microsurgery techniques allow the use of various free transferred flaps, so that the most suitable tissue can be chosen for the defect reconstruction, with minimal consequences in the donor site. For the aesthetic defect correction, the highly vascularized tissues are chosen to ensure that the volume of the graft remains as wide over time and they include the dermis, fascia, and fat. The following options can be used: a flap of subcutaneous fascia and dermis, harvested from the iliac region, using the deep iliac circumflex vessels as a pedicle [18]; the de-epithelialized flap of skin and subcutaneous tissue, harvested from the abdominal wall, which has as pedicle the paraumbilical perforating blood vessels of deep inferior epigastric origin [19]; the de-epithelialized lateral arm free transferred flap [20]; and the parascapular de-epithelialized flap (the flap size is perfect to fill the defect) [21]. For the extended parotidectomy cases resolved in our clinic, the aesthetic defect and Frey's syndrome risk following this type of surgery were counteracted by the use of myocutaneous free transferred flaps from the latissimus dorsi or pectoralis major, which demonstrated the best results for the aesthetic and functional issues. Usually, in cases of extended parotidectomies, the following complex plasty prevents Frey's syndrome. However, if Frey's syndrome occurs, a small amount of botulinum toxin injection resolves this complication.

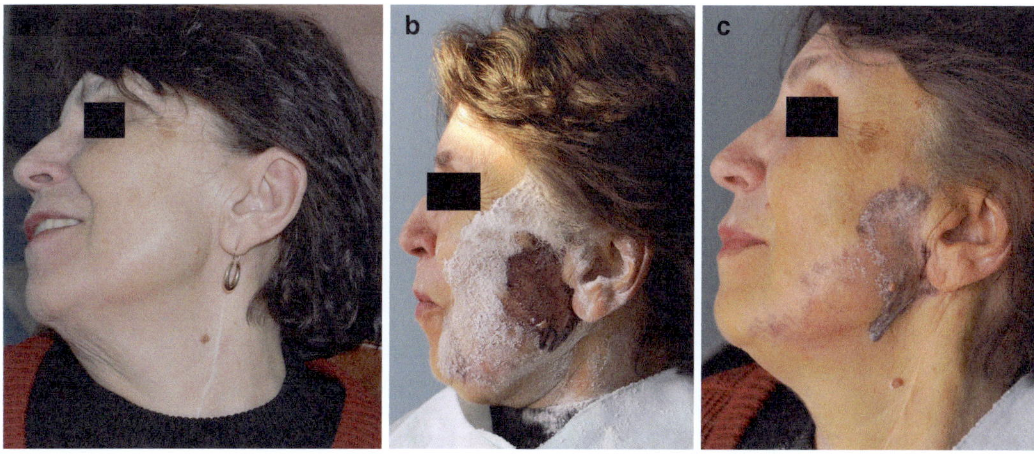

Fig. 14.5 (**a–c**) Frey's syndrome occurred in about 2 years after surgery. Optimal treatment involves botulinum toxin injection in the affected area. A Minor test ("starch-iodine" test) is performed by applying tincture of iodine and starch at the affected hemiface level, for greater accuracy. Masticatory movements cause a reaction between iodine and starch to the affected area, which can be well contoured in this way

14.5 The Problem of the Paralytic Lagophthalmos following the Extended Parotidectomy

Another important sequelae following extended parotidectomy is the lagophthalmos, secondary to facial nerve damage, and it requires prompt and effective treatment because prolonged corneal exposure can lead to keratopathy, abrasion, ulceration, or even blindness. It results from the unopposed action of the levator palpebrae superioris muscle on the upper eyelid normally contracted by the functioning orbicularis oculi muscle. The paralytic lagophthalmos consecutive to the facial nerve damage by parotid malignant tumor or its removal surgery can be corrected through a widely used technique of insertion, in the upper eyelid, of a predetermined gold wheight implant [22–25]. The lid closure is achieved by the gravitational action of the predetermined weight, while the functioning levator palpebrae superioris muscle is able to open the eyelid. Gold weights are the most commonly implanted material and have the advantage of being relatively inert, providing good color camouflage, high density, malleable, and nonallergenic. The complications of gold weight implants include migration, extrusion, soreness, and persistent lagophthalmos especially during sleep, and ptosis. The procedure is well accepted by patients, with satisfactory aesthetic results. But we should not overlook the fact that lagophthalmos is only a part of the spectrum of facial paralysis sequelae and that additional procedures are needed to rehabilitate these nerve deficiencies.

Conclusion

The extended parotidectomy is a complex surgery that is a complex surgery addressing malignant tumors that simultaneous involve the parotid tissue and the adjacent structures. The main problems are called into question in such operations are related to both surgical excision extent (which should provide a radical intervention) and also the correction of the main postoperative sequelae, which are aesthetic ones (depression of the parotid and upper laterocervical regions because of the missing tissues) and functional ones (the facial nerve palsy and Frey's syndrome).

References

1. De Vincentiis M, Magliulo G, Soldo P, Manciocco V, Pagliuca G, Del Gaizo R, et al. Extended parotidectomy. Acta Otorhinolaryngol Ital. 2005;25:169–73.
2. Hamper K, Lazar F, Dietel M, Caselitz J, Berger J, Arps H, et al. Prognostic factors for adenoid cystic carcinoma of the head and neck: a retrospective evaluation of 96 cases. J Oral Pathol Med. 1990; 19:101–7.
3. Ch'ng S, Ashford BG, Gao K, McGuinness J, Clark JR. Reconstruction of post-radical parotidectomy defects. Plast Reconstr Surg. 2012;129(2):275e–87.
4. Bianchi B, Ferri A, Sesenna E. Facial reanimation after nerve sacrifice in the treatment of head and neck cancer. Curr Opin Otolaryngol Head Neck Surg. 2012;20(2):114–9.
5. Tan ST. Anterior belly of digastric muscle transfer: a useful technique in head and neck surgery. Head Neck. 2002;24(10):947–54.
6. Fee WE, Tran LE. Functional outcome after total parotidectomy reconstruction. Laryngoscope. 2004;114:223–6.
7. Rosenthal EL, King T, McGrew BM, Carroll W, Magnuson JS, Wax MK. Evolution of a paradigm for free tissue transfer reconstruction of lateral temporal bone defects. Head Neck. 2008;30:589–94.
8. Elliott RM, Weinstein GS, Low DW, Wu LC. Reconstruction of complex total parotidectomy defects using the free anterolateral thigh flap. A classification system and algorithm. Ann Plast Surg. 2011;66:429–37.
9. Makitie AA, Beasley NJ, Neligan PC, Lipa J, Gullane PJ, Gilbert RW. Head and neck reconstruction with anterolateral thigh flap. Otolaryngol Head Neck Surg. 2003;129:547–55.
10. Sessions RB, Roark DT, Alford BR. Frey's syndrome: a technical remedy. Ann Otol. 1976;85:734–7.
11. Kornblut AD, Westphal P, Miehlke A. A reevalutation of the Frey syndrome following parotid surgery. Arch Otolaryngol. 1977;103:258–61.
12. Luna-Ortiz K, Sanson-RioFrio JA, Mosqueda-Taylor A. Frey syndrome. A proposal for evaluating severity. Oral Oncol. 2004;40:501–5.
13. Eckardt A, Kuettner C. Treatment of gustatory sweating (Frey's syndrome) with botulinum toxin A. Head Neck. 2003;25:624–8.
14. Bozzetti A, Biglioli F, Salvato G, Brusati R. Technical refinements in surgical treatment of benign parotid tumours. J Craniomaxillofac Surg. 1999;27:289–93.
15. Casler JD, Conley J. Sternocleidomastoid muscle transfer and superficial muscoloaponeurotic system plication in the prevention of Frey's syndrome. Laryngoscope. 1991;101:95–100.

16. Zaoli G. Le comblement des depressions residuelles apres parotidectomie par un lambeau compose arteriel sous-cutane. Ann Chir Plastic Esthet. 1989;34:123–7.
17. Kim SY, Mathog RH. Platysma muscle-cervical fascia-sternocleidomastoid muscle (PCS) flap for parotidectomy. Head Neck. 1999;21:428–33.
18. Baker DC, Shaw WW, Conley J. Microvascular free dermis-fat flaps for reconstruction after ablative head and neck surgery. Arch Otolaryngol. 1980;106:449–53.
19. Allen RJ, Kaplan J. Reconstruction of a parotidectomy defect using a paraumbilical perforator flap without deep inferior epigastric vessels. J Reconstr Microsurg. 2000;16:255–7.
20. Teknos TN, Nussenbaum B, Bradford CR, Prince ME, El-Kashlan H, Chepeha DB. Reconstruction of complex parotidectomy defects using lateral arm free tissue transfer. Otolaryngol Head Neck Surg. 2003;129:183–91.
21. Upton J, Albin RE, Mulliken JB, Murray JE. The use of scapular and parascapular flaps for cheek reconstruction. Plast Reconstr Surg. 1992;90:959–71.
22. Tower RN, Dailey RA. Gold weight implantation: a better way? Ophthal Plast Reconstr Surg. 2004;20:202–6.
23. Lavy JA, East CA, Bamber A, Andrews PJ. Gold weight implants in the management of lagophthalmos in facial palsy. Clin Otolaryngol. 2004;29:279–83.
24. Baheerathan N, Ethunandan M, Ilankovan V. Gold weight implants in the management of paralytic lagophthalmos. Int J Oral Maxillofac Surg. 2009;38:632–6.
25. Harrisberg BP, Singh RP, Croxson GR, Taylor RF, McCluskey PJ. Long-term outcome of gold eyelid weights in patients with facial nerve palsy. Otol Neurotol. 2001;22:397–400.

Direct Closure After Extended Parotidectomy

15

Eugenia I. Popescu, Constantin-Cătălin Ciocan-Pendefunda, and Victor-Vlad Costan

Abstract

The extended parotidectomy does not necessarily imply large defects but also complex defects that involve more than the parotid gland itself.

A wide variety of defects after extended parotidectomy, considering size and content, can be closed directly with acceptable cosmetic and functional outcomes, the only limitation being the availability of soft tissue for reconstruction. The surgeon needs to define the defect and assess closure possibilities together with expected results in comparison to the patient's expectations. We see in this procedure a choice for multimorbid patients with small- to medium-size defects, including the skin but without the involvement of bony structures or skull base, who cannot undergo a longer operation and for whom the aesthetic outcome is secondary. Postoperative follow-up and management of sequelae must be properly planned. Although there are both advantages and disadvantages to this method, direct suture closure is still a simple procedure that takes little time to perform, and it provides a direct view of any local tumour recurrence, with the downside of compromising on the aesthetic result in regard to the soft tissue deficit and facial asymmetry.

E.I. Popescu, MD, PhD
Department of Morpho-Functional Sciences (Anatomy Discipline), Faculty of Medicine, "Grigore T. Popa" University of Medicine and Pharmacy, Iasi, Romania

C.-C. Ciocan-Pendefunda, MD, M.D., PhD (✉)
Department of Oral and Maxillofacial Surgery, Fachklinik Hornheide Münster, Münster, Germany
e-mail: catalinciocan2004@yahoo.com

V.-V. Costan, MD, DMD, PhD
Department of Oral and Maxillo-Facial Surgery, Faculty of Dental Medicine, "Grigore T. Popa" University of Medicine and Pharmacy, "St. Spiridon" University Hospital Iasi, Iasi, Romania
e-mail: victorcostan@gmail.com

15.1 Introduction

The extended parotidectomy defines total or partial removal of the parotid gland together with surrounding structures infiltrated by tumour. This procedure does not necessarily include the facial nerve in the surgical specimen. This nerve will be resected only when the tumor affects it and we have to achieve clear margins.

We should not confuse this technique with total parotidectomy in which we may resect the nerve, but the nearby structures, other than

© Springer International Publishing Switzerland 2016
V.-V. Costan (ed.), *Management of Extended Parotid Tumors*, DOI 10.1007/978-3-319-26545-2_15

parotid tissue, remain intact. Furthermore, the extended parotidectomy is performed usually for malignant tumours.

The extended parotid tumours can be primary, when the neoplasia originates in the gland, or secondary, such as lymph node metastasis, or through direct involvement from an overlying skin malignancy. The common structures affected by extended parotid tumours are the skin, most frequently, muscles, malar, temporal and/or sphenoid bone, mandible, zygomatic arch and external and/or middle ear. So depending on the affected tissues, after the tumour resection, the postoperative defect may vary from a small cutaneous deficit, which could be closed directly, to a large exposure of the skull base, in which case we need complex three-dimensional plastic techniques. The reconstruction also has to take into consideration the need to perform neck dissection, the possible postoperative irradiation, complications and sequelae, the comorbidities and expectations of the patients.

From our point of view, the direct closure after extended parotidectomy has limited applications because these tumour resections lead in most cases to complex defects that cannot be addressed with this technique. Since the postoperative outcome is not very good due to facial asymmetry, we recommend this procedure in multimorbid patients who cannot undergo a longer operation.

An advantage is that most of the time, the tumour determines also an expansion of the surrounding soft tissues. If we corroborate this with a larger elasticity and excess of the skin in elderly cases, we may find enough substance to close the defect directly.

15.2 Anatomy

The parotid gland itself lies in the parotid lodge between the ramus of the mandible, mastoid process and external auditory conduct [1]. It has a capsule and it is covered by SMAS (superficial muscular aponeurotic system) and skin; it comes into contact with zygomatic arch, external ear, masseter and sternocleidomastoid muscles and ascending ramus of the mandible [2]. The extracranial part of the facial nerve goes through the parotid, giving its branches and dividing the gland into two parts.

Keeping in mind all these topographical relations, an extended parotid tumour may involve one or more of these tissues, leading to a variety of defects and postoperative sequelae.

15.3 Indications and Limitations

Direct closure after extended parotidectomy may be used when the tumour infiltrated only a small part of the overlying skin, but structures, like bones or skull base, are not involved.

The typical patient, who would not need local, regional or free flaps, presents a parotid mass that spreads to overlying skin, to adjacent muscles and/or to lateral aspect of the malar bone or zygomatic, or patients with skin tumors which infiltrate the parotid gland and the other structures mentioned previously. It is not mandatory for the facial nerve to be affected. We may use this to our advantage in the need to perform neck dissection, so when we outline the skin incision for tumour resection and lymph node surgery, we may design it in such a way that after the complete removal, we can use the elasticity of the skin to close the postoperative defect directly.

A different situation is a postoperative three-dimensional defect, extended to skin and bony structure. In order to achieve the best functional and aesthetical outcomes a free flap is recommended. But due to the general status of the patient, we have to stand back and choose a simpler technique that is not time-consuming and with satisfactory results.

We do not recommend a simple wound closure when the tumour infiltrates the sphenoid or the skull base because, in order to prevent a cerebral fluid fistula, we have to seal it "water-tight" using a locoregional flap, such as major pectoralis, trapezius or rotation flaps of the scalp. If the general status allows it, we recommend the use a microvascular technique, such as radial, latissimus dorsi or anterolateral thigh (ALT).

When we have to perform resection of the temporomandibular joint or of the ascending ramus of the mandible, direct closure is not enough to achieve an optimal functional outcome because it is necessary to rehabilitate the occlusion and masticatory function. An exception could be the case with poor general status when, due to histopathological type, grading tumor agressivenes the patient requires immediate postoperative irradiation and we have to close the defect as quickly as possible.

In cases where the external or middle ear or extensive parts of the skin are involved from tumour, we need to think of another option, because the defect is too large to be closed directly. If the ear is resected, we recommend the use of an epithesis, or, if the general conditions of the patients allow it, we may reconstruct the ear at a second time using, for example, rip cartridge or silicone implants.

The most common problem after direct closure is the postoperative facial asymmetry. In order to reduce its impact, we may use pedicled muscle flaps, for example, sternocleidomastoid muscle, or temporoparietal fascia to fill the defect. The superficial muscular aponeurotic system is suitable when the tumour developed in the deep lobe and extended to masseter, but the overlying skin is left intact. Other advantages of these interposition and lining techniques are prevention of Frey's syndrome or salivary fistula, if the gland is not completely removed, and the protection of the facial nerve, where it is preserved, against postoperative radiation, since most of the patients with extended parotid tumours receive radiotherapy. This irradiation is useful also for treating these salivary problems.

To prevent the salivary disorders, we recommend the injection of Botox intraoperatively in order to reduce these symptoms, and if they persist, we may repeat this procedure postoperatively.

In cases where the facial asymmetry persists after irradiation or after a long follow-up, tumour-free period, we may use lipostructure for defect augmentation.

If the tumour resection and the neck dissection involved the preauricular skin and the sternocleidomastoid muscle, we have to ensure the protection of the cervical vessels using locoregional or free flaps.

To summarise, direct closure is suitable for patients where the postoperative defect involves only the superficial structures or muscles, or, despite an extensive defect, they cannot undergo a complex reconstructive procedure due to their poor general status. This technique is adequate to close quickly the defect, a very important aspect in cases which need postoperative irradiation because we do not delay it.

It is difficult to establish a standard size of the defect which could be covered through direct closure, because this depends on many factors:

- Involvement of underlying tissues – when vital structures, such as skull base or neck vessels, must be protected, it is necessary to choose another technique.
- Local condition, like skin elasticity and capital. In elderly patients, the amount of available skin is higher.
- The need to perform neck dissection – sometimes this is an advantage because we may use the same incision, but we have to be careful and to protect the neck vessels.
- In some cases, despite their histological type, the tumour progression is not quite that aggressive, so during their evolution until they infiltrate the skin, they behave like an expander increasing the amount of soft tissues which could be used for defect coverage.

15.4 Clinical Application

Figure 15.1 presents a multiple morbid patient with an adenoid cystic carcinoma of the left parotid gland with infiltration of the overlying skin and facial nerve (Fig. 15.1a, b).

After extended parotidectomy with the resection en bloc of the tumour, facial nerve, the masseter and cranial part of sternocleidomastoid muscle, the vertical extension of the incision is allowed through direct closure (Fig. 15.2a, b). In this case, no muscle was used in order to fill the defect.

The general status of the patient and a relative small and not complex defect could be indications for direct closure conferring satisfactory aesthetic and functional outcome.

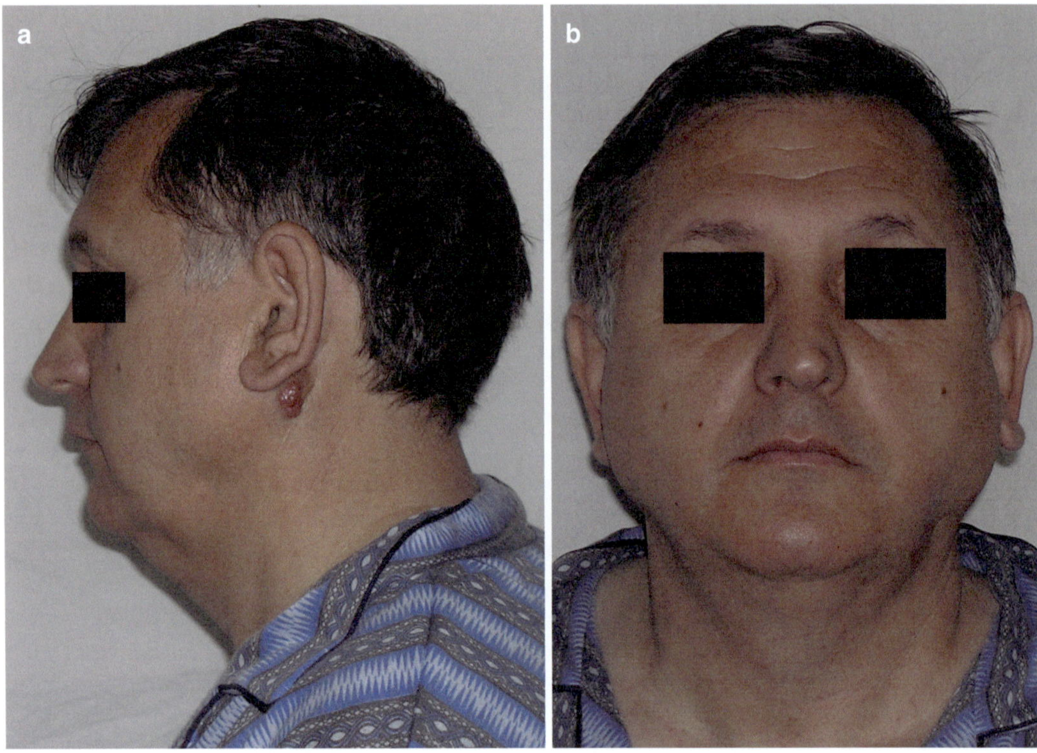

Fig. 15.1 (**a**, **b**) Extended parotid tumour of the left parotid with infiltration of the skin. We may also notice the distension effect upon the overlying skin

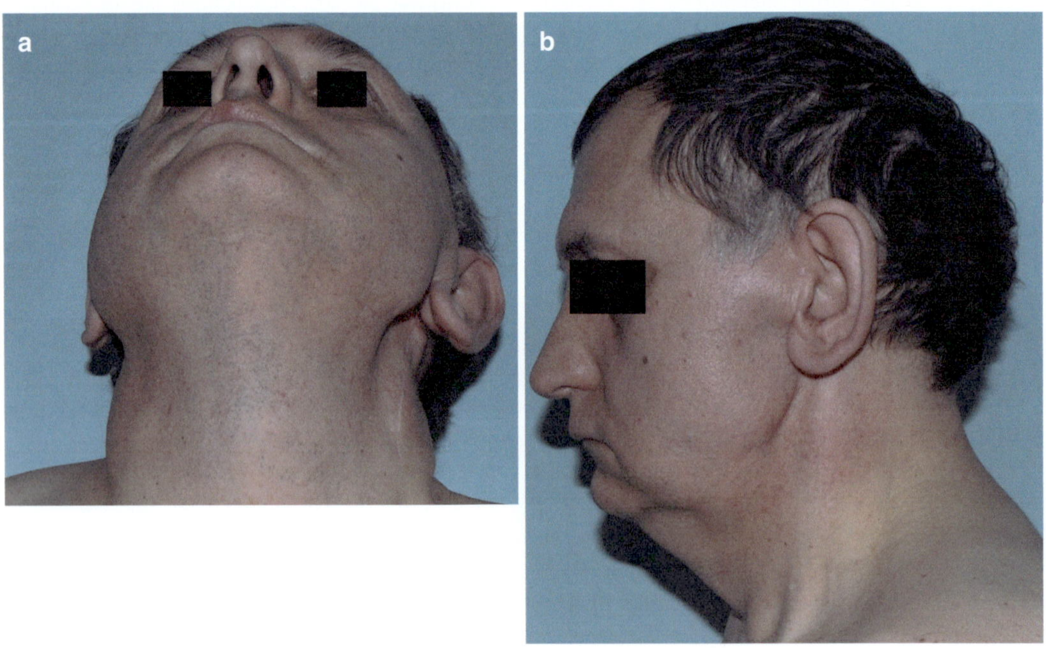

Fig. 15.2 (**a**, **b**) Postoperative outcome after direct closure of the defect using the advantage of the skin capital and elasticity. The disadvantage is the subsequent facial asymmetry which can be addressed later using lipofilling techniques

Postoperatively he presented with facial asymmetry and total paralysis. The asymmetry was ameliorated with lipostructure. The paralytic lagophthalmos was treated with lid loading using a golden plate. This stepwise management of these sequelae ensured a satisfactory outcome with a good quality of life.

This is another case with an extended parotid tumour which infiltrates the surrounding skin but without the involvement of facial nerve (Fig. 15.3a, b). Due to general status of the patient and to a limited superficial postoperative defect (Fig. 15.4), the closure was performed directly using the skin excess (Fig. 15.5a, b) without leading to a significant facial asymmetry (Fig. 15.5c).

15.5 Complication and Sequelae

Since we close the defect directly and in some cases there might be still the deep part of the gland on site, postoperatively we may encounter hematoma, wound dehiscence, sialocysts, Frey's syndrome and salivary fistula. To prevent the last two complications, we may use liners [3], described above. The postoperative irradiation reduces these symptoms.

Most frequent sequel is facial asymmetry which can be corrected with lipostructure, but this is the subject of other chapter.

If the facial nerve was affected, the patients will present lagophthalmos, ectropion, ptosis of the eyebrow and angle of the mouth.

The paralytic lagophthalmos may be treated with lid loading using golden plates or platinum chains. Ectropion may be addressed with the horizontal shortening of the lower lid, lateral canthopexy or tarsorrhaphy. For eyebrow ptosis we may perform direct or indirect eyebrow lifting. The angle of the mouth can be corrected using a string of fascia lata, by suspension sutures onto the temporal fascia or by the simple removal of a skin triangle. But the static or dynamic facial rehabilitation is not the subject of this chapter.

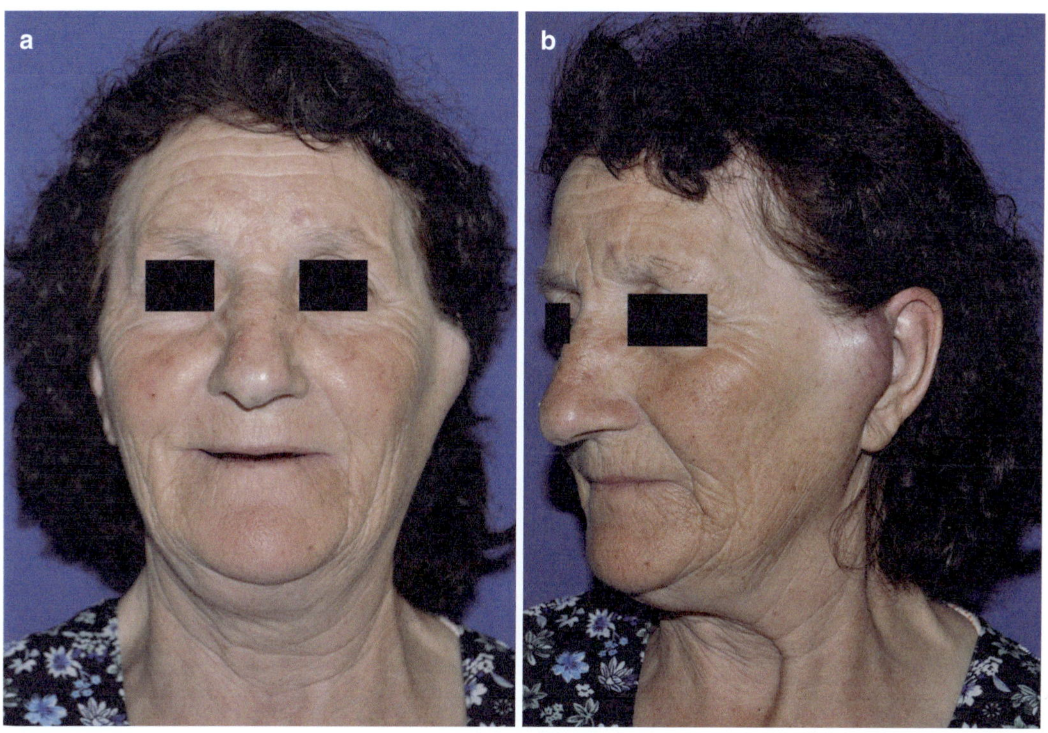

Fig. 15.3 (**a**, **b**) Mucoepidermoid carcinoma of the left parotid extended to preauricular skin. No signs of facial paralysis

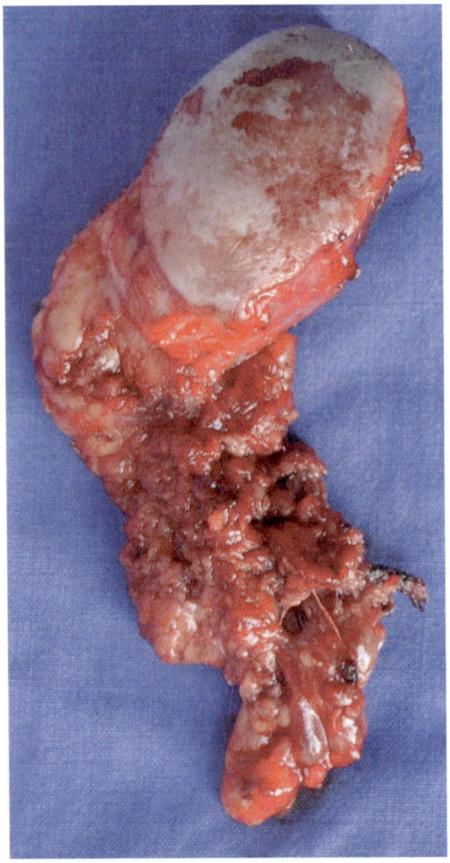

Fig. 15.4 Resection specimen including the parotid and the infiltrated skin, so the postoperative defect was not too complex

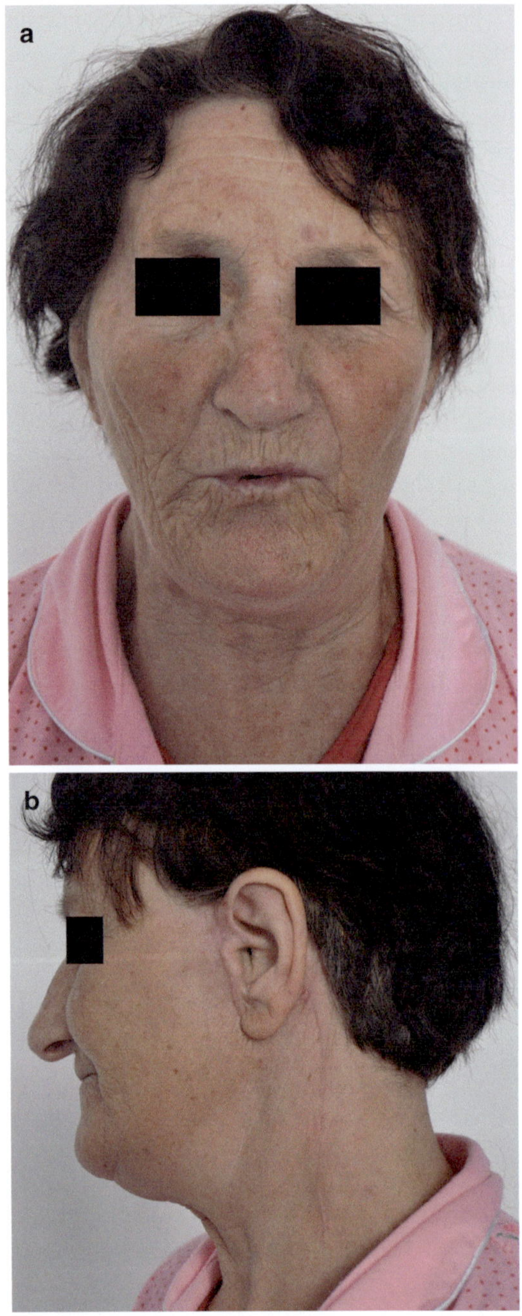

Fig. 15.5 (**a**, **b**) The incision allowed us to perform the neck dissection. After tumour removal with the preservation of the facial nerve, the skin excess was pulled to close directly the defect. No other reconstructive techniques were needed. Despite this simple procedure, the postoperative outcome is satisfactory, without a remarkable facial asymmetry

References

1. Carroll WR, Morgan CE. Ballenger's otorhinolaryngology head and neck surgery. 16th ed. Toronto: B. C. Decker; 2003.
2. Shah J. Head and neck surgery and oncology. 3rd ed. New York: Mosby; 2006.
3. Hoff SR, Mohyuddin N, Yao M. Complications of parotid surgery. Oper Technol Otolaryngol. 2009;2:123–30.

16 The Use of Local and Loco-regional Muscular Flaps

Felix P. Koch, Rober A. Sader, and Victor-Vlad Costan

Abstract

Patients in need of extended parotidectomy often present with significant comorbidities, and this is why one of the main concerns to keep in mind is the fact that the duration of the surgery should be reduced to a minimum. In this aspect, a therapeutic possibility for performing the plasty of the postoperative defect is the use of local and loco-regional muscular flaps. Although these techniques often do not allow achieving a great aesthetic result, they should be considered in order to avoid the occurrence of some postoperative complications (the most important one being Frey syndrome); since there is no need for a new operating field, they do not significantly prolong surgery time, and they are not associated with important morbidity in the donor area. Among these flaps, the one most often performed is the sternocleidomastoid flap, but the temporal flap, the temporoparietal, or digastric flaps are also useful. The disadvantage of these flaps is that the dissection performed during the removal of the primary lesion or during the neck dissection should be thoroughly performed in order not to injure the vascular pedicles. Additionally, the usual volume or surface of the flaps is generally limited and can only ensure a satisfactory reconstruction of the postoperative defects.

F.P. Koch, MD, DMD, MBA, PhD •
R.A. Sader, MD, DDS, PhD (✉)
Department of Oral, Cranio-Maxillofacial and Facial Plastic Surgery, University Hospital Frankfurt, Frankfurt, Germany
e-mail: Koch@facialplastics.de; r.sader@em.uni-frankfurt.de

V.-V. Costan, MD, DMD, PhD
Department of Oral and Maxillo-Facial Surgery, Faculty of Dental Medicine, "Grigore T. Popa" University of Medicine and Pharmacy, "St. Spiridon" University Hospital, Iasi, Romania
e-mail: victorcostan@gmail.com

16.1 Introduction

Motor nerves reach skeletal muscles accompanied always by vascular pedicles, and for this reason, it is possible to design various pedicled muscular flaps for filling postoperative defects. There are multiple patterns of vascularisation for different muscles, and this influences the choice of flap to be used considering the location of the donor site, the type of pedicle, the length of tissue that can be harvested and the arc of rotation. The vascularisation of a certain muscle is mainly

© Springer International Publishing Switzerland 2016

V.-V. Costan (ed.), *Management of Extended Parotid Tumors*, DOI 10.1007/978-3-319-26545-2_16

ensured by a single pedicle or multiple pedicles of a dominant, minor or segmental type [1]. Perforator vessels are also important since they pass through the muscle to supply the overlying skin meaning that this area of the skin can thus be used for reconstructive purposes, either separately or together with the muscle flap forming a myocutaneous flap. The advantages of using muscle flaps are represented by the possibility to cover important structures and fill defects with functional innervated tissue that is well vascularised and resists infection. In addition, the skin is preserved at the donor site, avoiding cosmetic deformity.

This chapter elucidates the local and regional muscular flaps that can be taken to cover defects in the parotid gland region.

16.2 Indications, Advantages and Disadvantages of Local and Loco-regional Muscular Flaps

One of the most frequently performed musculocutaneous flaps is the pectoralis major flap [2]. From a technical point of view, there is no significant difference between the raising of a musculocutaneous flap and the one of a muscle flap. In the latter, the indications of use are represented by volume defects of the parotid region, without a skin defect at this level. These flaps are described in detail in other chapters of this book. Also, the latissimus dorsi free flap will be described in detail in other chapters of this book. In this chapter, only the difference in dissection between the pedicled version and the free flap will be described. This chapter will focus on other muscular flaps, like the trapezius flap, the sternocleidomastoid flap, the digastric flap, the temporoparietal flap and the temporal muscle flap.

16.3 The Flaps

The *latissimus dorsi flap* has been known for a long time: Tansini described it first [3]. Mainly used as a free, microvascular flap, it can also be used as a pedicled flap and reach the clavicular region, the neck and the lower border of the mandible. The longer the distance to be bridged by the pedicle, the more likely the flap suffers from venous insufficiency. As there are other, more reliable flaps to cover the lower parotid area, the latissimus flap is a reconstructive option of the second or third choice, if other flap reconstructions are not available anymore. The latissimus muscle reaches from the humerus and the upper six thoracic vertebrae to the iliac crest and lower four ribs. The flap is pedicled by the thoracodorsal artery and vein, which are both branches of the subscapular artery. The most common position to harvest this flap is the lateral decubitus position, but prone and supine positions are also possible. It is important to reach the anterior border of the muscle. In patients with a thick subdermal layer, an ultrasound can confirm the correct incision. This is important because an incision too far back could miss the muscle part and that is decisive for a sufficient blood supply by the thoracodorsal vessels. After incision, the anterior border of the latissimus muscle is prepared. The dorsal extension of the flap is defined and incised including the fascia, first lifting the latissimus dorsi muscle and separating it from the serratus anterior muscle in order to identify the thoracodorsal vessels. Further dissection into the axilla reveals a branch to the serratus anterior muscle, and by further careful dissection, the thoracodorsal artery, vein and nerve are identified at this level. Cranially to the point of entry of the thoracodorsal vessels into the muscle, the pedicle is further dissected into the axilla, since the flap mobility is dependent on the length of the pedicle.

To reach the parotid region, a tunnel for the flap pedicle has to be prepared. In the neck, this tunnel is performed subplatysmal and proceeds to the anterior incision under or above the pectoralis major muscle. If placed over the pectoralis major muscle, the pedicle will be shorter. Care needs to be taken not to injure the internal jugular vein during the preparation of the tunnel and while passing the flap through the cervical tunnel. Kinking and stretching of the pedicle has to be avoided during the pull-through manoeuvre.

Pulling by a thick silk suture fixed to the lower edge of the flap in combination with pushing, the latissimus flap is brought through the tunnel [5]. The donor site is closed primarily and drained, if the defect size does not exceed 10×12 cm. Otherwise skin grafts will be needed. The latissimus dorsi pedicled flap often serves as a salvage flap when other choices of reconstruction, like the pectoralis major flap, have failed [2].

Another muscular flap from the dorsal donor site, suitable for coverage of defects in the neck, the oral cavity, the mandible and the temporal region is the *trapezius flap*. Similar to the latissimus flap, it is dedicated to patients with comorbidities and in cases that lack alternatives. In the 1970s, several versions have been described: the superior [3], the lateral island trapezius flap, the vertical trapezius flap and the lower island flap. The transverse cervical vessels and branches of the posterior intercostal vessels supply the triangular muscle. The overlying skin receives its blood supply from the dorsal scapular artery, the intercostal arteries and the transverse cervical artery, as well as branches of the occipital artery [4]. The transverse occipital artery, which is a branch of the thyrocervical trunk in 75–80 %, reaches the muscle at the base of the neck and runs down in a deeper layer. The muscle is spanned between the occipital bone, the spina of the seventh cervical vertebra, all thoracic spinal processus and to the lateral third of the clavicle, the acromion and scapula.

For harvesting, the patient is positioned prone or alternatively in a lateral decubitus position. The length of the pedicle is estimated by constructing a pivot point in the groove between the trapezius muscle and sternocleidomastoid muscle. The flap can be muscular or myocutaneous. An incision along the assumed pedicle is done in the skin, and the back is prepared to the lateral side to elevate the trapezius muscle flap. Medially the skin is also lifted from the muscle. Then the trapezius is incised in the desired dimensions. Incision of the trapezius muscle is done inferiorly to extend it upwards by preserving the paraspinal perforators. Reaching the rhomboid major muscle, the dorsal scapular artery is identified, which offsprings in between the rhomboid major and minor muscles. The descending branches can be ligated; the main branch needs to be preserved. In order to get more flexibility, the rhomboid minor muscle can be divided. The pedicled flap is transpositioned through a skin tunnel or an open incision to be positioned within the facial and parotid region [2].

The digastric muscle does not have a significant volume, but it can have interesting indications in the case of extended parotidectomy. The indications are represented by the filling of postoperative defects but also the treatment of facial nerve paralysis [5]. The two indications apply to either one of the two bellies of the digastric, the anterior and the posterior respectively. It is interesting to note that the embryologic origin of the two bellies differs, with the posterior belly originating in the second pharyngeal arch, innervated by the facial nerve and vascularised by branches of the occipital artery, while the anterior belly of the muscle originates in the first pharyngeal arch and is innervated by a branch of the trigeminal nerve and vascularised by means of the submental artery.

One of the most important steps in the surgery of the parotid gland is represented by the uncovering of the posterior belly of the digastric muscle (Fig. 16.1a–c). The entire superficial surface of this muscle is revealed during dissection since it is of real help in identifying the facial nerve. Considering the fact that the nourishing vessels approach the muscle from its deep surface, they can usually be preserved without great difficulty. At the same time, the motor innervation can be preserved in most cases by careful dissection of the facial nerve. This aspect is important since it limits the postoperative atrophy of the muscle whose volume is not a significant one nevertheless. Considering this volume, the main indication is to protect the deep surface of the facial nerve when removing the deep parotid lobe. After the sectioning of the intermediate tendon (see Fig. 16.1a–c), the muscle is displayed (see Fig. 16.1d) and modelled as a "bed" for the trunk of the facial nerve which it protects and improves the functional recovery of nerve (see Fig. 16.1e).

The technique is simple and quick, performed in the same surgical field. Still, it does not provide

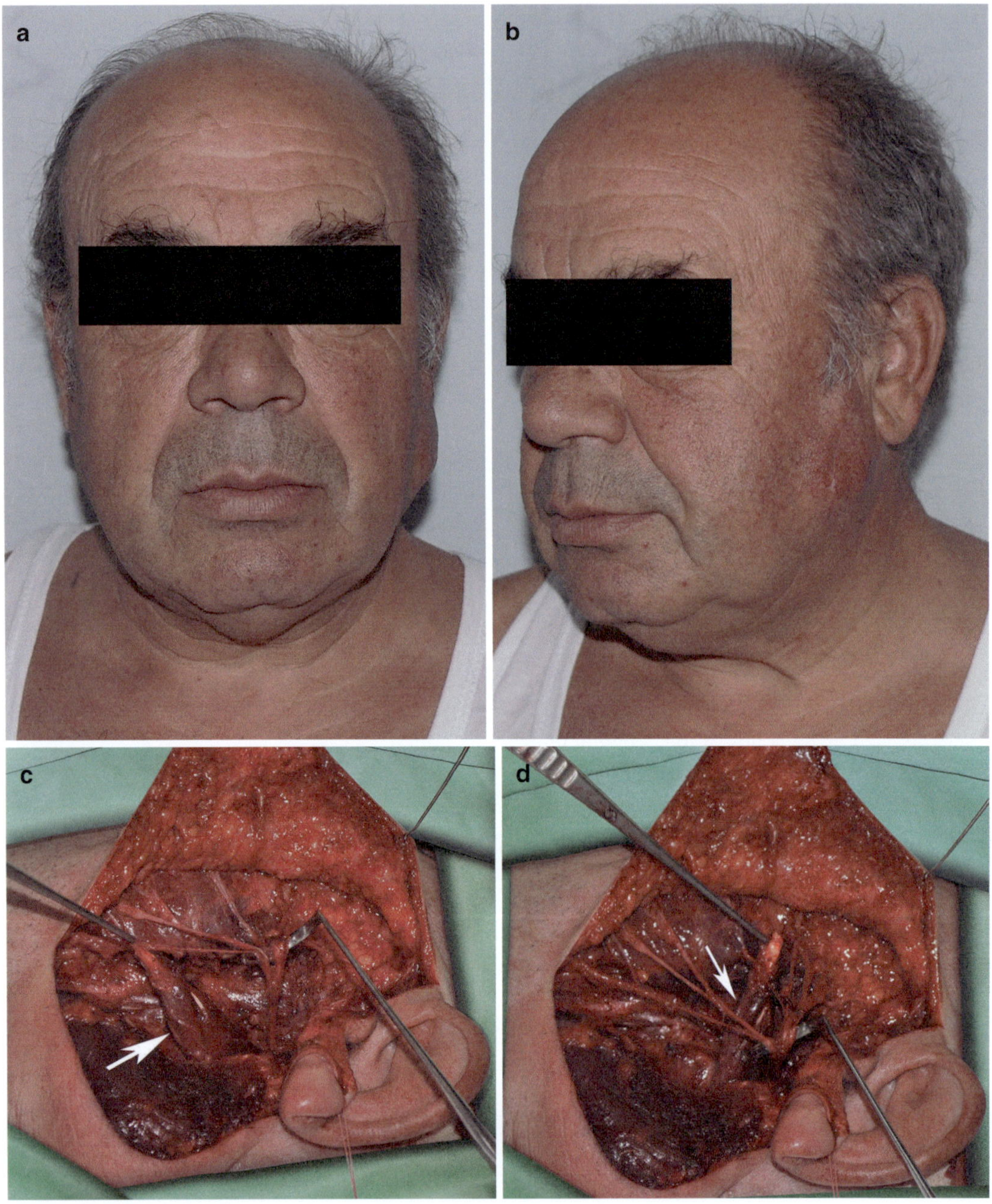

Fig. 16.1 (**a**, **b**) Adenoid cystic carcinoma of the right parotid gland previously operated and relapsed. (**c**) A muscular flap consisting of the posterior belly of the digastric muscle was used for the plasty of the postoperative defect. The raising of the flap is simple with the dissection of the muscle after the parotidectomy. The muscular flap is raised (*arrow*) after the sectioning of the intermediate tendon. (**d**) Following the raising of the flap, it is introduced under the facial nerve (*arrow*). (**e**) The flap is displayed and sutured under the facial nerve, thus restoring the lost volume of the deep lobe of the parotid gland. Afterwards, a sternocleidomastoid muscular flap is raised, by sectioning the muscle from the level of the clavicle. (**f**) The sternocleidomastoid flap covers the trunk of the facial nerve and its main divisions, restoring to a certain degree the volume of the superficial parotid lobe. (**g**–**i**) Appearance at 2 years postoperatively proving good restoration of the facial symmetry but with the presence of asymmetry of the cervical region because of the missing contour of the sternocleidomastoid muscle

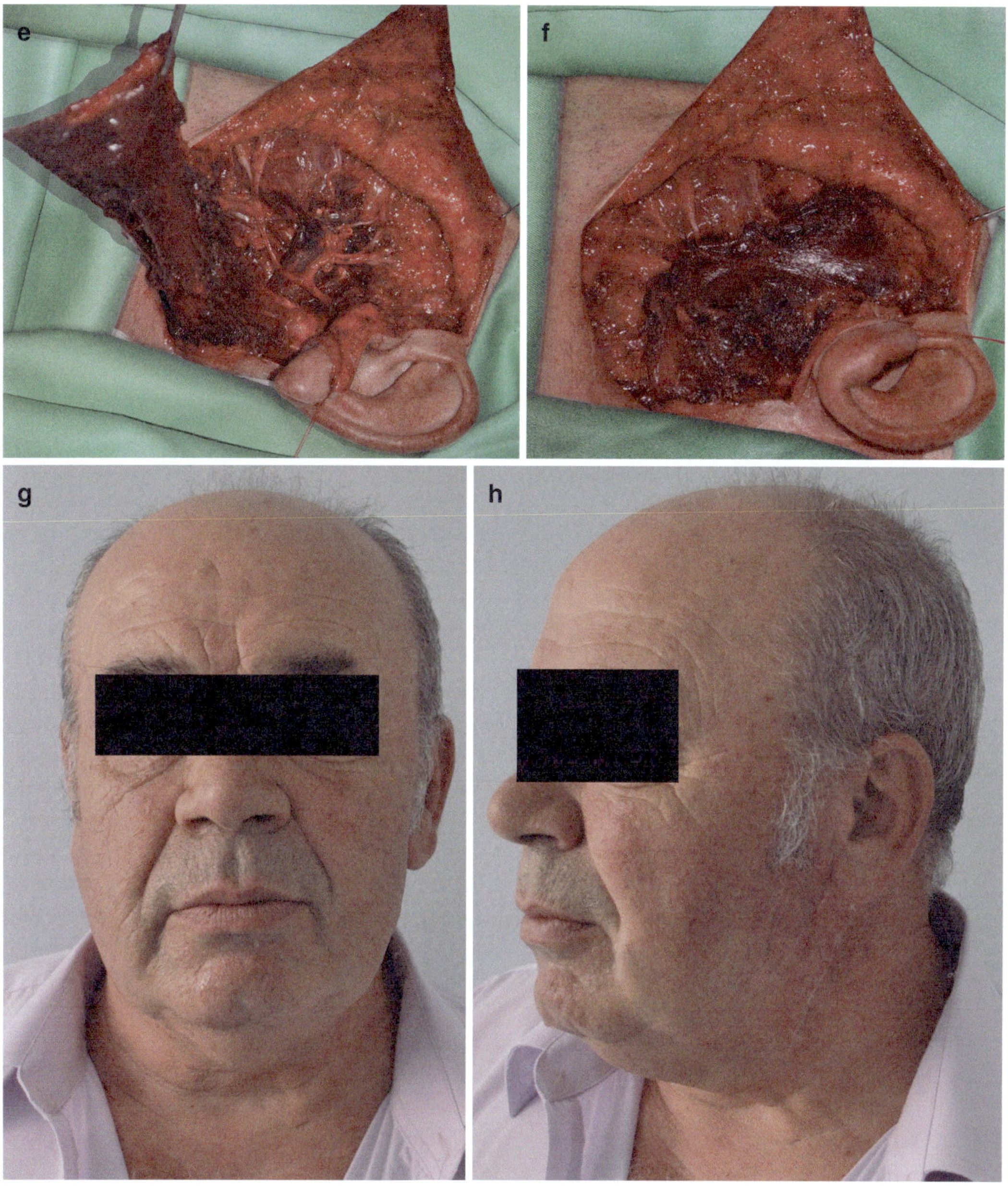

Fig. 16.1 (continued)

i

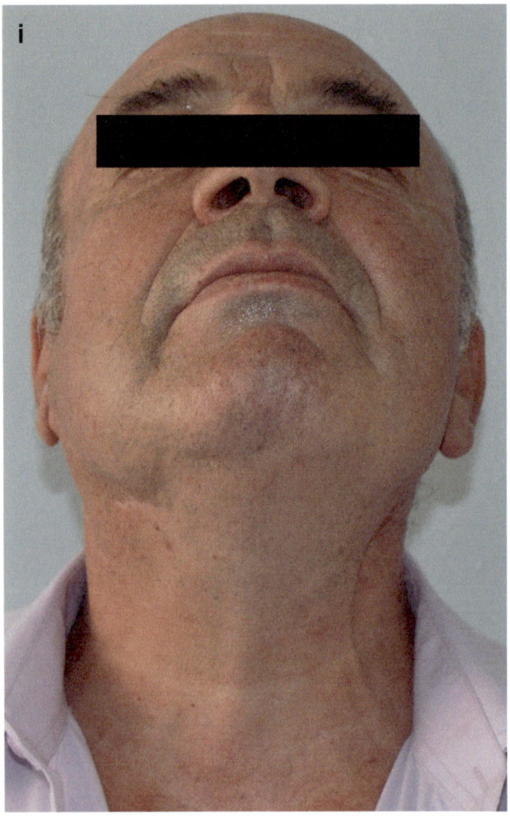

Fig. 16.1 (continued)

a significant muscular volume, but it achieves a well-vascularised protective bed, especially for the main trunk of the facial nerve and for the origin of the main branches. Generally a second muscular flap is needed. Usually, the sternocleidomastoid flap is used in association.

The *sternocleidomastoid flap* provides muscle volume to cover the parotid region without extending the surgical approach to a different body region. If this flap is planned for reconstruction, care has to be taken for the blood supply during neck dissection. The blood supply of the sternocleidomastoid flap is divided in the superior, middle and inferior part. In order to flip the muscle flap upwards, only the superiorly pedicled type can be used. Owens described this flap 1955 with all the length covered by skin, whereas Aryan suggested to leave just the lower third of the skin attached to the muscle [6, 7]. As the vessels reach the sternocleidomastoid muscle by multiple perforators arising from different arteries, a neck dissection easily compromises the flap nutrition. The occipital artery nurtures the upper part of the muscle, while branches of the superior thyroid artery and external carotid artery supply the middle third part. In extended parotidectomy, the access is often provided by a Blair-type incision modified in order to allow removal of additional structures. This access allows a good visualisation of the jugular-carotid space so that whenever there is need for a neck dissection, the vascularisation of the sternocleidomastoid muscle can be preserved, at least when concerning the superior pedicle. The same type of incision allows the smooth dissection of the deep surface of the muscle, as well as the superficial one, and it is therefore possible to descend to the level of the clavicle and sternum where the muscle is sectioned (see Fig. 16.1e). By ligating the vessels arising from the transversa colli artery and superiorly the branches deriving from the superior thyroid artery, the sternocleidomastoid muscle is mobilised. Keeping the branches of the occipital vessels intact, it can be turned upward to cover the parotid region [2].

The display of this flap allows filling of the parotid region so that most of the length of the facial nerve branches that have been dissected can be covered by muscular mass, thus protecting them from trauma (see Fig. 16.1f). The presence of the flap brings well-vascularised tissues to the level of the facial nerve thereby hastening the optimal functional recovery. Last but not least, this approach of the reconstruction techniques allows the prevention of the development of the auriculo-temporal nerve syndrome (Frey's syndrome): the sternocleidomastoid muscle can be placed between the skin and the resection cavity to prevent a nerve anastomosis [8].

The advantages of using the sternocleidomastoid muscle are represented by the ease of raising the flap, allowing the restitution of facial symmetry in the case of less significant postoperative defects (see Fig. 16.1g, h), practically without an increase in surgical time. The role of this muscle in preventing Frey syndrome is well known.

On the other side, the sternocleidomastoid muscle does not bring a significant volume of soft tissues, and this is why this technique is to be avoided in patients in which the postoperative aesthetic result is important, even more so when the main disadvantage is represented by the disappearance of the muscular contour followed by the occurrence of a cervical asymmetry (see Fig. 16.1i).

In case a radical neck dissection is not necessary, the *temporoparietal flap* can be harvested together with the temporalis muscle as a muscular-fascial flap with the advantage of increasing the length of the otherwise short temporalis muscle flap, by including additional temporoparietal fascia and dissecting more along the superficial temporal artery. The condition is to preserve all the supplying arteries, deriving from both the internal maxillary artery and the superficial temporal artery, since it includes both muscle and fascia. Another option is to raise different versions of the flaps in this area, creating a temporalis muscle flap to fill one part of the defect and a distinct temporoparietal fascial flap to cover a different part of the defect. The temporoparietal flap can be raised as a fascial, fasciocutaneous, myofascial or osteomyofascial flap for the reconstruction of cheek or ear defects [9, 10].

Another flap of the donor region, similar to the temporoparietal flap, is the *temporalis muscle* flap. The flap receives its blood supply from the anterior and posterior deep temporal arteries, branches of the internal maxillary artery [11]. A minor part of the temporalis muscle also receives blood supply from branches arising from the superficial temporal artery [12]. After a skin incision starting in the preauricular skin fold and extended to the vertex of the head has been performed, the scalp is prepared superficial to the temporal fascia. The branches of the facial nerve should be treated with care. The anterior border of the muscle is incised and released from the fossa temporalis. Flipped over or under the zygomatic arch (in this case, the zygomatic arch needs to be osteotomised temporarily), the m. temporalis flap can be taken to cover the skull base, the orbit after exenteration or the palate and the oral, buccal plane [2]. It can be used to lift the corner of the mouth after facial paralysis [13]. A disadvantage is the hollowing of the temporal region and the shrinking of this muscular flap.

The most important limitation of pedicled temporalis and temporoparietal flaps is represented by the fact that, by definition, an extended parotidectomy implies the interruption of the vascularisation at this level. On the other hand, the use of these flaps accentuates facial asymmetry leading to a skeleton-like appearance of the area as a result of temporalis muscle dissection.

Conclusion

The use of local and loco-regional muscular flaps is not an ideal solution for the plasty of the postoperative defects and the diminishing of postoperative sequelae in extended parotidectomy. Still, considering the associated morbidity of the patients necessitating this type of parotidectomy, the local muscular flaps provide a well-vascularised tissue without additional surgical trauma, with the purpose of protecting the facial nerve and promoting the more rapid restoration of its functions. At the same time, they allow the more or less correct restoration of facial symmetry while also diminishing the chances of developing Frey syndrome.

References

1. Mathes SJ, Nahai F. Classification of the vascular anatomy of muscles: experimental and clinical correlation. Plast Reconstr Surg. 1981;67(2):177–87.
2. Fernandes R. Local and regional flaps in head and neck reconstruction. A practical approach. Hoboken: Wiley; 2015.
3. Conley J. Use of composite flaps containing bone for major repairs in the head and neck. Plast Reconstr Surg. 1972;49(5):522–6.
4. Chen WL, Li J, Yang Z, Huang Z, Wang J, Zhang B. Extended vertical lower trapezius island myocutaneous flap in reconstruction of oral and maxillofacial defects after salvage surgery for recurrent oral carcinoma. J Oral Maxillofac Surg. 2007;65(2):205–11.
5. Aszmann OC, Ebmer JM, Dellon AL. The anatomic basis for the innervated mylohyoid/digastric flap in facial reanimation. Plast Reconstr Surg. 1998;102(2):369–72.
6. Ariyan S. One-stage reconstruction for defects of the mouth using a sternomastoid myocutaneous flap. Plast Reconstr Surg. 1979;63(5):618–25.
7. Owens N. A compound neck pedicle designed for the repair of massive facial defects: formation, development and application. Plast Reconstr Surg (1946). 1955;15(5):369–89.

8. Kornblut AD, Westphal P, Miehlke A. The effectiveness of a sternomastoid muscle flap in preventing post-parotidectomy occurrence of the Frey syndrome. Acta Otolaryngol. 1974;77(5):368–73.
9. Cesteleyn L. The temporoparietal galea flap. Oral Maxillofac Surg Clin North Am. 2003;15(4):537–50, vi.
10. Tellioglu AT, Tekdemir I, Erdemli EA, Tuccar E, Ulusoy G. Temporoparietal fascia: an anatomic and histologic reinvestigation with new potential clinical applications. Plast Reconstr Surg. 2000;105(1):40–5.
11. Edwards SP, Feinberg SE. The temporalis muscle flap in contemporary oral and maxillofacial surgery. Oral Maxillofac Surg Clin North Am. 2003;15(4):513–35, vi.
12. Nakajima H, Imanishi N, Minabe T. The arterial anatomy of the temporal region and the vascular basis of various temporal flaps. Br J Plast Surg. 1995;48(7):439–50.
13. McLaughlin CR. Permanent facial paralysis; the role of surgical support. Lancet. 1952;2(6736):647–51.

17 Platysma Myocutaneous Flap: A Solution for Reconstruction of Defects After Extended Parotidectomy

Constantin-Cătălin Ciocan-Pendefunda, Eugenia I. Popescu, and Victor-Vlad Costan

Abstract

In order to cover postoperative defects after removal of extended parotid tumors, the surgeon can use local flaps (rotated or translated random fasciocutaneous flaps or platysma myocutaneous flap), locoregional (major pectoralis myocutaneous flap), or microvascular free flaps (radialis or latissimus dorsi). The most suitable technique depends on local factors, such as size of the defect, structures involved by tumor resection, previous neck surgery or irradiation, the need to perform neck dissection, and general factors, such as preoperative status and treatment compliance of the patients.

In cases with poor general condition, in which tumor involved the overlying skin, a good and reliable option to cover the postoperative defect is a platysma myocutaneous flap. The advantages are low donor site morbidity, the flap can be harvested at the time of tumor resection, and rising of it facilitates neck dissection. The main disadvantage is represented by the vascularity problems. The esthetic result is satisfactory, but in these patients, local control of the tumor comes in front of cosmetics. The postoperative sequelae are not due to flap harvesting, but secondary to extended parotidectomy, and can be addressed later.

C.-C. Ciocan-Pendefunda, MD, DMD, PhD (✉)
Department of Oral and Maxillofacial Surgery, Fachklinik Hornheide Münster, Münster, Germany
e-mail: catalinciocan2004@yahoo.com

E.I. Popescu, DMD, PhD
Department of Surgery (Dentoalveolar Surgery, Oral and Maxillofacial Surgery), Faculty of Dental Medicine, "Grigore T. Popa" University of Medicine and Pharmacy, Iasi, Romania

V.-V. Costan, MD, DMD, PhD
Department of Oral and Maxillo-Facial Surgery, Faculty of Dental Medicine, "Grigore T. Popa" University of Medicine and Pharmacy, "St. Spiridon" University Hospital, Iasi, Romania

17.1 Introduction and Indications

Reconstruction of large and complex facial defects, such as after extended parotidectomy, remains a challenge for plastic and oral and maxillofacial surgeons due to the limitation in obtaining adequate color and texture [1]. Extensive parotid tumors may involve nearby tissues, including the skin, muscles, middle and external ear, temporal mandibular joint, bones (mandible, zygomatic arch, temporal, and malar bone), so the subsequent defect may be very large in sur-

© Springer International Publishing Switzerland 2016

V.-V. Costan (ed.), *Management of Extended Parotid Tumors*, DOI 10.1007/978-3-319-26545-2_17

face, in depth, or in both dimensions and composite. Furthermore, these tumors arise in elderly patients with poor general condition (diabetes, high blood pressure, heart disease, blood vessel diseases), which make treatment plan even more difficult. In these cases, we have to choose the most appropriate technique which is the least aggressive to reconstruct the missing tissues. The best reconstruction is to replace like with like when possible.

Other important problem is represented by the postoperative sequelae, such as facial paralysis, paralytic lagophthalmos, ectropion, and facial asymmetry, which are difficult to deal with.

These extensive parotid tumors may originate from parotid tissue and invade surrounding structures (primary), or they can be secondary from carcinomas of the skin which extend to parotid, or intraparotid metastatic lymph nodes from squamous cell carcinomas which drain into parotid lymph nodes.

There are many techniques to cover the postoperative defects. The most common tissues involved by these tumors are the overlying skin and muscle, such as the masseter or sternocleidomastoid muscle, and the chosen reconstructive method must take into consideration the defect size, type of structures involved by tumor resection, and the presence of neck dissection and pre- or postoperative irradiation.

In elderly patients with medium-sized defects and which underwent neck dissection, deep plane cervicofacial flaps are very useful [2]. In order to have a viable flap, some authors consider the preservation of facial artery mandatory [3, 4].

Platysma myocutaneous flap is a good alternative to reconstruct small to midsize defects after extended parotidectomy in patients with poor general status to whom esthetics come into second place.

The first description was made in 1887 by Gersuny who used this flap to reconstruct a cheek defect [5] but only in 1978 was introduced in the English literature by Futrell and recommended for intraoral malignancies [5–7]. In 1999 Kim used the platysma muscle flap [PMF] to reconstruct defects after parotidectomy [8].

This flap can also be used for defects of the lower part of the face, neck, hypopharynx, trachea, esophagus [9], chin, and lips [10, 11] and reimplantation of severed ears [12, 13].

17.2 Advantages and Disadvantages

PMF is easy to harvest and has almost the same color and texture as the facial skin and a low morbidity of the donor site, and it and can provide up to 90 cm^2 (6 × 15 cm) of skin for resurfacing [5, 14]. In patients who underwent neck dissection, this flap doesn't need any additional preparation time, so the operative act is not increased due to no new dissection fields, and the cosmetic appearance is optimized by primary closure of the neck incision [5, 9]. The large intraoperative exposure of the neck vessels and lymph nodes during the harvesting of PMF gives a great advantage to perform a very good neck dissection with a small amount of time, important in cases where general condition is an impediment to postoperative irradiation and in which operation must not last too long.

Tumor resection can be generous with tumor-free margins, and the platysma flap excludes the need for special microsurgical expertise [5].

Another advantage is adequate protection of facial nerve grafting in patients who underwent this procedure.

The main disadvantage is related to vascularization problems. The blood supply and drainage may be compromised during flap harvesting or neck dissection or by preoperative irradiation.

Previous neck surgery, facial artery ligation, and ipsilateral facial nerve paralysis may also have a negative impact upon flap viability [5, 15] and also to the underlying structures. But other studies [16, 17] and from our experience ligation of facial artery during the operation had not influenced the flap vascularization. The removal of the sternocleidomastoid muscle may be considered a relatively contraindication because the neck vessels will be covered only by skin.

Prior irradiation of the neck has as result a potential postradiation arteritis and skin changes.

Despite these, performing the dissection in a plane underneath the platysma is not very difficult. Also, the blood supply of the flap remains satisfactory, so the irradiation after previous ipsilateral neck dissection is not a contraindication for the use of PMF. However, other authors [18] reported that patients from their study, who have undergone previous neck dissection, had no postoperative complications due to the placement of the neck incision and to multiaxial blood supply of the flap.

Some authors report vascularization problems in patients who received neoadjuvant chemotherapy [19, 20].

In large and composite defects with the involvement of bony structures and the skull base, the PMF is too thin and does not bring enough volume to replace the resected tissues and to establish the facial symmetry. In these cases, major pectoralis or free flaps are recommended.

17.3 Anatomy

The platysma muscle itself lies under the subcutaneous tissue of the neck, superficial to the muscular fascial sheath, and it is a remnant of the panniculus carnosus.

Platysma may present anatomical variations. It arises from the fascia covering major pectoralis and deltoid muscles, and the fibers ascend medially from lateral side of the neck, across the clavicle and to the midline behind the symphysis menti.

Innervation of the muscle comes from cervical branch of the facial nerve.

The blood supply is multiaxial and comes from the submental branch of facial artery, superior thyroid artery, and occipital and posterior auricular artery [21].

Venous drainage uses external jugular and submental veins, and it appears to have a predominantly vertical orientation [22, 23]. Because of these considerations, there are some authors who recommend harvesting of the flap together with the external jugular and anterior communicating veins [22].

PMF can have three pedicles. The superior and posterior pedicles bring enough soft tissue to reconstruct small to midsize intraoral or cutaneous defects. The third pedicle lies inferior, and vascularization comes from superior thyroid artery, so its applications in oral and facial plastic surgery are limited [24].

The platysma myocutaneous flap used to cover defects after extended parotidectomy has a design more like a medial pedicle flap, so it has a multiaxial vascularization. The arterial blood supply is reliable from facial and submental arteries and, therefore, enjoys a high success rate. Venous drainage is less efficient and uses anterior communicating veins which drain into facial or superior thyroid veins [25] and external jugular vein.

17.4 Operative Technique, Pre- and Intraoperative Cautions

This procedure is chosen especially in elderly patients, with poor general status, where extended parotidectomy is performed alongside with ipsilateral neck dissection. The presence of large metastatic lymph nodes, adherent to skin, is a contraindication for this flap.

Due to its random vascularization, when we plan the extended parotidectomy, we have to keep in mind and imagine the incisions for flap harvesting. In order to avoid postoperative necrosis, the PMF needs a sufficient width of the base. Because of this consideration, after tumor resection en bloc with overlying skin, the first incision goes along the clavicle, and the second is placed 2 cm below and parallel to inferior border of the mandible. Commonly, these two incisions come together on the anterior margin of the trapezius muscle (Fig. 17.1). In some patients, the posterior incision needs to be placed up to 3–5 cm further on the trapezius, but also in these cases the risk of flap necrosis is low.

A very important issue is when we have to perform also a contralateral neck dissection. In order to preserve the flap blood supply, the incision starts approximately 5 cm from the anterior cervical midline and continues 1 cm below hyoid, parallel to inferior border of the mandible. In order to avoid the risks of compromising flap's viability, we can perform contralateral neck dis-

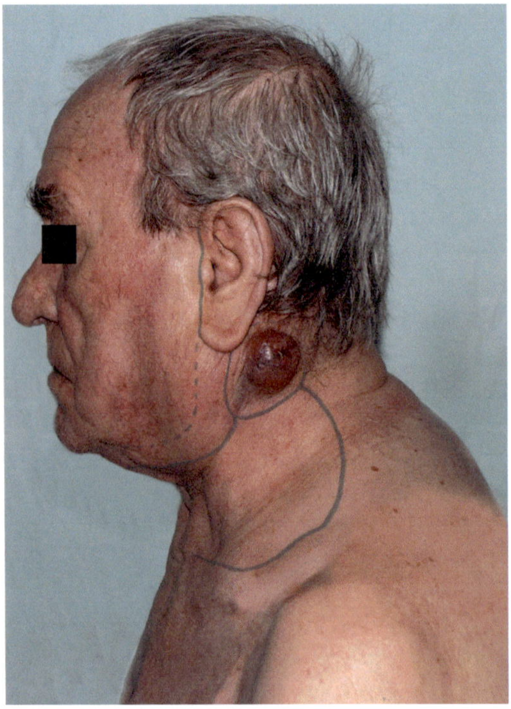

Fig. 17.1 Skin incisions for platysma myocutaneous flap. The posterior incision needs to be placed up to 3–5 cm further on the trapezius

section in a second operative time after 1 week from the first procedure.

In all patients, after skin and muscle incision, the dissection must be performed underneath platysma plan. This operation step requires special attention because the neck dissection needs to respect oncological considerations and it must be as radical as possible. If possible, it is recommended to keep the external jugular vein at is caudal point, so the blood drainage into the internal jugular would not be affected, preventing postoperative flap congestion. Since lymph nodes metastases are not common along this vein, we are able to respect the oncological considerations. Sometimes we cannot dissect the external jugular at its junction with internal jugular vein because of massive supraclavicular or level V lymph nodes involvement. A special attention must be addressed to preservation, when possible, of the cervical branch of facial nerve. The dissection of the flap must be performed until the midline so we can have a wide angle to rotate it onto the defect.

The flap can now be elevated, and neck dissection can be easily performed because of wide exposure of lymph node levels and anatomical structures. After this step, the platysma can be translated and rotated over the defect after extended parotidectomy (Fig. 17.2).

Because the flap is thin, it takes easily the shape of the defect. The downside is that the postoperative facial asymmetry can be significant, which in these patients with poor general status is not very important, but the upside is the lack of dead spaces which could collect hematoma or seroma and might delay the healing process and postpone any eventual adjuvant radiotherapy.

The donor site can be easily closed primarily without using special plastic procedures. Sutures can be placed so postoperative scars would not interfere with head movements (Fig. 17.3).

There are cases in which after tumor resection, there is still a large amount of skin inferior from defect. This happens mainly when the mass lies at the anterior part of the parotid or a skin tumor of the cheek spread and involved secondary the gland. In these patients, after tumor resection en bloc with the parotid (total or superficial), the first incision goes caudal and posterior of sternocleidomastoidian muscle, or on the anterior border of trapezius, and continues 3–5 cm inferior of the clavicle, where we make a 5- to 7-cm back cut. Cranially, the dissection is performed under the skin until the border of the mandible from where the dissection plane lies under the platysma muscle. Posteriorly the flap is elevated with the skin until the sternocleidomastoidian muscle, from where the dissection goes under the platysma. We must be careful to preserve, when possible, the accessorius nerve. Further, the dissection must respect the considerations from the other technique. After the flap is elevated, we carry on with the neck dissection. After this step, the platysma is rotated over the defect like a cervicofacial rotation flap. In its anterior part will result a Burow corner which we have to remove carefully not to damage the blood supply of the PMF. The postoperative defect can now be easily closed.

When possible, it is very important to "hang" the flap with a few 2-0 nonresorbable, positioning/suspension sutures onto the periosteum of the

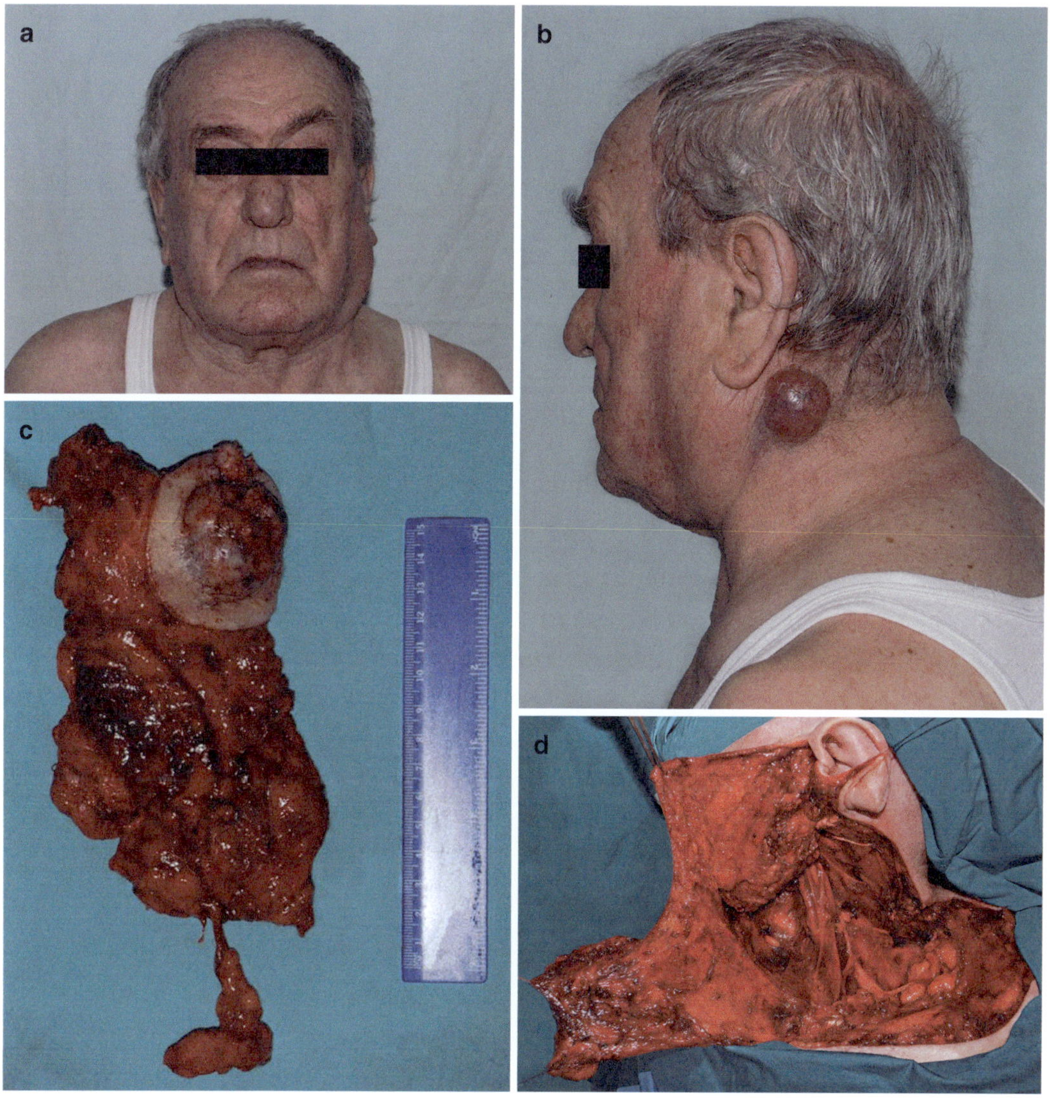

Fig. 17.2 (**a**) Patient with adenoid cystic carcinoma of the left parotid. (**b**) The mass infiltrates the overlying skin in the retroauricular region, without any sign of facial paralysis. (**c**) Resection specimen who includes the tumor, skin, and lymph nodes levels II–V left side. (**d**) The myocutaneous platysma flap is elevated, and the neck dissection is very easy to perform due to the large operation field exposure

malar bone or zygomatic arch in order to prevent traction-induced ectropion.

Two drainages are placed, one medial from sternocleidomastoidian muscle and the second posterior from it but inferior of marginal border of the mandible to prevent flap necrosis.

Postoperatively, there might be some tension in the flap. This can be reduced if the patient's head is turned toward the donor side.

17.5 Complications and Sequelae

The reported rate of complications in literature is 14–55 % [5, 7, 26].

The most common include partial or total flap necrosis, wound dehiscence, and injury to the mandibular branch of facial nerve.

Marginal necrosis can lead sometimes to wound dehisces. In these cases the conservative

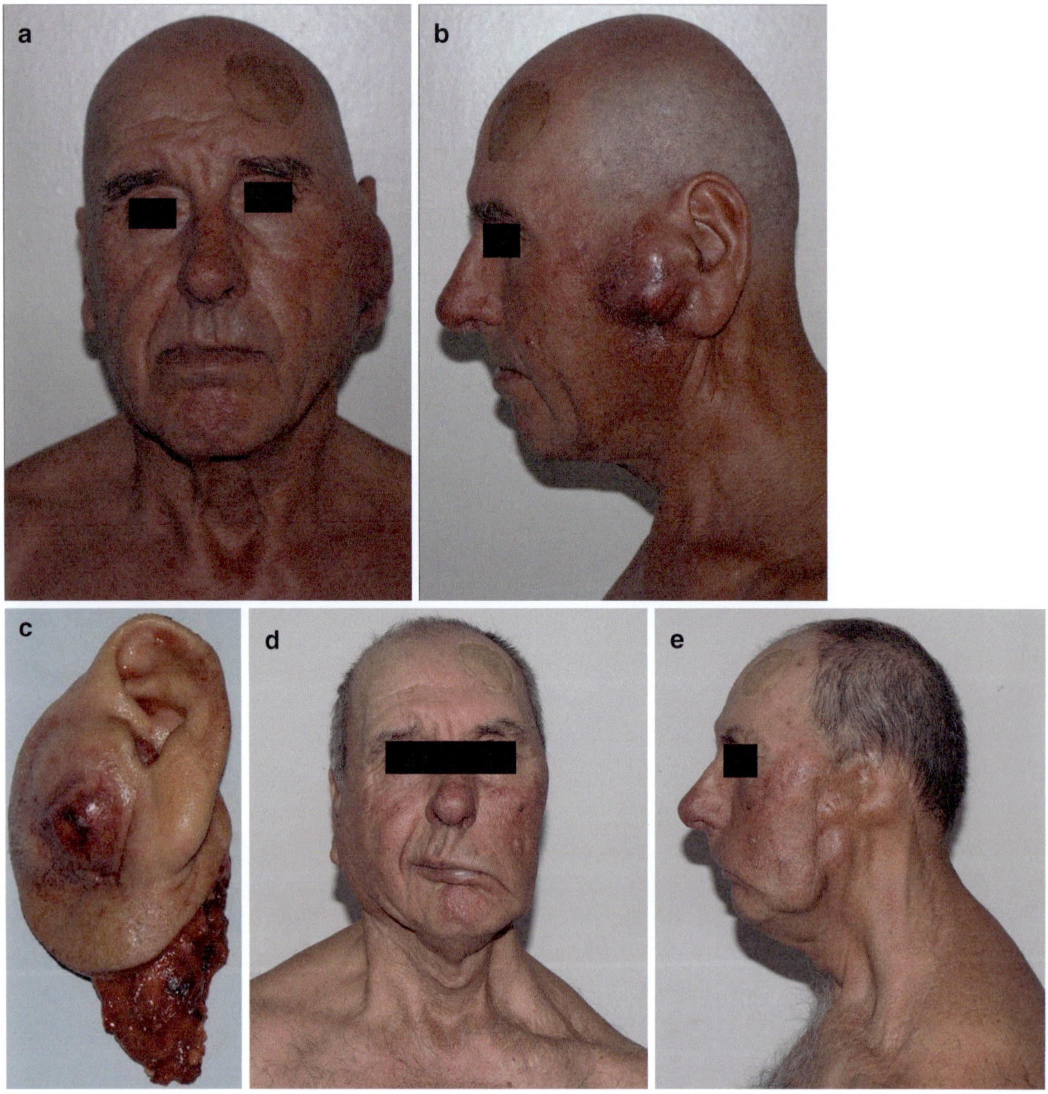

Fig. 17.3 (**a**) Patient with lymph node metastases in the left parotid from a squamous cell carcinoma of the forehead. (**b**) The mass infiltrates the skin and external ear. (**c**) The resection specimen with the left ear, parotid, and lymph nodes level II–V left side. (**d**, **e**) Postoperative status after defect reconstruction with platysma myocutaneous flap. The scars are not very visible, movements of the head are not limited, there is no traction, and facial asymmetry is not significant (except the missing ear). The patient presented a facial paralysis that was treated with static reanimation procedures, but facial rehabilitation is the subject of another chapter

treatment is adequate, and the functional and esthetic outcomes are satisfactory (Fig. 17.4).

Total flap necrosis is rare but very difficult to treat due to poor general status of the patient. We have to remove the livid platysma and use locoregional flaps, such as major pectoralis or scalp rotated flap, depending on the size, depth, and localization of the final defect.

In patients in whom we do not remove the entire parotid because the tumor arises from the skin and involves only the capsule or superficial lobe, an important complication is salivary fistula. This can be addressed during the operation by injection of botulinum toxin in the deep lobe of the parotid.

An important sequel is facial asymmetry, which can be addressed later with lipofilling.

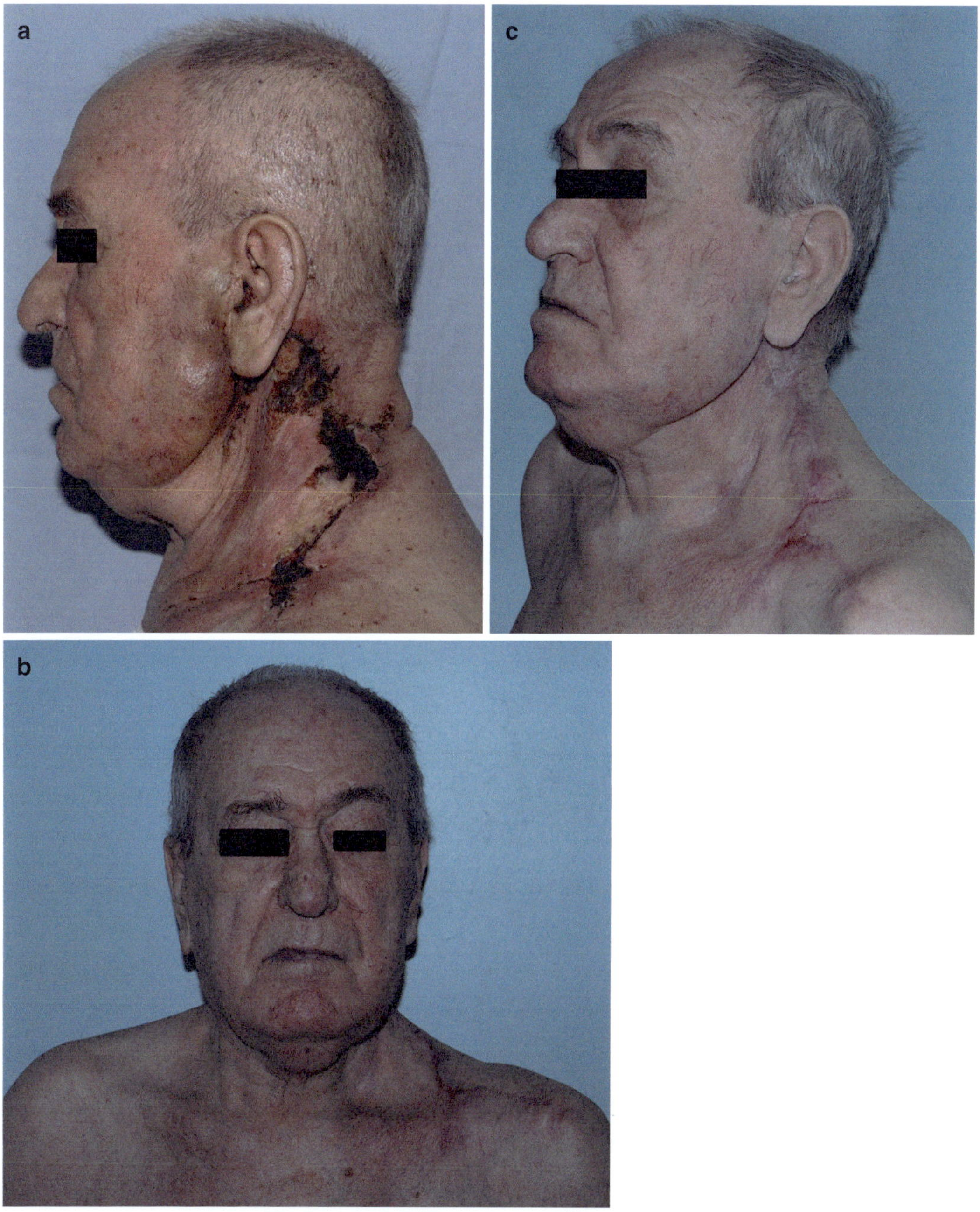

Fig. 17.4 Marginal necrosis of the platysma myocutaneous flap (**a**), but under conservative, treatment esthetic and functional outcomes are satisfactory, without any traction scars on neck (**b**, **c**)

Sometimes, because of the traction, gravity, facial paralyses, and healing process, patients can present ectropion. When possible, the best way is to prevent it by using suspension sutures of the flap onto the periosteum of malar bone or zygomatic arch. But if ectropion appears even after these prophylactic measures, we can address it through specific correction described in other chapters, such as lateral canthopexy or shortening of the lower eyelid.

The other complications or sequelae, such as facial paralysis with lagophthalmos, are due to extended parotidectomy and not to reconstructive technique and are treated in other chapters.

References

1. Chen W, Li Y, Wang N. The need for a complete platysma component for platysma myocutaneous flaps: an introduction of the expanded cutaneous dominant platysma flap for facial defect reconstruction. J Plast Reconstr Aesth Surg. 2010;63(12):2172–6.
2. Tan ST, MacKinnon CA. Deep plane cervicofacial flap: a useful and versatile technique in head and neck surgery. Head Neck. 2006;28(1):46–55.
3. Myers NE, Ferris RL, Clark J, Sneddon L, O'Brien C, Laramore GE, et al. Salivary gland disorders. New York: Springer; 2007. p. 237–57, 257–76; 378–90; 436–92.
4. Conley JJ, Lanier DM, Tinsley Jr P. Platysma myocutaneous flap revisited. Arch Otolaryngol Head Neck Surg. 1986;112:711–3.
5. Nitzan D, Bedrin L, Yahalom R, Talmi PY. The platysma myocutaneous flap. Oper Tech Otolaryngol. 2005;16:270–4.
6. Tosco P, Garzino-Demo P, Ramieri G, Tanteri G, Pecorari G, Caldarelli C, et al. The platysma myocutaneous flap (PMF) for head and neck reconstruction: a retrospective and multicentric analysis of 91 T1–T2 patients. J Craniomaxillofac Surg. 2012;40(8):e415–8.
7. Futrell JW, Johns ME, Edgerton MT, Cantrell RW, Fitz-Hugh GS. Platysma myocutaneous flap for intraoral reconstruction. Am J Surg. 1978;136:504–7.
8. Kim SY, Mathog RH. Platysma muscle-cervical fasciasternocleidomastoid muscle (PCS) flap for parotidectomy. Head Neck. 1999;21:428–33.
9. Puxeddu R, Dennis S, Ferreli C, Caldera S, Brennan PA. Platysma myocutaneous flap for reconstruction of skin defects in the head and neck. Br J Oral Maxillofac Surg. 2008;46:383–6.
10. Yeo JF, Egyedi P. Reconstruction of soft tissues of the chin and lower lip region following excision of a basal cell carcinoma. J Craniomaxillofac Surg. 1988;16:337–9.
11. Moschella F, Cordova A. Platysma muscle cutaneous flap for large defects of the lower lip and mental region. Plast Reconstr Surg. 1998;101:1803–9.
12. Ariyan S, Chicarilli ZN. Replantation of a totally amputated ear by means of a platysma musculocutaneous "sandwich" flap. Plast Reconstr Surg. 1986;78:385–9.
13. de Mello-Filho FV, Mamede RC, Koury AP. Use of a platysma myocutaneous flap for the reimplantation of a severed ear: experience with five cases. Sao Paulo Med J. 1999;117:218–23.
14. Ariyan S. The transverse platysma musculocutaneous flap for head and neck reconstruction: an update. Plast Reconstr Surg. 2003;111:378–80.
15. Coleman JJ, Nahai F, Mathes SJ. Platysma musculocutaneous flap: clinical and anatomic considerations in head and neck reconstruction. Am J Surg. 1982;144:477–81.
16. Ruark DS, McClairen WC, Schlehaider UK, Abdel-Misih RZ. Head and neck reconstruction using the platysma myocutaneous flap. Am J Surg. 1993;165:713–9.
17. Talmi PY, Wolf M, Badrin L, Horowitz Z, Dori S, Chaushu G, et al. Preservation of the facial artery in excision of the submandibular salivary gland. Br J Plast Surg. 2003;56:156–7.
18. McGuirt WF, Matthews BL, Brady JA, May JS. Platysma myocutaneous flap: caveats reexamined. Laryngoscope. 1991;101:1238–44.
19. Rogers JH, Freeland AP. Arterial vasculature of cervical skin flaps. Clin Otolaryngol Allied Sci. 1976;1:325–31.
20. Verschuur HP, Dassonville O, Santini J, Vallicioni J, Poissonnet G, Laudoyer Y, et al. Complications of the myocutaneous platysma flap in intraoral reconstruction. Head Neck. 1998;20:623–9.
21. Uehara M, Helman JI, Lillie JH, Brooks SL. Blood supply to the platysma muscle flap: an anatomic study with clinical correlation. J Oral Maxillofac Surg. 2001;59:642–6.
22. Rabson JA, Hurwitz DJ, Futrell JW. The cutaneous blood supply of the neck: relevance to incision planning and surgical reconstruction. Br J Plast Surg. 1985;38:208–19.
23. Hakim SG, Jacobsen HC, Aschoff HH, Sieg P. Including the platysma muscle in a cervicofacial skin rotation flap to enhance blood supply for reconstruction of vast orbital and cheek defects: anatomical considerations and surgical technique. Int J Oral Maxillofac Surg. 2009;38:1316–9.
24. Su T, Zhao YF, Liu B, Hu YP, Zhang WF. Clinical review of three types of platysma myocutaneous flap. Int J Oral Maxillofac Surg. 2006;35:1011–5.
25. Agarwal A, Schneck CD, Kelley DJ. Venous drainage of the platysma myocutaneous flap. Otolaryngol Head Neck Surg. 2004;130:357–9.
26. Koch WM. The platysma myocutaneous flap: underused alternative for head and neck reconstruction. Laryngoscope. 2002;112:1204–8.

The Use of Muscular or Musculocutaneous Pectoralis Major Flap

18

Orlando Guntinas-Lichius

Abstract

Reconstruction of large parotid defects after extended parotidectomy is common in the field of head and neck surgery. After wide local excision of the primary tumor, regional island flap can often not be used because the defect is too large. In such a situation, reconstruction with a muscular or musculocutaneous pectoralis major flap is a good alternative to free tissue transfer. The pectoralis major flap provides a reliable and ample vascularized soft tissue bulk with skin coverage for defect filling in the parotid area. Its location on the chest wall, the favorable vascular anatomy, and its arc of rotation that is unmatched by any other local flap are other advantages. The pectoralis major flap might also be indicated in cases with failure of a primary reconstruction with a free muscle transfer. After radical parotidectomy needing facial nerve reconstruction, the pectoralis major flap offers a perfect recipient bed to stabilize the facial nerve reconstruction. The special features of defect reconstruction using the pectoralis major flap after extended parotidectomy are presented in this chapter.

18.1 Introduction

After ablative extended parotid surgery for parotid cancer, a large defect can occur in the parotid area and surrounding structures. Parts of the mandible and of the temporomandibular joint might be exposed. An additional skin defect might exist because the primary tumor infiltrated the regional skin. Even when the skin is not affected, it might be difficult to close the defect because a bedding layer is missing to hold the skin. In such a situation, it has to be considered if the patients might profit from a regional or a microvascular flap for defect closure and esthetical reconstruction of the parotid region and the lateral face.

The pectoralis major flap is one of the important working horses for regional reconstruction in the armamentarium of the head and neck surgery [1–3]. It is often said that the pectoralis major flap is one of the best or even the best myocutaneous flap utilized in the head and neck region. If a regional flap is needed, the pectoralis major flap

O. Guntinas-Lichius, MD
Department of Otorhinolaryngology, University Hospital Jena, Jena, Germany
e-mail: orlando.guntinas@med.uni-jena.de

© Springer International Publishing Switzerland 2016

V.-V. Costan (ed.), *Management of Extended Parotid Tumors*, DOI 10.1007/978-3-319-26545-2_18

is frequently used to repair defects in the floor of the mouth or of the tongue. As a musculocutaneous flap, i.e., with dermal graft, it is often selected for defects of the hypopharynx or oropharynx. Here, the use of this flat muscle flap is presented to reconstruction defects after ablative and extended parotid surgery (Figs. 18.1 and 18.2).

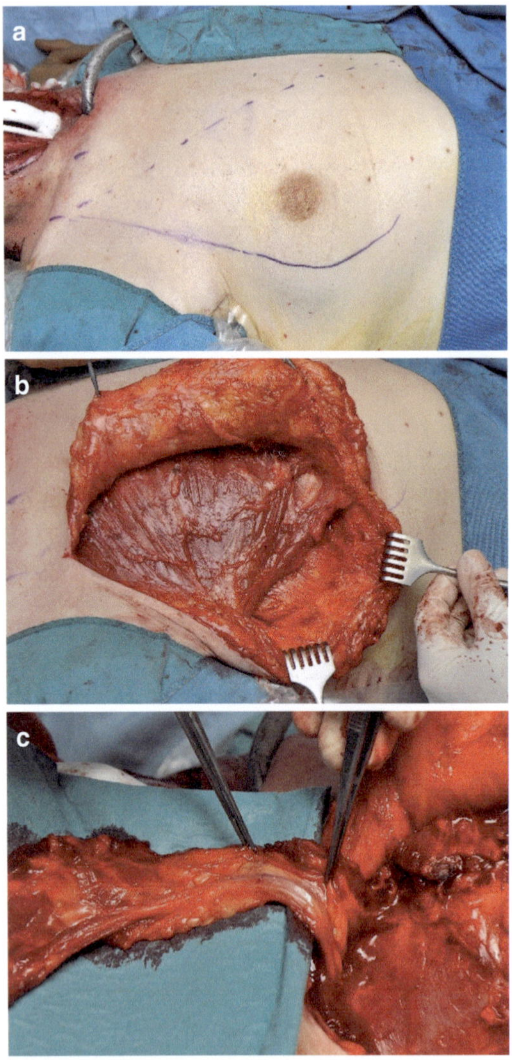

Fig. 18.1 Preparation of a muscular or musculocutaneous pectoralis major flap. (**a**) Skin incision marked for a flap on the left side. (**b**) Elevation of the skin (no skin island used in this case) exposing the pectoralis major muscle. (**c**) Situs after elevating the muscle flap showing the vessel pedicle of the flap

18.2 Indication for a Muscular or Musculocutaneous Pectoralis Major Flap

The pectoralis major flap can be selected for to reconstruct skin and parotid loss after resection of these structures [4]. A rotated medial cheek flap might be thought to be an alternative [5]. But if radiotherapy is planned later on, such a skin flap might not survive. If the patient already had radiotherapy for primary treatment and one is confronted with a recurrent tumor, a simple skin flap might not heal in an irradiated recipient area. Or there are other risk factors for complicated wound healing like a patient with diabetes or severe arteriosclerosis. In all these situations, a pectoralis muscle flap should be preferred. A general advantage of the muscle flap is the transplanted muscle itself allowing a defect filling and pretentious reconstruction of the original contour of the parotid area and surface.

One should be aware of the limitation of a pectoralis major flap in the parotid region. Such a flap lacks function. If extended parotidectomy included resection of parts of the masseter muscle or of the pterygopalatine muscles, the regional flap will not restore chewing function or decrease dysphagia. Muscle bulk can be a limitation but in the parotid region rather helpful than disturbing.

When the primary even completely resected parotid tumor has a high rate of local recurrence, a complete coverage of the primary defect in the parotid region by a pectoralis major flap is contraindicated if surgery was performed in curative intent. When a parotid tumor recurrence occurs in such a situation, the muscle flap will hinder an early detection of the recurrence. The recurrent tumor might grow underneath the muscle flap and will be palpable only when reaching a large tumor size and advanced stage.

18.3 Diagnostics

General diagnostics are presented in detail in Chaps. 10 and 11. Special preoperative investigations such as computed tomographic angiograms and perforator localization by means of Doppler devices are

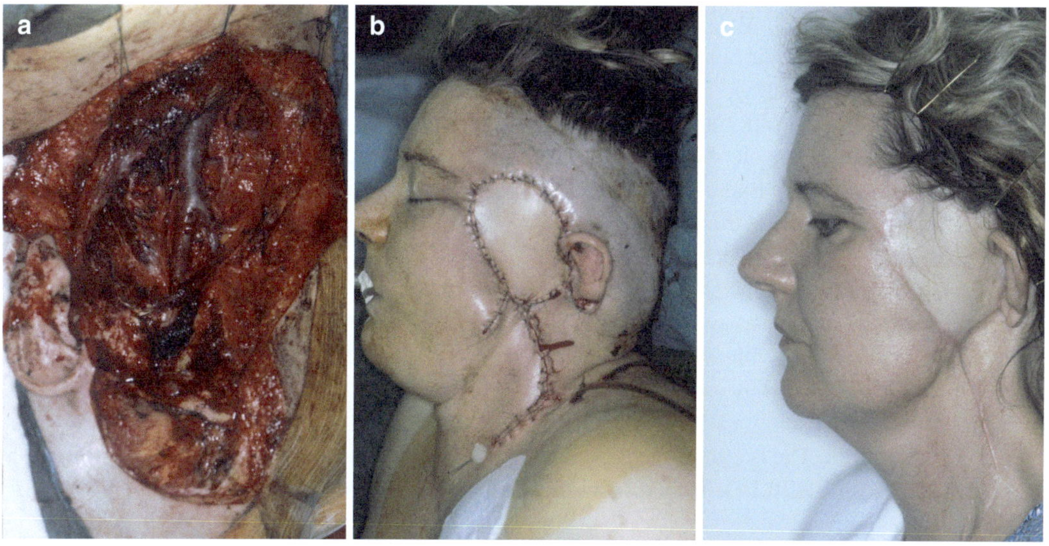

Fig. 18.2 The use of a musculocutaneous pectoralis major flap for the reconstruction of a large parotid defect after resection of a recurrent adenoid cystic carcinoma of the left side. (**a**) Situs after extended parotidectomy and neck dissection. (**b**) Situation after reconstruction with the musculocutaneous muscle flap. (**c**) Appearance 6 months later

normally not necessary for planning a pectoralis major flap. Imaging that has been performed for the primary tumor staging should, of course, rule out tumor infiltration or metastasis at the donor site.

18.4 Surgery

The techniques for extended parotidectomy are presented elsewhere (see Chaps. 5, 6, 7, and 8). Typically the preparation of the pectoralis muscle flap is started when the ablative tumor surgery is finished. Secondary surgery might be indicated after necrotic loss of a local flap used for primary reconstruction [3]. The preparation of the pectoralis muscle flap can be combined with a deltopectoral flap preparation. This double-flap usage is not presented here.

18.4.1 Informed Consent for a Pectoralis Major Muscle Flap

Surgery is usually performed in general anesthesia. Informed consent discussing the surgical steps of the pectoralis muscle preparation and of its complication is mandatory. The most important complications are [2]:

- Necrosis and loss of the flap.
- Infection.
- Bulk of the flap might be cosmetically disturbing.
- Hematoma and seroma of the donor site.

Furthermore, the patient has to be informed that the flap might hinder an early detection of recurrent disease.

18.4.2 Preparation of the Flap

1. Outline the probable course of the pectoral branch of the thoracoacromial artery feeding the pectoralis major muscle on the patient's skin. A first line is sketched from the shoulder tip to the xiphoid process. A second line is sketched from the midportion of the clavicle in a right angle to the first line. The pectoral branch runs from the cross point of both lines downward along the first line. The pectoral branch of the thoracoacromial artery is the main axial artery for the muscle flap. Seldom

is the pectoral branch not well developed. In such a situation the major blood supply to the flap is from the lateral thoracic artery. Therefore, it is very important to check the underportion of the muscle during the subsequent preparation of the flap. Additionally, the muscle size and if needed the skin size that is required to fill the defect are outlined. Alternatively, and especially in female patients, it is better to use a curvilinear incision line inferior to the breast exactly in the breast crease [6]. Thereby, one can camouflage the otherwise obvious scarring on the anterior chest wall. The breast tissue has to be preserved. It can easily be elevated from the pectoralis major muscle.
2. The first incision follows along the lateral border of the outlined skin (or muscle size if no skin is needed) down to the muscle. If this incision is near the lateral border of the pectoralis major muscle, this lateral border is used as dissection plane along the pectoralis minor muscle.
3. If the lateral border of the pectoralis major muscle is too far lateral to the incision line, the muscle is split about 2 cm medial to the lateral border along its inferior oblique fibers. It is very important that the pectoral branch of the thoracoacromial artery is lying medial to the splitting line.
4. A blunt dissection is performed. Take care that the fascia of the deep side of the pectoralis major muscle is kept to the muscle.
5. Have a view on the vessels during the entire muscle preparation. For the next step, the edges of the skin are sutured to the underlying muscle to prevent separation of skin and muscle flap.
6. The flap is mobilized further. The medial skin incision is completed together with the dissection of the medial parts of the muscle flap. The attachments to the rectus fascia and to the costochondral cartilages are transected. The attachments of the superior and horizontal fibers of the muscle are transected lateral to the lateral thoracic artery.
7. After complete mobilization, a skin tunnel is prepared over the clavicle. The flap is passed over the clavicle. Be careful not to dissect the vessel bundle from the surrounding fascia during this preparation step.
8. A separate suction drainage is used for the donor site on the chest. In most cases, the donor site can be closed by additional dissection of the medial and lateral skin. Seldom is a skin graft needed.

18.4.3 Reconstruction of the Extended Parotidectomy Defect

The pectoralis muscle flap is elevated after resection of the parotid tumor. Defect filling with the pectoralis muscle flap can also be combined with a second flap from the sternocleidomastoid muscle to be transferred to the former area of the deep lobe of the parotid gland [4]. During reconstruction, avoid rotating the vessel bundle of the pectoralis muscle flap. This might obstruct the veins and arteries. After extended parotidectomy, typically the zygoma arch and mandible are widely exposed in the parotid bed. If a facial nerve reconstruction is planned, it is at best performed lateral to a first defect filling of the deep lobe region. Hence, at best a first flap is placed in the deep lobe region before the nerve reconstruction is started. If the sternocleidomastoid muscle is available, it can be used. Otherwise, the muscle body part of the pectoralis muscle flap is used. After finishing the nerve reconstruction on the surface of the muscle flap, the nerve reconstruction is covered by either the complete pectoralis muscle flap or, if already used for the deep lobe filling, by the skin island from the pectoralis major musculocutaneous flap.

References

1. Ariyan S. The pectoralis major myocutaneous flap. A versatile flap for reconstruction in the head and neck. Plast Reconstr Surg. 1979;63(1):73–81. PubMed.
2. McLean JN, Carlson GW, Losken A. The pectoralis major myocutaneous flap revisited: a reliable technique for head and neck reconstruction. Ann Plast Surg. 2010;64(5):570–3. PubMed.

3. Schneider DS, Wu V, Wax MK. Indications for pedicled pectoralis major flap in a free tissue transfer practice. Head Neck. 2012;34(8):1106–10. PubMed.
4. Motomura H, Yamanaka K, Maruyama Y, Sakamoto M, Harada T. Facial nerve reconstruction using a muscle flap following resection of parotid gland tumours with thorough recipient bed preparation. J Plast Reconstr Aesthet Surg. 2011;64(5):595–601. PubMed.
5. Behan FC, Lo CH, Sizeland A, Pham T, Findlay M. Keystone island flap reconstruction of parotid defects. Plast Reconstr Surg. 2012;130(1):36e–41. PubMed.
6. Jena A, Patnayak R, Sharan R, Reddy SK, Manilal B, Rao LM. Outcomes of pectoralis major myocutaneous flap in female patients for oral cavity defect reconstruction. J Oral Maxillofac Surg. 2014;72(1):222–31. PubMed.

19 The Use of Latissimus Dorsi Free Flap

Felix P. Koch, Robert A. Sader, and Victor-Vlad Costan

Abstract

The free latissimus dorsi flap covers large defects involving the skin, malar, mandible, temporal and sphenoid bone, external and medium ear and zygomatic arch. The muscle is very helpful to isolate the epidural space from the surrounding tissue. In cases a neck dissection is demanded, vessels for the flap anastomosis should be already prepared, shortening the surgery time. By connecting the thoracodorsal nerve to the facial nerve, a facial reanimation is possible. For reconstructions in the area of the head, it is preferable to change the classical positioning of the patient from a prone or supine decubitus to a position allowing elevation of the flap by a second team at the same time with the tumour excision. On the other hand, the flap can be too bulky compared to the volume of the defect, especially in those cases with an association between an important surface and a relative superficial defect. Additionally, there are differences between the skin texture of the flap and of the facial skin.

19.1 Introduction

The first description of a pedicled latissimus dorsi flap was performed by Tansini in 1896 [1]. Quill et al. described in 1978 the application of a pedicled latissimus dorsi flap for head and neck reconstruction for the first time [2]. One year later Watson used it as a free flap [3]. The latissimus dorsi flap can fill even deep defects by its soft tissue volume. Therefore it leads to favourable results to fill the resected parotid gland's region by transferring muscle, fat and skin. Even defects reaching the oral side can be reconstructed by a second skin paddle if the supplying

F.P. Koch, MD, DMD, MBA, PhD •
R.A. Sader, MD, DDS, PhD (✉)
Department of Oral, Cranio-Maxillofacial and Facial Plastic Surgery, University Hospital Frankfurt, Frankfurt, Germany
e-mail: Koch@facialplastics.de; r.sader@em.uni-frankfurt.de

V.-V. Costan, MD, DMD, PhD
Department of Oral and Maxillo-Facial Surgery, Faculty of Dental Medicine, "Grigore T. Popa" University of Medicine and Pharmacy, "St. Spiridon" University Hospital Iasi, Iasi, Romania
e-mail: victorcostan@gmail.com

© Springer International Publishing Switzerland 2016
V.-V. Costan (ed.), *Management of Extended Parotid Tumors*, DOI 10.1007/978-3-319-26545-2_19

arteries of the transverse and vertical branch of the thoracodorsal artery are isolated. Alternatively the whole skin paddle can be partially deepithelized to flip the caudal part inside the mouth and cover the buccal plane. Due to its size, the latissimus dorsi flap is able to cover the cheek and the temporal region, the orbits and the skull base. Especially for defects of the parotid region, which include a facial nerve resection, the motoric branches of the thoracodorsal nerve can be connected to the facial nerve branches to rehabilitate its function [4, 5].

19.2 Anatomy

Latissimus dorsi muscle lies between the VI and XII thoracic, lumbar and sacral vertebra, the posterior iliac crest and the humerus, where it inserts between the m. teres major and m. pectoralis major. The blood supply arises from the dorsal thoracic artery which originates from the subscapular artery. The pedicle is situated beneath the m. latissimus dorsi near its lateral border. Therefore the lateral border of the muscle and its covering skin needs to be identified. The length of the pedicle is 9 cm in average, but can be as short as 6 cm. The thoracodorsal pedicle supplies a branch to the anteriorly situated m. serratus anterior and another one to the tip of the scapula at the posterior side. This branch can be used to take a bone graft of the scapula with a pedicle length of 15 cm [6]. The thoracodorsal artery has been described with a diameter of 1.5–4 mm [7]. This variety of diameters often causes several recipient cervical or temporal arteries to be prepared, to get a suitable vessel of similar diameter. After the thoracodorsal vessels have entered the latissimus muscle, it divides in two branches, one running parallel to the proximal muscle rim and another parallel to the anterior muscle border. This quite regular anatomy makes a flap with two skin paddles possible. Care should be taken with the caudal and medial part of the muscle, as it is nutritioned by the intercostal perforators arising from the paravertebral region. As the main vessel at the anterior muscle rim safely perfuses also distal parts of the muscle through muscular perforators, the latissimus flap can be extended to a size of about 20 cm width and 40 cm length [8]. The size of the flap harvest is, however, limited by the intension to provide a primary closure.

If a facial reanimation is necessary, the thoracodorsal nerve should be harvested as a motoric branch arising from the plexus brachialis. It runs parallel to the thoracodorsal vessels [4, 5].

19.3 Preparation of the Flap

The most important landmark in the initial planning of the flap is the accurate determination of the anterior border of the latissimus dorsi muscle. It can be easily palpated and marked preoperatively, with the patient standing up, hands positioned on the hips, tensing the muscles of the back (Fig. 19.1). We found intraoperative palpation, and marking of the anterior border can be difficult due to the lack of muscle tension and is especially challenging in overweight patients.

An additional marking can be performed for orientation purpose, starting at the middle of the iliac crest to the posterior axillary fold. It is estimated that approximately 12 cm below the axilla, along this line, the pedicle can be found entering the muscle. The flap will be designed to overlay this area. The superior border of the flap is represented by the initial skin incision performed on the outlined anterior border of the latissimus muscle. The size and shape of the skin paddle, as well as the amount of skin and muscle needed, can be marked and further adjusted intraoperatively following the surgery of the tumour, according to the size and depth of the postoperative defect.

Any side can be chosen as donor site, but we generally prefer elevating the flap from the opposite side to the tumour to ensure enough tissue is left on the tumour side to easily perform a pectoralis major flap with primary closure of the defect, in the event of free flap failure. Versatility in the reconstruction method is especially important in the case of extended parotidectomy that will lead to large defects and possible exposure of great vessels and bone surfaces. A small inconvenience to choosing the opposite side for

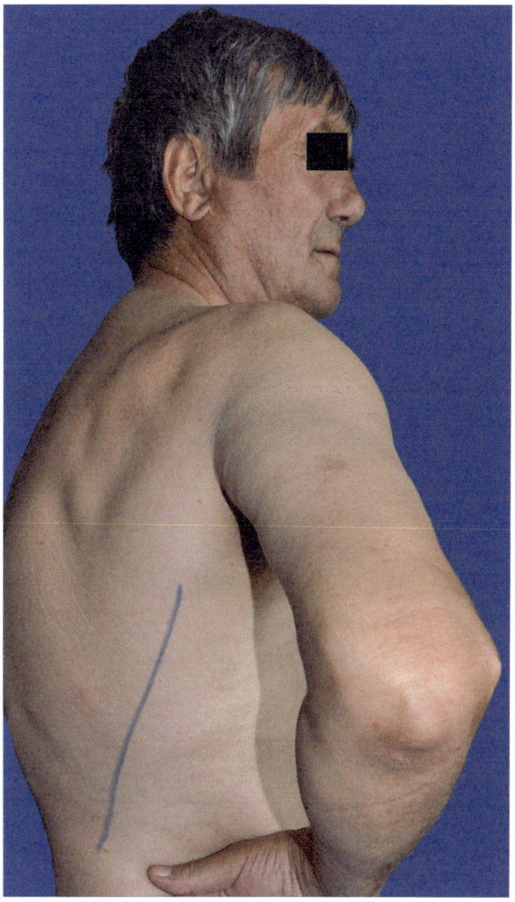

Fig. 19.1 Preoperatively the anterior border of the latissimus dorsi muscle was marked

elevation of the flap is that it becomes technically difficult although still possible to apply a two-team approach.

We position the patient in a supine position, slightly rotated to the opposite side, with the ipsilateral arm fixated in an elevated position to better expose the area of the muscle. The ipsilateral shoulder, axilla, arm, thorax and back are prepared and draped for accurate exposure of marked landmarks and free movement in the operating field considering also the undermining that will be necessary for primary closure of the donor site.

The skin incision is performed along the marked line representing the anterior margin of the axilla. An incision anterior to its border should be preferred to a more posterior incision. The muscle is exposed by bluntly dissecting in a superior direction, separating and lifting the subcutaneous tissue from the serratus muscle to expose the anterior border of the latissimus along the whole length of the incision.

This is one of the key moments of the surgery since along this line, 1–2 cm behind the anterior border, on the medial side of the muscle, the vertical branch of the thoracodorsal artery travels to form the intramuscular portion of the pedicle. We take great caution in dissecting the anterior border since this branch is located very close to the margin of the muscle and can be easily injured leading to the compromising of the flap.

When a musculocutaneous flap is desired, care is taken not to dissect the subcutaneous tissue inferior from the line of incision in order to avoid separating the overlying skin from the latissimus muscle.

While dissecting and retracting the tissues superiorly from the anterior edge of the muscle, a branch of the thoracodorsal artery that supplies the serratus anterior muscle is encountered penetrating between the serratus and latissimus muscles. Following the course of this artery will lead to the vascular pedicle that can usually be found travelling 1–2 cm behind the anterior border of the muscle.

The intramuscular pedicle must be visible on the whole length of the muscle in order to be protected during surgery. Further dissection will bring us to the point where the pedicle enters the muscle.

Then we separate the medial side of the latissimus muscle from the thoracic wall. There is a fairly avascular areolar tissue in between the serratus and latissimus muscles that facilitates dissection in this area. In the distal part of the muscle, we pay attention to carefully coagulate vessels from the chest wall entering the flap since they can retract and demand a difficult haemostasis.

The muscle fascia must be preserved on the medial side of the latissimus since it contains the vasculature. Furthermore, when a muscular flap is desired to fill a defect, the skin overlying the latissimus dorsi must be carefully separated from the muscle, leaving the fascia attached to the muscle.

Once the planes have been carefully separated, this allows for easy retraction of the tissues and further dissection of the vessels can be performed with ease.

At this point the neurovascular pedicle already exposed can be traced along its course towards the axilla, and further dissection in the axilla can continue depending on the desired length of the pedicle, but not above the circumflex scapula vessels. Haemostasis is carefully achieved in proximity to the thoracodorsal vessels. All other vessels of considerable calibre that are encountered during dissection should be preserved until the pedicle has been dissected and the elevation completed.

The skin incision is then completed along the caudal, proximal and inferior borders, according to the desired dimensions of the skin paddle and followed by the incision of the muscle. Passing suspension sutures through the muscle and overlying skin help to prevent the sliding of the subcutaneous tissue on the muscle and tearing of the blood supply to the skin paddle, while also aiding in retracting and lifting the muscle to facilitate the incision. Although the vessels should be protected all through the surgery, transection of the muscle at the cranial aspect of the flap in particular requires increased attention in order to avoid injuries to the pedicle. The amount of skin and muscle necessary for the reconstruction can be adjusted according to the characteristics of the postoperative defect.

Once we have isolated the flap in the desired shape and size and the recipient vessels are prepared for the anastomosis, careful haemostasis at the donor site must first be ensured, communicating vessels previously preserved around the pedicle are now ligated and then the pedicle can be divided at the desired length.

If increased length of the pedicle is needed, this can only be achieved in a caudal direction. The superior part of the pedicle is limited in its length, but adjustments can be made by dissecting the intramuscular pedicle away from the anterior border of the muscle in a caudal direction. In doing so, dividing the horizontal branch of the thoracodorsal artery is needed. Dissecting the pedicle caudally will result in increased pedicle length. Additionally, elevating the flap from the point where the pedicle enters the muscle will lead to a thicker flap, while descending along the pedicle and elevating at a lower level will ensure a thinner flap.

If a facial reanimation is planned, in case the facial nerve was also resected, the thoracodorsal nerve running parallel to the vessels is kept as well.

Closure of the postoperative defect at the donor site can usually be achieved by primary closure if extensive undermining of the surrounding tissues is performed. Two to three suction drains are placed and the wound is closed in layers in order to decrease wound tension.

19.4 Indications, Limitations, Advantages and Disadvantages

This flap is very useful to reconstruct large and composite defects after extended parotidectomy, which includes the skin, ear and bone (Figs. 19.2a, b and 19.3), and especially in cases where temporal bone was resected (Figs. 19.4a, b and 19.5). Due to its bulkiness (Fig. 19.6), this flap is ideal to seal the skull base in order to prevent cerebral fluid leakage.

As a limitation we may consider patients with comorbidities, which cannot undergo a long operation to cover the defect. Also cases with previous surgery or trauma in this area should be excluded from this type of reconstruction method.

The advantages of the latissimus flap are a constant anatomy with enough myocutaneous perforators [9]. Technically the flap is quite easy to harvest. The volume effect, however, is difficult to predict, because big percentage of the volume belongs to muscular tissue, which atrophies over time.

In case the facial nerve is infiltrated by the neoplasm as well and needs to be resected, the latissimus dorsi flap provides the possibility of a facial reanimation. Then the thoracodorsal nerve, which runs parallel to the thoracodorsal vessels, is harvested as well and disconnected after leaving the plexus brachialis. Before the anastomosis of donor nerve and facial nerve is done, a sample of the facial nerve should be sent to the pathol-

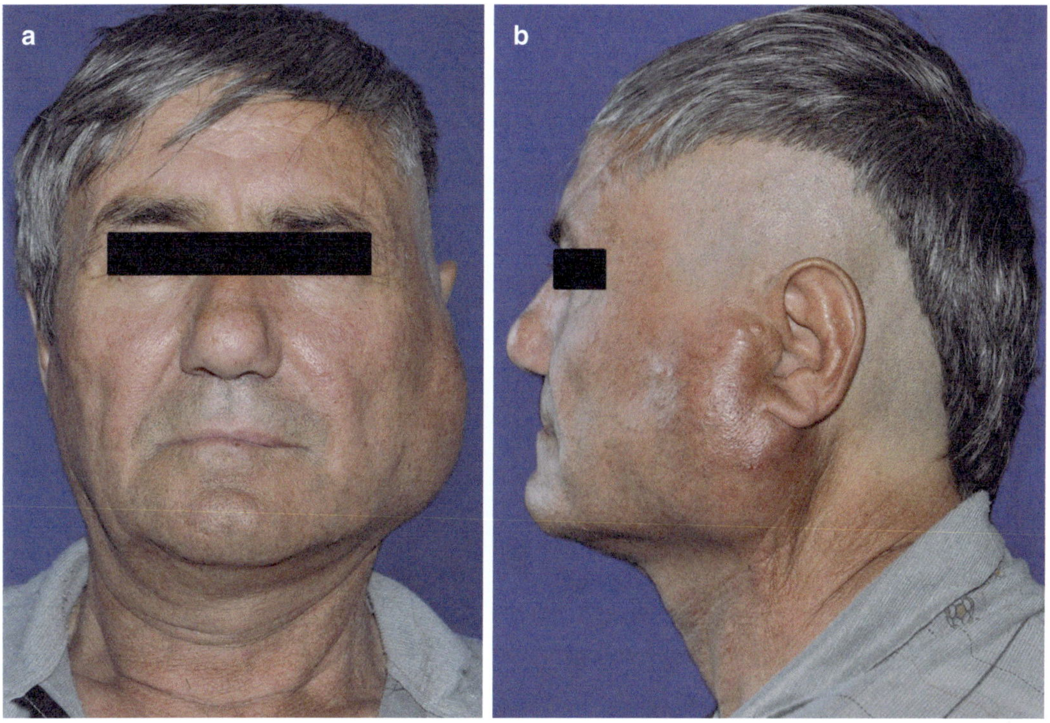

Fig. 19.2 (**a**, **b**) Poorly differentiated squamous cell carcinoma of the left parotid gland: frontal and lateral view. Notice the absence of obvious signs of facial nerve invasion. Given the clinically evident invasion of the external ear canal, a decision was made to use the musculocutaneous latissimus dorsi free flap

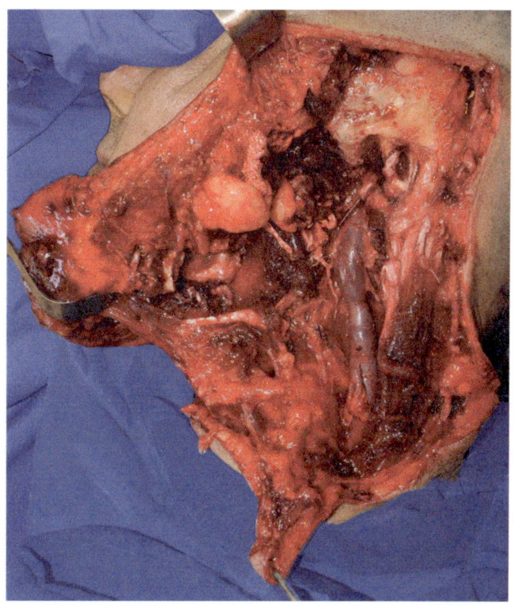

Fig. 19.3 The appearance of the postoperative defect after conducting the extended parotidectomy involving the left auricle and external ear canal and the skin of the occipital region and resection of the left mandible with disarticulation and complete resection of the masseter and pterygoid muscles, sacrificing the facial nerve. A left neck dissection extended to the trapezius muscle was also performed

ogy to get intraoperative information on cancer infiltration. Especially acinic cell carcinoma and adenoid cystic carcinoma tend to infiltrate nerves. In case the facial nerve is completely resected as well, a nerve *interponate* e.g. from the n. suralis is transferred and connected with

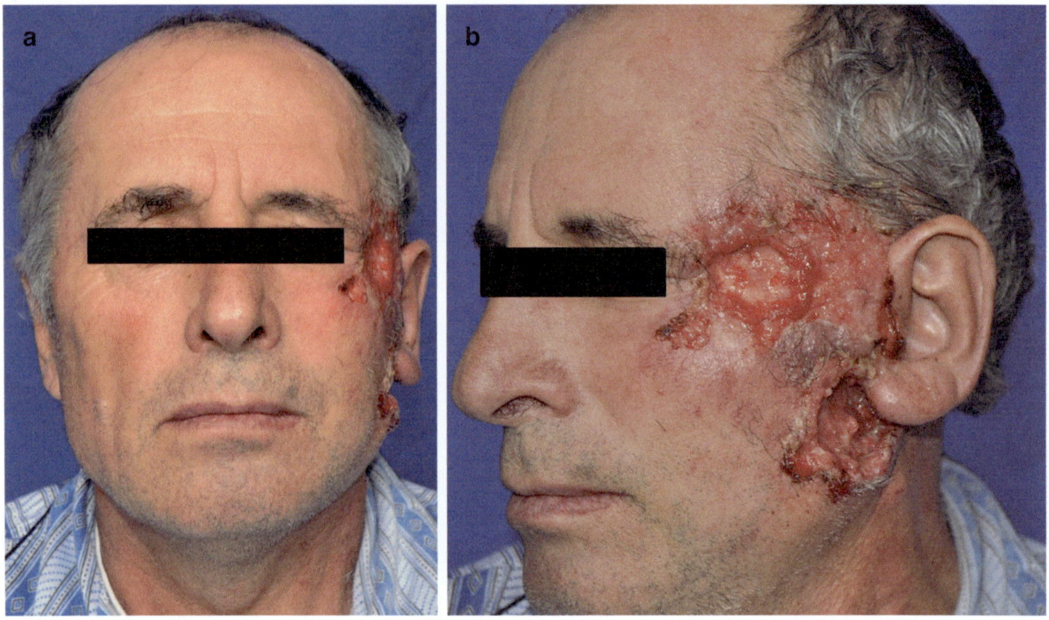

Fig. 19.4 (**a**, **b**) Morphea-type basal cell carcinoma of the left parotid region, previously operated, relapsed, with invasion of the parotid gland, pinna, external ear canal and skin of the temporal and zygomatic regions

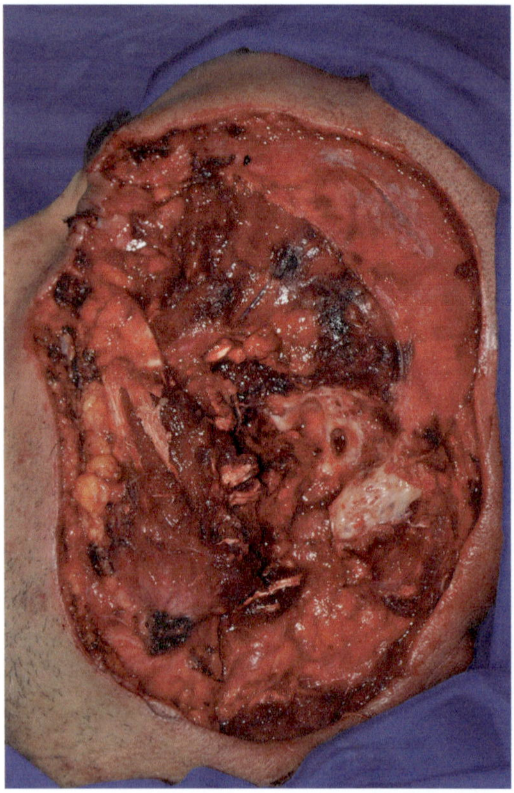

Fig. 19.5 The postoperative defect – following parotidectomy extended to the pinna, external auditory meatus and invaded skin, partially the temporal bone and zygoma, with division of the facial nerve – turned out to be a voluminous one, also involving a large surface area. The plasty was performed by the use of a musculocutaneous latissimus dorsi free flap

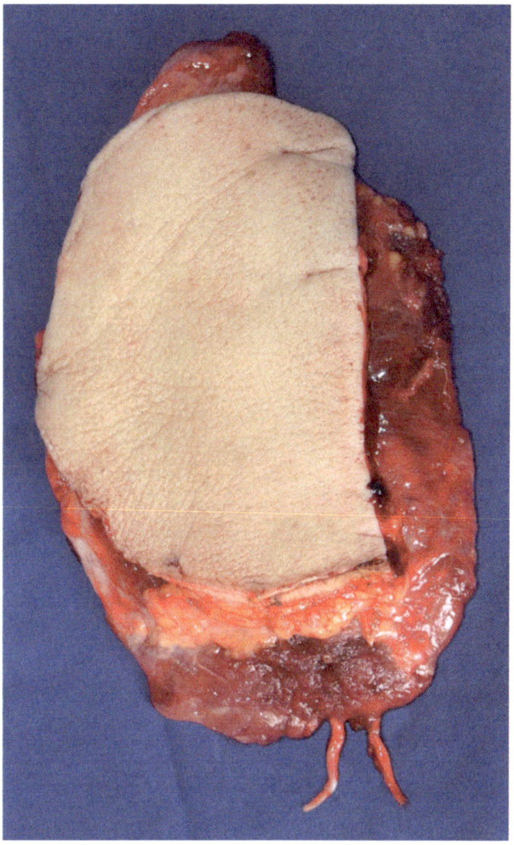

Fig. 19.6 Given the increased volume of the postoperative defect, the plasty was performed by the use of a musculocutaneous latissimus dorsi free flap

the contralateral side. To reconstitute the mimic functions, typically the angle of the mouth is lifted [4, 5]. Therefore the latissimus muscle is spanned between the zygomatic arch and the angle of the mouth. Therefore, a preauricular incision and a subcutaneous preparation similar to a rhytidectomy are performed to fix the muscle at the zygomatic arch by heavy, absorbable sutures; the distal part of the muscle fibres are split longitudinally and sutured into prepared tissue pockets of the upper and lower lips.

Some authors like the big diameter of the vessels, because they are easy to suture and anastomose. However, it is not easy to find suitable vessels of that size in the neck. Since a discrepancy between the vessels diameters could disturb the laminar flow and cause thrombosis, sometimes even the external carotid artery needs to be taken for the anastomosis. Also an end to side anastomosis to the external carotid artery is described [4]. Furthermore, the flap pedicle is often quite short. Another apparent disadvantage is the classical positioning of the patient in a prone or supine decubitus position, but the patient can be positioned in a way that allows the elevation of the flap to be performed at the same time with the tumour removal. The bulkiness and different skin texture of the flap compared to the surrounding skin lead to an aesthetic mismatch (Figs. 19.7 and 19.8a, b). In time, and especially after the radiotherapy sessions, the muscular volume decreases significantly, and by performing small corrective surgery, the facial asymmetry can be corrected. On the other hand, similar to the radial flaps, an increased survival of the patients makes the difference in the appearance of the skin of the flap compared to the surrounding facial skin to diminish significantly (Fig. 19.9a, b).

19.5 Sequelae and Complications

In some patients we need to perform corrective operations to obtain facial symmetry, not only to correct the volume of the flap that can be excessive.

Due to its weight, the flap can induce traction upon nearby tissues, especially the lower lid, leading to ectropion. Suspension sutures may prevent this inconvenience. If this occurs after all preventive measures, we may correct it in a second operation using tarsorrhaphy or lateral canthopexy.

As a complication we may count partial or total necrosis of the flap. In these cases we might need another flap to close the defect, so we may use an ALT or radial flap or major pectoralis flap. In elderly patients and patient with high comorbidity, the cervicofacial advancement flap is very useful and rather fast and technically easy to perform [10, 11].

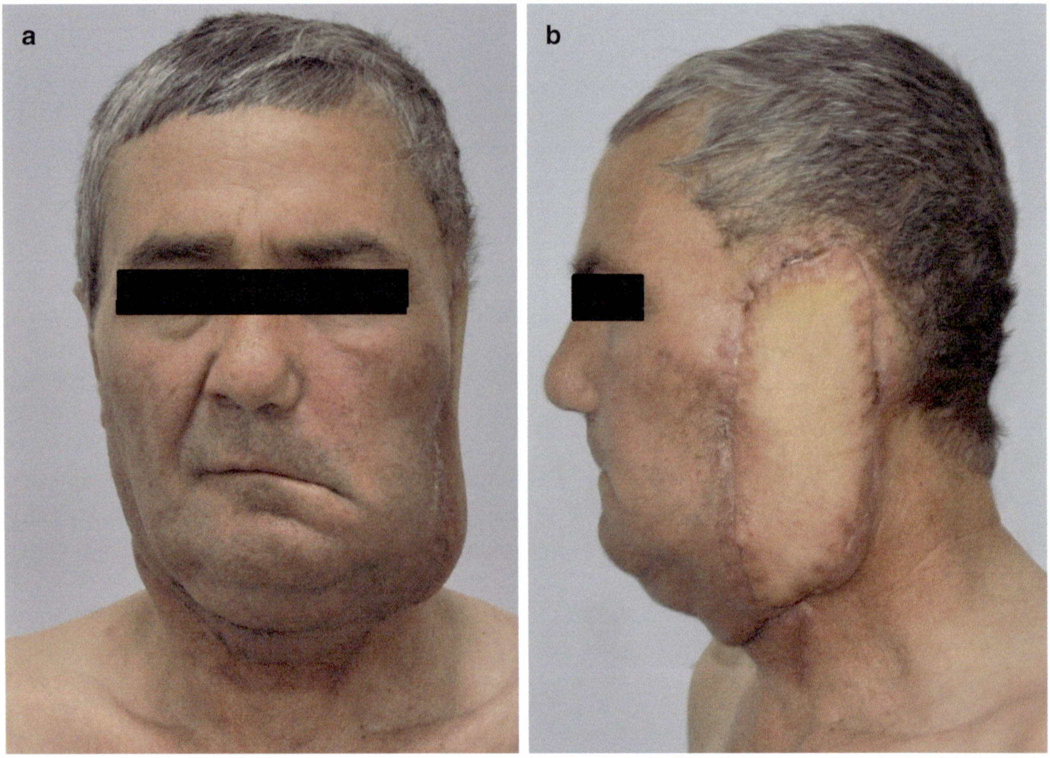

Fig. 19.7 Appearance of the patient 1 month postoperatively. Facial symmetry is satisfactory, although no mandibular reconstruction was performed. In spite of the increased volume of the flap that has been used, the area of reconstruction does not appear to have significant volume

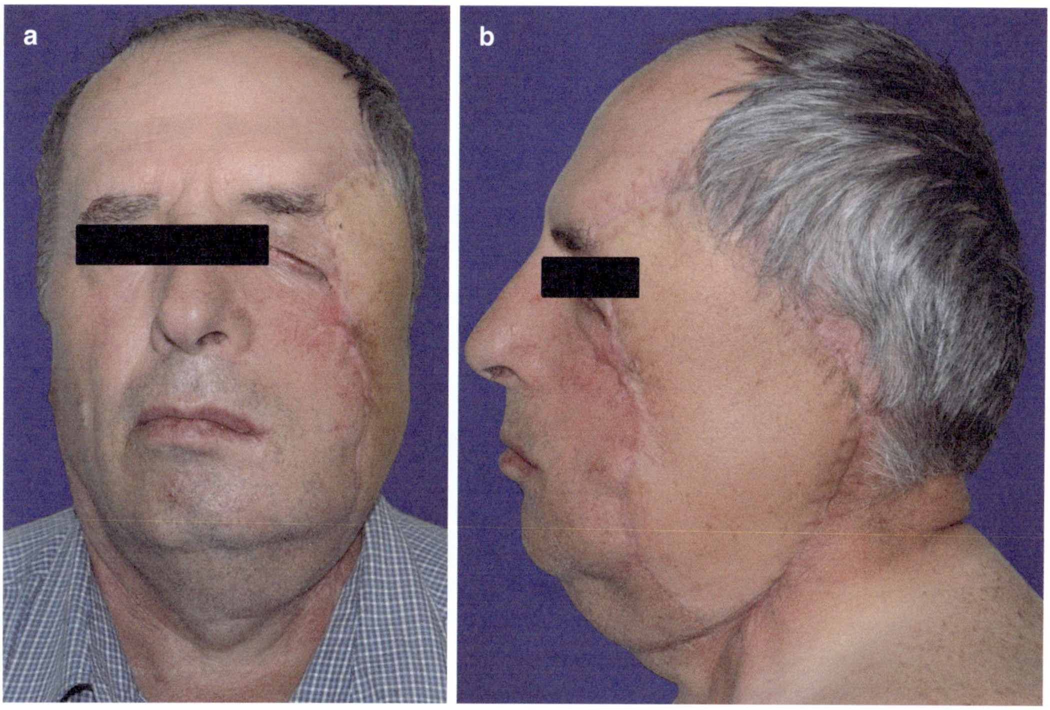

Fig. 19.8 (**a**, **b**) The appearance of the patient 2 years after surgery emphasizes the maintenance of symmetry achieved postoperatively, with a minimum reduction of the flap volume, since in this case radiotherapy was not recommended. Notice that, in this case, the weight of the flap was useful, allowing the occlusion of the eye on the side affected by paralysis of the facial nerve, without requiring additional surgery

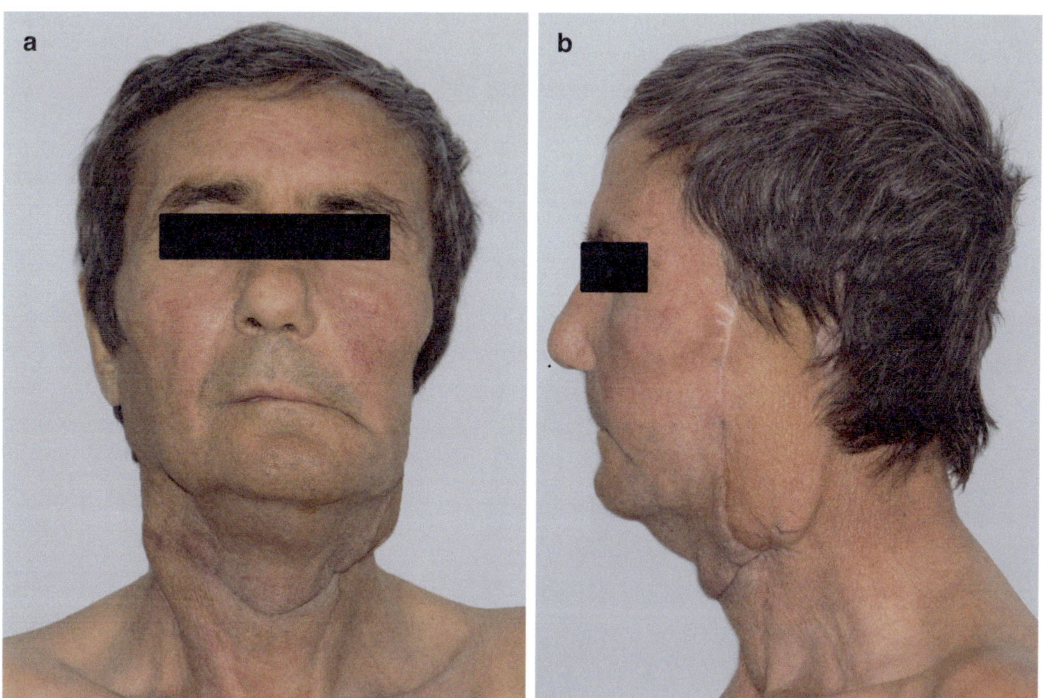

Fig. 19.9 (**a**, **b**) Appearance of the patient 2 months postoperatively, after external radiotherapy and associated chemotherapy. Note the atrophy of the latissimus dorsi flap. The symmetry of the chin is maintained although no mandibular reconstruction was performed following the resection of the left mandible

Conclusion

The latissimus dorsi provides the surgeon with great freedom and versatility in reconstructions following extended parotidectomy. The reliable anatomy of the area allows an easy and fast harvesting of large soft tissue volumes, of soft tissue, which is especially important in plasties following extended parotidectomy.

The inconveniences of this particular flap compared to other flaps can usually be overcome by small adjustments of the havesting techique and modifications to increase the length of the pedicle and adjust the thickness of the muscle.

The versatility is provided by the ability to plan and model the flap according to the size, amount and type of missing tissues to be reconstructed. The unique anatomy of the area allows for the elevation of composite flaps suited to a great variety of postoperative defects, especially complex ones involving different tissues. The amount of skin and muscle can also be modelled to fit the requirements of the defect. Large surfaces of the skin can be elevated, two skin paddles can be created, a simple muscular flap is possible, the bone from the scapula is available when appropriate and a functional reconstruction by nervous anastomosis is feasible. Although large skin paddles are elevated, due to the quality of the surrounding tissues, primary suture at the donor site is usually possible.

Whenever large volumes of tissue are necessary for the reconstruction, the latissimus dorsi flap is a reliable tissue source providing a good coverage and minimal postoperative sequelae.

References

1. Tansini I. Sopra il mio nuovo processo di amputazione della mammella. Gazz Med Ital Torino. 1906;57: 141–3.
2. Quillen CG, Shearin Jr JC, Georgiade NG. Use of the latissimus dorsi myocutaneous island flap for reconstruction in the head and neck area: case report. Plast Reconstr Surg. 1978;62(1):113–7.
3. Watson JS, Craig RD, Orton CI. The free latissimus dorsi myocutaneous flap. Plast Reconstr Surg. 1979;64(3):299–305.
4. Olvera-Caballero C, Hidalgo-Monroy P. Neurovascular musculocutaneous latissimus dorsi free-flap transfer for reconstruction of a major cheek defect with facial palsy in a 14-month-old child. Microsurgery. 2005; 25(5):373–7.
5. Safak T, Akyurek M. Primary one-stage reconstruction of cheek defect after a shotgun blast to the face: use of the latissimus dorsi musculocutaneous free flap for soft-tissue repair and facial reanimation. Ann Plast Surg. 2001;47(4):438–41.
6. Seitz A, Papp S, Papp C, Maurer H. The anatomy of the angular branch of the thoracodorsal artery. Cells Tissues Organs. 1999;164(4):227–36.
7. Wolff K-D, Hölzle F. Raising of microvascular flaps – a systematic approach. Berlin: Springer; 2005.
8. Maxwell GP, Stueber K, Hoopes JE. A free latissimus dorsi myocutaneous flap: case report. Plast Reconstr Surg. 1978;62(3):462–6.
9. Olivari N. Use of thirty latissimus dorsi flaps. Plast Reconstr Surg. 1979;64(5):654–61.
10. Becker Jr DW. A cervicopectoral rotation flap for cheek coverage. Plast Reconstr Surg. 1978;61(6): 868–70.
11. Becker FF, Langford FP. Deep-plane cervicofacial flap for reconstruction of large cheek defects. Arch Otolaryngol Head Neck Surg. 1996;122(9):997–9.

20 The Use of Radial Free Flap to Reconstruct Defects After Extended Parotidectomy

Victor-Vlad Costan, Eugenia I. Popescu, and Constantin-Cătălin Ciocan-Pendefunda

Abstract

The use of forearm free flap for reconstruction after extended parotidectomy is suitable for large superficial defects which may involve the skin, external and medial ear, zygomatic arch, and lateral part of malar bone. Due to its big surface and pliability, this flap is useful for extended and irregular skin defects. It is not ideal for deep defects with mandible or skull base resection in which cases we cannot achieve a good functional and aesthetic result. Not all patients with extended parotid tumors need resection of the facial nerve, but due to tumor status, such as extension, perineural spreading, histological pattern, and grading, most of them will undergo postoperative irradiation. For these cases, the flap ensures a good protection of the facial nerve against radiotherapy. A major disadvantage of this flap is the aesthetical appearance of donor site. In some cases, depending on the resected structures, such as bones, there might be postoperative facial asymmetry, which can be addressed later with lipostructure, leading to good aesthetic and functional outcome. Another immediate postoperative inconvenience is the color difference between the flap and recipient site, but later this will fade away.

V.-V. Costan, MD, DMD, PhD
Department of Oral and Maxillo-Facial Surgery, Faculty of Dental Medicine, "Grigore T. Popa" University of Medicine and Pharmacy, "St. Spiridon" University Hospital Iasi, Iasi, Romania
e-mail: victorcostan@gmail.com

E.I. Popescu, DMD, PhD
Department of Surgery (Dentoalveolar Surgery, Oral and Maxillofacial Surgery), Faculty of Dental Medicine, "Grigore T. Popa" University of Medicine and Pharmacy, Iasi, Romania
e-mail: jenypopescu@yahoo.com

C.-C. Ciocan-Pendefunda, MD, DMD, PhD (✉)
Oral and Maxillofacial Surgery, Fachklinik Hornheide Münster, Münster, Germany
e-mail: catalinciocan2004@yahoo.com; constantin-catalin.ciocan-pendefunda@fachklinik-hornheide.de

20.1 Introduction

Forearm free flap based on the radial artery, also known as the Chinese flap, was described for the first time by Yang in 1978 [1]. In 1982, Song et al. have published more than 100 successful transplanted flaps [2]. In 1981, Mühlbauer presented in the European literature the advantages of this flap: its pliability, thinness, long pedicle, easy to harvest, and relative constant anatomy [3, 4]. Later other authors had used this flap to reconstruct head and neck intraoral and skin defects [5]. The rich blood supply allows its use for

© Springer International Publishing Switzerland 2016
V.-V. Costan (ed.), *Management of Extended Parotid Tumors*, DOI 10.1007/978-3-319-26545-2_20

closure of perforating defects of the oral cavity [6]. Due to its big surface and pliability, this flap is useful for extended and irregular defects involving the skin and underlying tissues, for example, muscles and zygomatic arch [7, 8], such as after extended parotidectomy.

20.2 Anatomy

The pedicle of the flap is based on the radial artery, which together with cubital artery forms the deep palmar arch of the hand. This vessel lies in the lateral intermuscular septum, between the brachioradialis and flexor carpi radialis muscles [5, 9]. It gives between 9 and 17 collaterals to the antebrachial fascia, most of them lying in the distal third of the forearm [5]. These numerous branches form a dense fascial plexus which nourishes the entire antebrachial skin and that is why this is considered a fasciocutaneous flap [5].

Besides the radial artery, the blood supply of the skin of the hand and forearm comes also through the ulnar artery and anterior and posterior interosseous arteries. Bearing this in mind, we may harvest a forearm flap based on the ulnar artery in cases where this artery is damaged at the beginning of radial flap harvest [5]. But the disadvantage comes from a not reliable blood supply of the skin through these last vessels.

The drainage is made through the deep radial veins or superficial venous system and between these are many anastomoses [5]. In our cases we had extended dorsally the flap design in order to include the cephalic vein, and based on the anastomoses with the comitant veins, we were able to use it as drainage vessel.

20.3 Indications, Limitations, Advantages, and Disadvantages

The use of forearm free flap for reconstruction after extended parotidectomy is suitable for large superficial defects which may involve the skin, external and medial ear, and zygomatic arch.

Not all patients with extended parotid tumors need resection of the facial nerve, but due to tumor status, such as extension, perineural spreading, histological pattern, and grading, most of them will undergo postoperative irradiation. In cases where the nerve is left intact, the radial flap assures a good protection against radiotherapy.

It is not ideal for deep defects with mandible or skull base resection in which cases we cannot achieve a good functional [restoration of the mandible or preventing cerebral liquid fistulas] and aesthetic result.

There are authors who described the harvesting of this flap as an osteocutaneous flap including a bony segment of the radius in order to reconstruct bony defects [4, 10, 11]. But from our experience, we consider there are other more suitable reconstructive options for these bulky composite defects, such as latissimus dorsi, ALT in combination with fibula, or iliac crest free flap, depending on resected structures.

If we use forearm flap to reconstruct a deep defect after extended parotidectomy, we can have a postoperative facial asymmetry which can be corrected later with Coleman lipostructure technique. Usually this happens after partial resection of the malar bone along with the parotid tumor.

Another limitation is the general status of the patient, but this is a general pullback for all kinds of free flaps. If the patient cannot undergo such a complex reconstructive operation, we have to decide to a less consuming time covering technique, such as local flaps [rotation of the scalp, platysma myocutaneous flap] or local regional flaps [major pectoralis flap]. But in patients where we have to perform neck dissection together with tumor resection, the operation time is not that prolonged if a second team harvests the flap at the same time.

The advantages of this flap are [5]:

- It is thin and pliable with a large surface.
- Vessels have a large-caliber artery, 2–3 mm; comitant veins, 1–3 mm; and cephalic vein, 3–4 mm, and the anatomy is relative constant.
- Pedicle is long, so we are able to perform easily the anastomosis in the neck.

- The nourishing of the flap is variable and has ortho- and retrograde flow, and the venous drainage is made equally through superficial or profound system. The enlargement of anastomosis possibilities increases the indications of this flap, because we may choose recipient veins with different caliber. This aspect is very useful since a large number of cases undergo extended parotidectomy for lymph nodes metastases.
- Subcutaneous fatty tissue is poor and it does not tend to accumulate fat.
- We do not need to reposition the patient, so the harvesting can be performed at the same time with tumor surgery.
- This flap is easy to harvest so it is a good flap to begin free flap surgery.

Depending on the area which has to be reconstructed, we may design a flap with more or less hair. Usually we do not have to perform corrective surgeries, except the situation when there is a persistent facial asymmetry. Because this is a fasciocutaneous flap, it is very stable in time and even after irradiation does not tend to reduce its volume, such as a myocutaneous flap. The good blood supply reduces postoperative complications, such as wound dehiscence or partial necrosis.

Immediately postoperatively there is usually a considerable color difference between the flap and receiving area, but in time this will not be obvious anymore.

In our department we had never performed an anastomosis of a branch of the antebrachial cutaneous nerve to a sensory nerve of the recipient site in order to obtain the sensory recovery of the radial forearm flap. According to some authors and also from our experience, the sensation will be partially reestablished spontaneously after some years by secondary nerve sprouting [5].

This flap has also disadvantages, mainly regarding donor site. The interruption of radial artery means that the hand nourishing will be assured only through ulnar artery and anterior and posterior interosseous vessels. In order to prevent postoperative ischemia of the hand, it is mandatory to perform the Allen test preoperatively.

A major disadvantage is the aesthetic appearance of donor site. Some publications report a complication rate of 30–50 % for the donor site, most of them due to a poor site to integrate a skin graft [12–18]. Some authors had recommended various techniques for wound closure on the forearm, such as V-Y plasty, transposition flaps, and the use of tissue expanders [12–18]. But from our experience, the fabrication of a good receiving bed for skin graft is the best solution to reduce donor-site complications. In order to help the healing of the graft, we immobilize the hand for 10–14 days postoperatively.

Other disadvantages regarding donor-site morbidity are edema, paresthesia, and cold intolerance. Despite the lack of functional limitations, we prefer to harvest from the nondominant hand.

Postoperatively, the radial flap tends to have an edema due to the change of the vascularity from "flow-through" to "flow-in" [5].

If we compare this thin flap with latissimus dorsi or ALT, in some patients with extended composite defects, we may end up with facial asymmetry which can be later corrected.

Because harvesting of forearm flap means the interruption of one main vascular axe of the hand, an alternative would be the use of perforator-based free flaps, such as ALT, which brings more volume and has a less donor-site morbidity.

20.4 Clinical Application

To use a flap, free or pedicled, to cover a defect after extended parotidectomy means that it is mandatory to have clear margins. The only exception, when we may reconstruct such a defect with microscopically residual tumor, is a neoplasia which involves the skull base, but its complete resection is not achievable, such as squamous cell carcinomas with neurotropism. In these cases we have to close the defect quickly as possible so the patients could receive postoperative irradiation. The forearm free flap is very useful mainly for large defects after extended parotidectomy, but without the involvement of deeper structures, such as the mandible or skull base. For these, an option is latissimus dorsi free flap.

Most of the patients suitable for this reconstruction had undergone extended parotidectomy including resection of the skin (Fig. 20.1a, b), external ear, muscles [masseter, sternocleidomastoid, and temporal muscle], and zygomatic arch and partial resection of the malar bone (Fig. 20.2a–c). If intraoperatively only one ramus of the facial nerve is infiltrated by tumor, we have to resect it in order to obtain free margins, but we must preserve the other branches.

The covering of the defect may be performed at the same time with tumor resection, including neck dissection, where necessary, or in a second time if we are not certain of clear margins. In order to reduce the operating time, two-team approach is recommended. After a positive Allen test on both hands, it is better to choose as donor the nondominant side (Fig. 20.3a, b). Our experience recommends harvesting of the flap without a gauge, because the collateral branches can be easily identified, so dissection of the pedicle is carried out safe and the risk of bleeding from the flap after anastomoses is reduced.

Despite a longer harvesting time, we preferred to include for all cases the cephalic vein in the flap, and the anastomoses were performed at facial or superior thyroid artery and internal or, sometimes, external jugular vein. There were some situations when the drainage through the cephalic vein was not viable, so the venous anastomosis was performed using both comitant veins.

To close the donor site, we recommend split-thickness skin graft from the thigh, due to low morbidity of donor site and acceptable aesthetic and functional outcome of the forearm (Fig. 20.4).

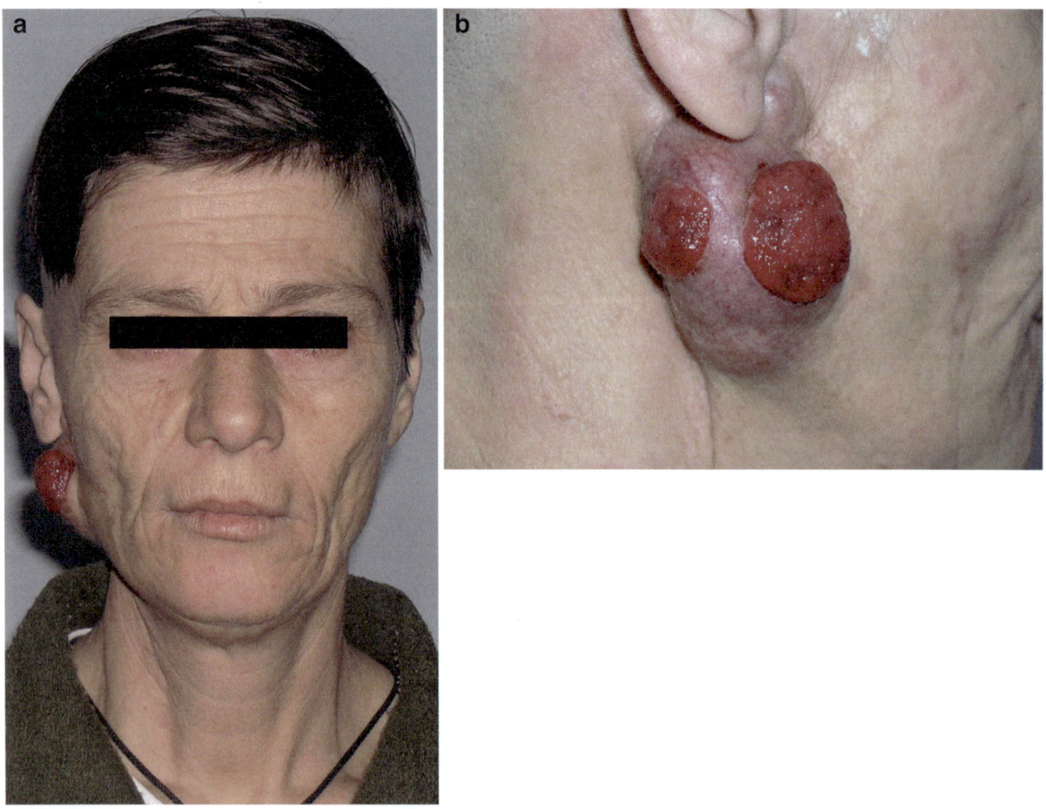

Fig. 20.1 (**a**, **b**) Relapse of an adenoid cystic carcinoma of the right parotid gland. The tumor infiltrated the overlying skin. The patient showed no involvement of the facial nerve. The treatment included extended parotidectomy en bloc with the affected skin, with the preservation of the nerve VII. At the same time a radical neck dissection modified was performed. After ensuring clear margins, the defect was covered using a radial free flap

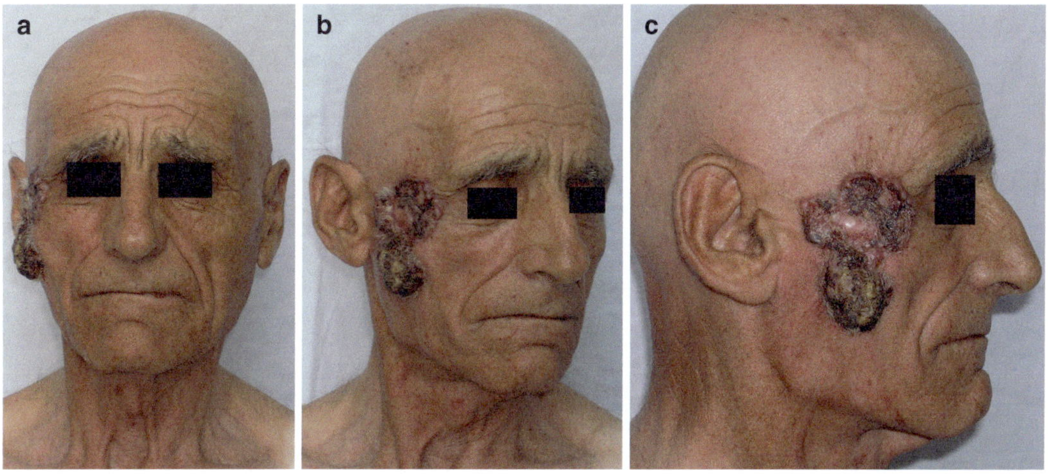

Fig. 20.2 (**a–c**) Patient with extensive adenoid cystic carcinoma of the skin with the infiltration of parotid gland, zygomatic arch, and malar bone right side. There was no preoperative facial paresis

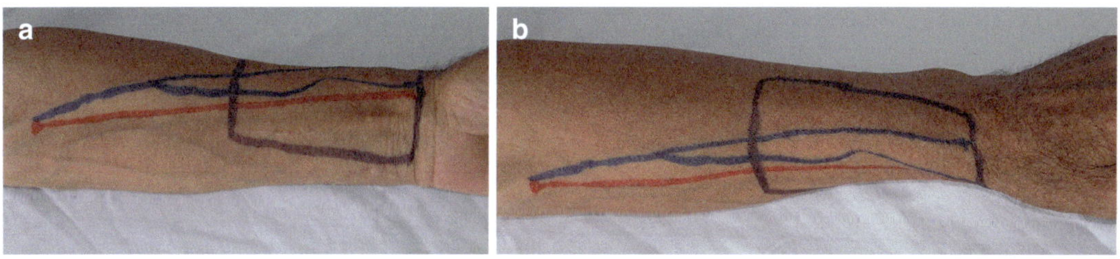

Fig. 20.3 (**a**, **b**) Due to large surface infiltration of the tumor, we may consider the radial flap the most suitable choice to cover the defect. Allen test was performed preoperatively. Anatomical landmarks and design of the forearm flap on the left hand. Dorsal extension of the skin paddle is noticeable in order to include the cephalic vein in the flap, so the venous drainage could be achieved through this vessel

The immediate postoperative result is good, with a slight facial asymmetry and paresis in cases where facial nerve was partially (Fig. 20.5) or totally sacrificed. The difference of color and texture between the flap and facial skin is easy to be noticed in the first postoperative months (Figs. 20.5 and 20.6). Later, the asymmetry may persist, but these color differences will fade away (Figs. 20.7a, b and 20.8a, b). The persistence of the facial asymmetry may be due to resection of the bony structures, or to postoperative radiotherapy, although the forearm free flap is relatively stable during irradiation with minimum change of volume.

In order to prevent traction on the nearby structures, such as the lower eyelid leading to ectropion, a suspension of the flap with some non-resorbable sutures to the bony structures is advisable. Despite this, some cases may present a light traction due to healing process. For these patients, we can perform in a second stage correction of ectropion using lateral canthopexy and loosening of the scar with insertion of a skin graft. In some cases lipostructure of the lower eyelid is also useful.

If we bear in mind that most of the patients need postoperative irradiation but not in all of them the nerve was resected, the forearm flap is a very good structure to protect the facial nerve and its branches against radiotherapy by forming a good vascularized barrier, reducing the incidence of sequelae.

In cases where tumor surgery involved resection of the external ear, partial or total, we may combine radial flap with an ear epithesis to obtain the best aesthetic outcome. This prosthesis is

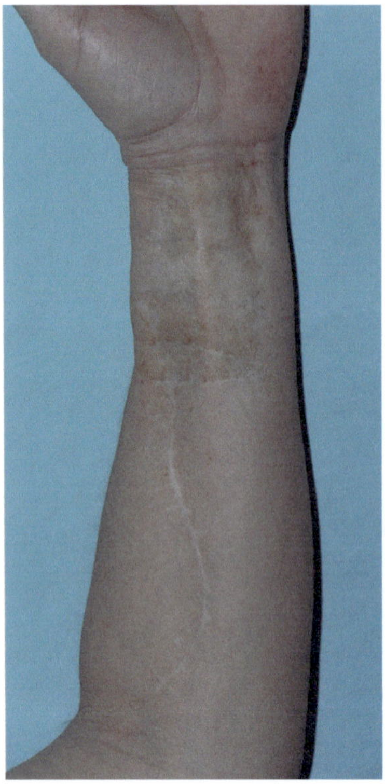

Fig. 20.4 Postoperative outcome of the donor site: the most common disadvantage is the aesthetic appearance of the inner side of the forearm, without any functional limitations. The patients may report increased sensitivity by cold of the forearm

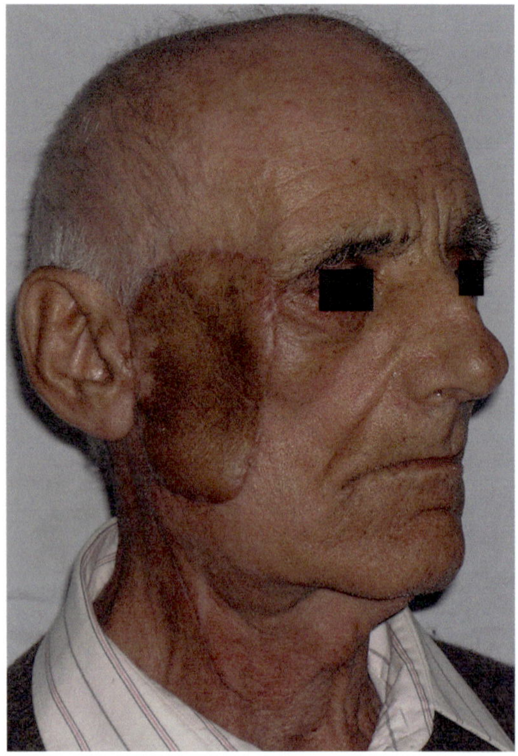

Fig. 20.5 Immediate postoperative result with a significant color difference comparative to facial skin. Intraoperatively the branch for the upper eyelid of the facial nerve was infiltrated from the tumor; so in order to obtain free margins we had to sacrifice it leading to paralytic lagophthalmos

fabricated in a second time, after the insertion of the implants and integration of the flap. We have to maintain permeable or to reopen the external conduct of the ear.

20.5 Sequelae and Complications

Sequelae and complications regarding the donor site have already been described earlier.

If we do not remove the entire parotid gland because the tumor arises from the skin and involves only the capsule or superficial lobe, some patients may have salivary fistula and/or salivary cyst. This can be addressed during the operation by injection of botulin toxin in the deep lobe of the parotid. Postoperative irradiation has its own role in reducing the incidence of salivary fistula.

When we use this flap for medium deep defects and the patients have no fatty tissue on the forearm, postoperatively they will have facial asymmetry (see Fig. 20.7a, b), which can be addressed later with lipostructure leading to good aesthetic and functional outcome.

Sometimes, because of the traction due to gravity, facial paralyses, and healing process, patients can present ectropion. When possible, the best way is to prevent it by using suspension sutures of the flap onto bony structures. But if ectropion appears even after these prophylactic measures, we can address it through specific correction described in other chapters, such as lateral canthopexy or shortening of the lower eyelid.

The other complications or sequelae, such as facial paralysis with lagophthalmos, are due to extended parotidectomy and not to reconstructive technique and are treated in other chapters.

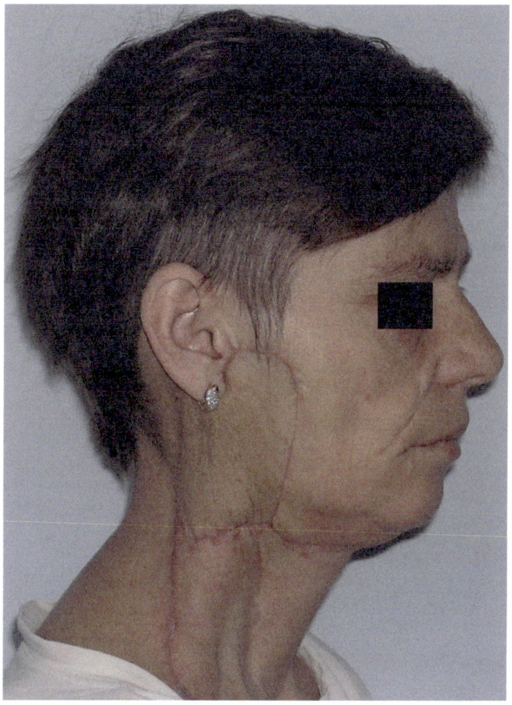

Fig. 20.6 One month postoperatively, we can notice a difference in color and texture between the flap and surrounding facial skin

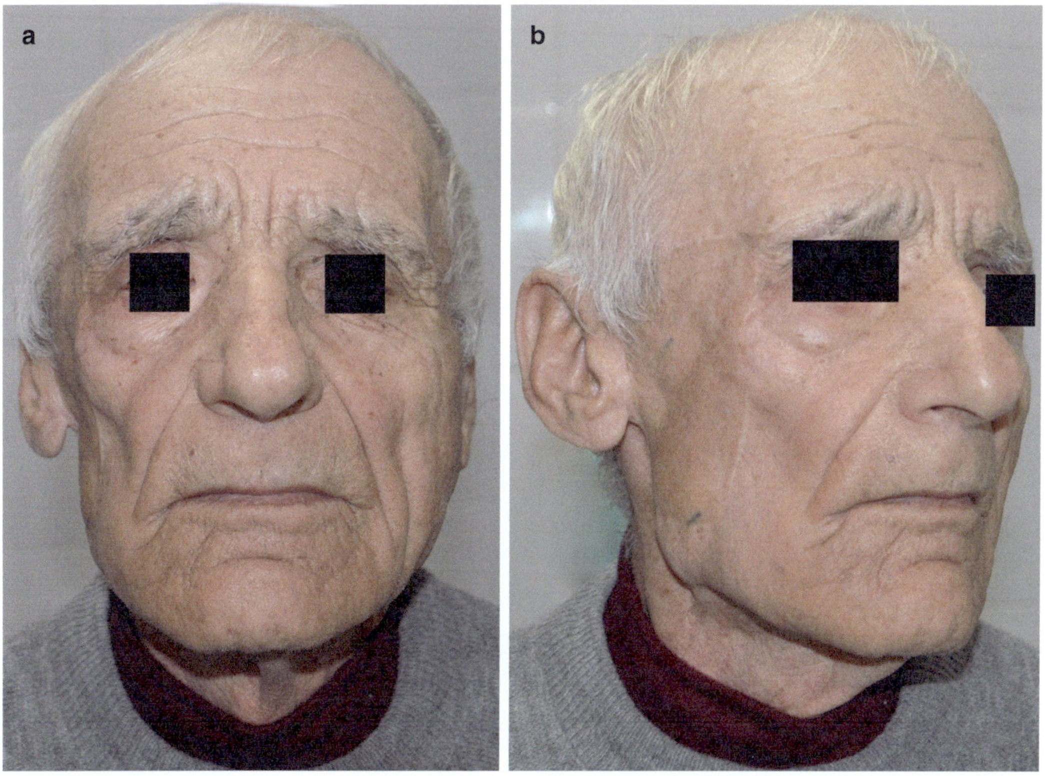

Fig. 20.7 (**a**, **b**) At 6 years of tumor-free survival. The patient has a slight facial asymmetry, which can be corrected with lipostructure, but we address this issue in other chapters. The color and texture differences compared to nearby skin are very hard to notice

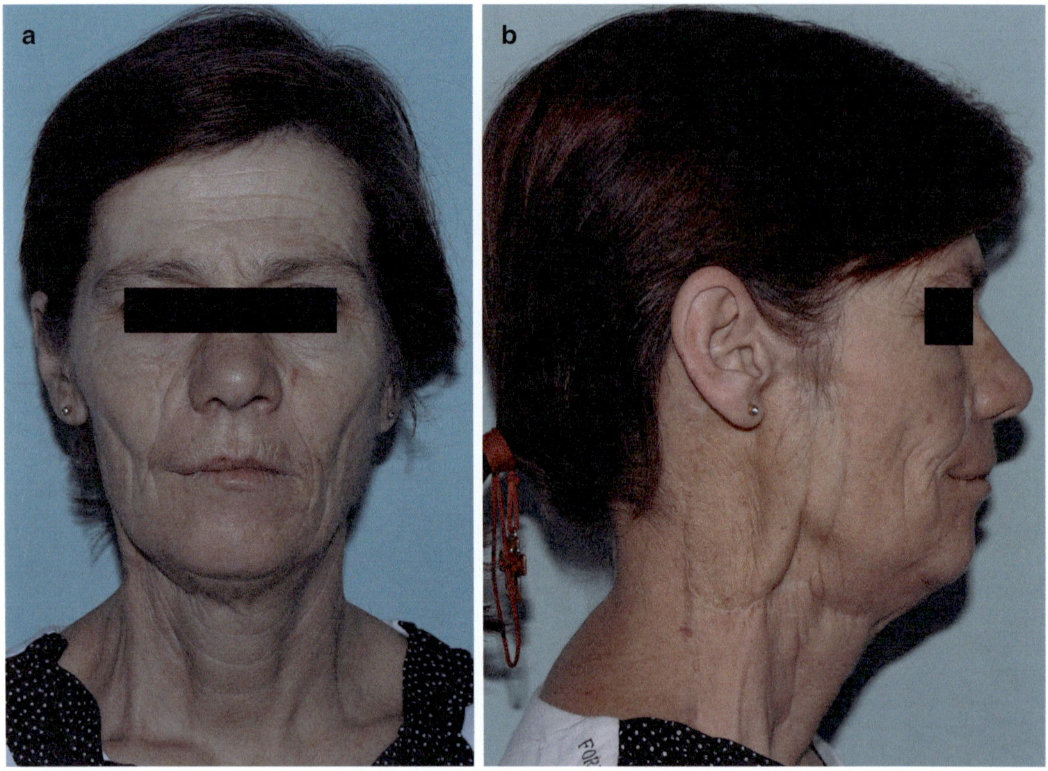

Fig. 20.8 (**a**, **b**) At 5 years of tumor-free survival. The previous difference of color and texture is diminished. Compared to the other case, despite the postoperative adjuvant therapy, there is no facial asymmetry. This may be due to the preservation of underlying bony structures. The function of the facial nerve is intact

References

1. Yang G, Chen B, Gao Y, Liu X, Li J, Jiang S, He S. Forearm free skin transplantation. Natl Med J China. 1981;61:139.
2. Song R, Gao Y. The forearm flap. Clin Plast Surg. 1982;9:21.
3. Mühlbauer W, Olbrisch RR, Herndl E, Stock W. Die Behandlung der Halskontraktur nach Verbrennung mit dem freien Unterarmlappen. Chirurg. 1981; 52:635.
4. Mühlbauer W, Herndl E, Stock W. The forearm flap. Plast Reconstr Surg. 1982;70:336.
5. Wolff KD, Hölzle F. Raising of microvascular flaps. Berlin: Springer; 2005. p. 1–20.
6. Boorman JG, Green MF. A split Chinese forearm flap for simultaneous oral lining and skin cover. Br J Plast Surg. 1986;39:179.
7. McGregor IA, McGregor FM. Cancer of the face and mouth. Philadelphia: Churchill Livingstone; 1986.
8. Coessens A, Van Geertruyden J, De Mey A. Surgical tattooing as an aesthetic improvement in facial reconstruction with a free radial forearm flap. J Reconstr Microsurg. 1993;9:331–4.
9. Urken ML, Cheney ML, Sullivan MJ, Biller HF. Atlas of regional and free flaps for head and neck reconstruction. New York: Raven; 1990.
10. Soutar DS, Widdowson WP. Immediate reconstruction of the mandible using a vascularized segment of the radius. Head Neck Surg. 1986;39:176.
11. Stock W, Stock M. Der osteokutane Unterarmlappen. Handchirurgie. 1983;15:49.
12. Bardsley AF, Soutar DS, Elliot D, Batchelor AG. Reducing morbidity in the radial forearm flap donor site. Plast Reconstr Surg. 1990;86:287.
13. Elliot D, Bardsley AF, Batchelor AG, Soutar DS. Direct closure of the radial forearm flap donor defect. Br J Plast Surg. 1988;41:358.
14. Fenton OM, Roberts JO. Improving the donor site of the radial forearm flap. Br J Plast Surg. 1985;38:504.
15. Hallock GG. Refinement of the radial forearm flap donor site using skin expansion. Plast Reconstr Surg. 1988;81:21.
16. Hallock GG. Complications of 100 consecutive local fasciocutaneous flaps. Plast Reconstr Surg. 1991;88:264.
17. Masser MR. The preexpanded radial free flap. Plast Reconstr Surg. 1990;86:295.
18. Timmons MJ, Missotten FEM, Poole MD, Davies DM. Complications of radial forearm flap donor sites. Br J Plast Surg. 1986;39(2):176–8.

21 Attitude Toward the Facial Nerve in Extended Parotidectomy

Eugenia I. Popescu, Constantin-Cătălin Ciocan-Pendefunda, and Victor-Vlad Costan

Abstract

The facial nerve crosses the parotid tissue and considering the initial location malignancies can grow to engulf one or several branches of the nerve on different lengths or even the main trunk of the nerve, and removal of the involved segments must be performed together with the tumor. The functional sequelae following interruption can be quite debilitating for the patient, and reconstruction of the nerve should be performed whenever possible in order to ensure a good quality of life. The outcomes of the reconstruction are different depending on the moment of reconstruction and the chosen method. A wide range of reconstructive techniques are available and must be carefully selected in order to suit each case and ensure acceptable restoration of nerve function.

21.1 Introduction

Tumors frequently associated with facial nerve invasion are the ones arising in the deep lobe of the gland, salivary duct malignancies, and tumors of increased size [1]. The characteristic of deep lobe malignancies is the invasion of the main trunk of the nerve, making the reconstruction problematic, in contrast to tumors of the superficial lobe that most often invade one or more branches of the nerve. Different from the simple invasion from an adjacent tumor, perineural spread is a characteristic exhibited by certain histological types like cutaneous squamous cell carcinoma and adenoid cystic carcinoma, and it can lead to the malignancy skipping to structures situated at a certain distance from the primary tumor [2]. This can lead to incomplete tumor removal

E.I. Popescu, DMD, PhD
Department of Surgery (Dentoalveolar Surgery, Oral and Maxillofacial Surgery), Faculty of Dental Medicine, "Grigore T. Popa" University of Medicine and Pharmacy, Iasi, Romania

C.-C. Ciocan-Pendefunda, MD, DMD, PhD
Department of Oral and Maxillofacial Surgery, Fachklinik Hornheide Münster, Nordrhein-Westfalen, Germany

V.-V. Costan, MD, DMD, PhD (✉)
Department of Oral and Maxillo-Facial Surgery, Faculty of Dental Medicine, "Grigore T. Popa" University of Medicine and Pharmacy, "St. Spiridon" University Hospital Iasi, Iasi, Romania
e-mail: victorcostan@gmail.com

© Springer International Publishing Switzerland 2016
V.-V. Costan (ed.), *Management of Extended Parotid Tumors*, DOI 10.1007/978-3-319-26545-2_21

and continuation of evolution. An example is the invasion of intracranial structures by the malignancy spreading along the course of the facial nerve, following its entrance into the skull base.

21.2 Diagnosis of Facial Nerve Invasion

Preoperative assessment of facial nerve function is imperative in deciding the fate of the nerve. Absence of paresis or paralysis does not guarantee the absence of tumor infiltration, but the presence of paralysis certifies the necessity for facial nerve resection even when there is no intraoperative macroscopic evidence of malignant invasion.

The assessment of the extent of tumor infiltration of the facial nerve and the presence of perineural spread can be performed by the use of imagistic techniques, collaborated with good knowledge of the local anatomy. Since the facial nerve has both an intraosseous and a soft tissue course, there is usually the need to combine imaging techniques for best results. Although the presence of paralysis incriminates the invasion of the facial nerve, the extent of the invasion, particularly the intracranial invasion, either direct or by perineural spread, is best determined by the use of CT scan. The intracranial course of the nerve is best visualized by the use of high-resolution temporal bone CT. For the extracranial course of the nerve, soft tissue invasion is best determined with the help of contrast-enhanced MRI. Perineural tumor spread is considered possible when there is evidence of enlargement of the nerve contour, contrast enhancement, and obliteration of the fat pad surrounding the nerve [3].

21.3 Surgical Management

When facial nerve weakness is not clinically obvious but intraoperatively we notice a nerve branch entering or crossing the tumor, it is a clear sign that the concerned branch cannot be preserved. Considering the starting point of the tumor and the extent of invasion of the neighboring tissues, one or more branches of the nerve can become involved by malignancy, even the main trunk. The branches that do not appear to be infiltrated intraoperatively, and in the absence of clinical signs of paralysis, can and should be preserved whenever possible in order to minimize the sequelae. This is especially important regarding the temporofacial division of the facial nerve. Very often it is possible to preserve this branch by careful dissection and avoid the postoperative lagophthalmos, one of the most bothering consequences.

When the main trunk of the facial nerve is engulfed by tumor, ensuring free surgical margins can imply an additional mastoidectomy. Intracranial invasion must also be considered both due to the proximity of the skull base and the possibility of perineural spread exhibited by certain histologic types.

Even when desired, preservation of the nerve is not always an easy task in the case of extended parotid masses that tend to invade or obstruct the usual surgical landmarks used to identify the nerve. If the facial nerve is free of tumor but difficult to expose due to the size or location of the malignancy, retrograde dissection can come in handy. If we are able to identify clearly just one of the peripheral branches, it can be traced back to the main trunk. The temporal branch is usually thicker and can be identified with greater ease, but in other cases the marginal mandibular branch can be easily spotted crossing the facial vein in the submandibular region and followed backward. In rare cases, mastoidectomy can also help expose the main trunk of the nerve.

When the tumor belongs to the deep lobe of the gland, the nerve can be dissected off both sides and lifted to expose and remove the tumor, but due to increased size of the mass, it is sometimes necessary to transect certain branches, most often the buccal ones, in order to remove the entire tumor safely. A neurorrhaphy of the transected nerve can then be performed.

21.4 Facial Nerve Reconstruction

By the use of multimodal treatment, the survival of patients with parotid gland malignancy is increasing, and at the same time, the quality of life of these patients should be ensured. It used to be considered that for elderly patients suffering from malignancy, static procedures of facial reanimation should be preferred due to the disadvantage of increasing the operation time without certainty of a real long-term benefit, but it is now desired that the dynamic reconstruction of the facial nerve performed at the same time with the removal of the tumor should be attempted in all cases [4].

Whenever possible, it is best to perform the reconstruction of the nerve during the initial surgery [5], in order to increase the chances of achieving acceptable nerve function but also to avoid the difficult dissection in case of a second surgery with distortion of the local anatomy, presence of fibrous tissue, adherences, and increased risk of facial nerve injury during the dissection.

When the reconstruction of the facial nerve is performed during the initial surgery for tumor removal, most likely patients will further undergo multimodal treatment, especially postoperative radiotherapy. The results of the reconstruction of the facial nerve do not seem to be altered by postoperative radiotherapy [5].

The simplest option for nerve reconstruction is when, by increase in tumor size, there is also an elongation of the nerve branches or even of the trunk of the nerve. In this manner it is possible for the intratumoral course of the nerve to be removed together with the tumor, and at the same time the continuity of the nerve can be restored by end-to-end anastomosis (Fig. 21.1a–e).

If facial nerve reconstruction is to be performed at a later time, the interrupted nerve ends can be marked during the initial surgery using surgical sutures in order to facilitate their finding in the following operation. When facial nerve repair surgery could not be performed at the same time with tumor ablation, the best results can be achieved the first 2 months postoperatively. After this time a slowly progressing denervation process begins together with muscle atrophy and fibrosis, and it is considered that after 2 years the reconstruction of the nerve must be associated with muscle transfer in order to obtain significant results [6].

When the facial nerve branches have been transected for access to the tumor, they can be immediately anastomosed after the removal of the mass, but when a certain length of the branch has been resected, direct suture between nerve ends is not possible without increased tension that would compromise the outcome, and therefore it is necessary to select an appropriate reconstruction method.

Various dynamic and static methods of reconstruction have been imagined to suit the variety of clinical situations considering the level of nerve interruption, the length to be reconstructed, and availability of regional or distant tissues for reconstruction, the general condition of the patient, and the time passed from the initial surgery [7].

The most popular technique is nerve grafting using the greater auricular nerve or sural nerve and interposition of the graft in between the proximal and distal ends of the facial nerve. The greater auricular nerve is easy to harvest since it is located near to the surgical field and has the advantage of splitting in several arms that can be used to reconstruct more than one branches of the facial nerve. Unfortunately, in some cases of extended parotid tumors, due to the proximity of the nerve, it can become infiltrated by the tumor, and another reconstructive technique becomes necessary. Due to the length available for harvesting, the sural nerve is especially useful in cross-facial grafting. But increased length of the graft, especially longer than 4–5 cm, is associated with poor postoperative functional results. The main reason is that in longer grafts it takes axons a longer time to reach the distal anastomosis and fibrous tissue will form in the meantime [8]. In older patients, the potential for facial regeneration after the use of interposition grafts is decreased, and it is stated that end-to-end anastomosis techniques can lead to more reliable postoperative results [8].

When the proximal end of the nerve is either too short or not available, the reconstruction can be performed either by cross-facial grafting or by anastomosing the distal end of the facial to a local nerve, like the hypoglossal nerve when it is available.

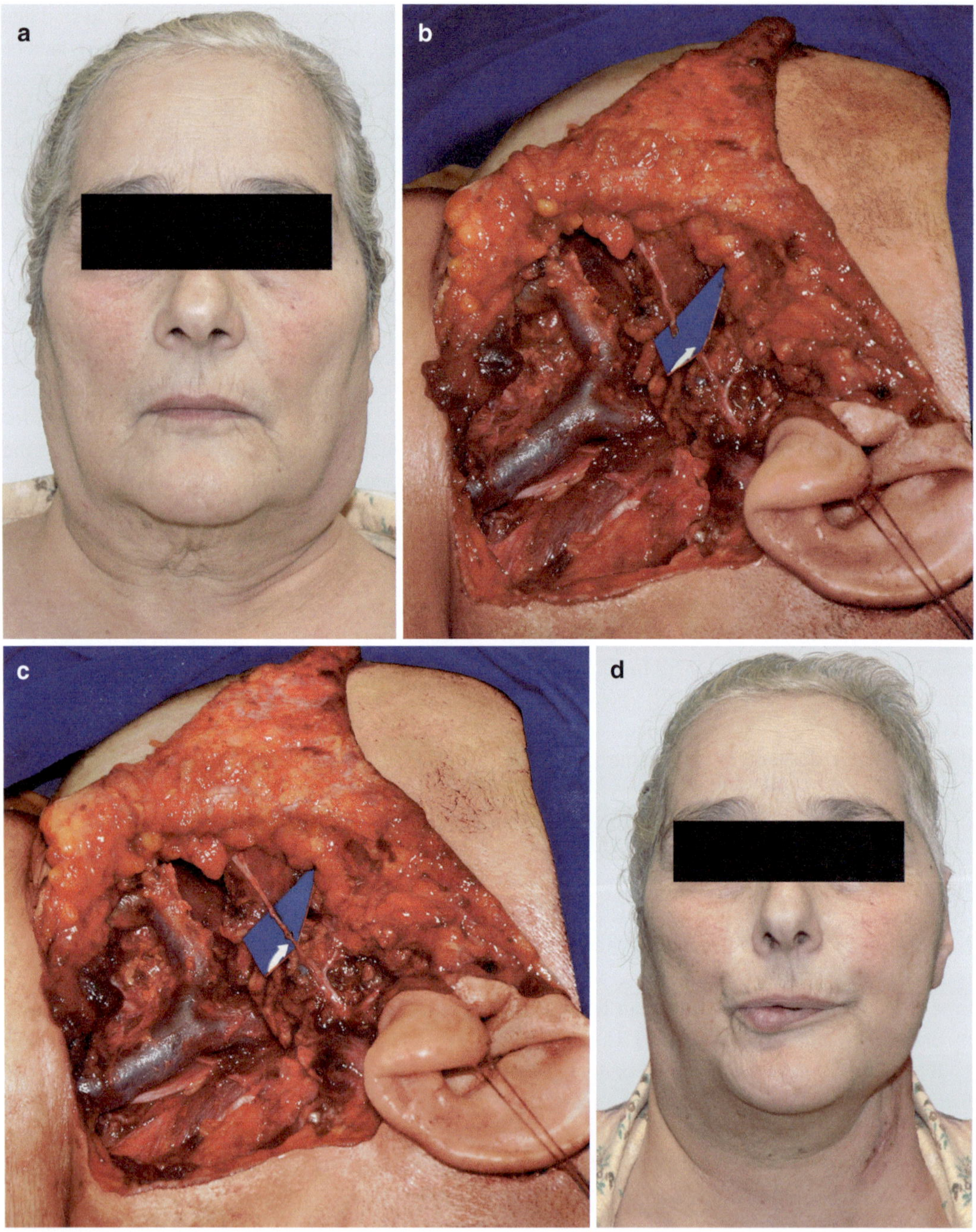

Fig. 21.1 (**a**) Tumor of the left parotid gland; no signs of facial nerve paralysis. (**b**) The intratumoral course of the cervicofacial branch of the facial nerve made it necessary to remove the intratumoral segment of the nerve. (**c**) The increase in tumor volume led to the increase in length of the facial nerve so that after tumor removal it was possible to perform an end-to-end anastomosis of the cervicofacial branch. (**d**) Obvious signs of paralysis of the cervicofacial ramus 1 month postoperatively. (**e**) Six months postoperatively, the nervous regeneration can be considered complete with restoration of facial symmetry

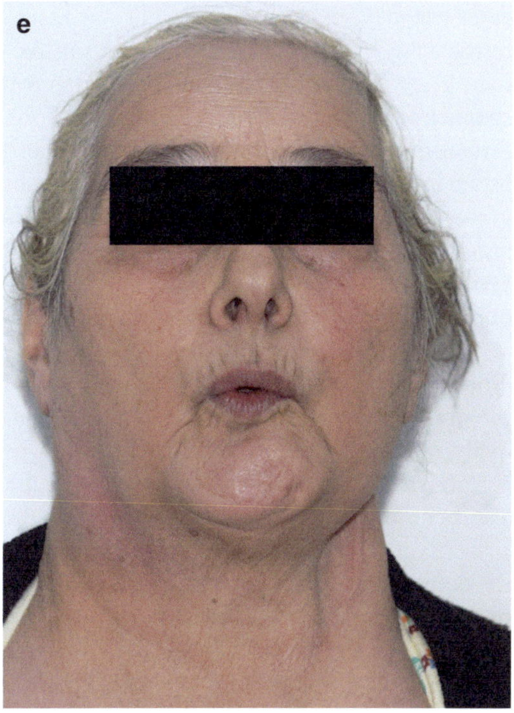

Fig. 21.1 (continued)

Cross-facial grafting comes with the disadvantage of a mild transient facial nerve paresis on the contralateral side that must be accepted by the patient. End-to-end anastomosis to the hypoglossal nerve will lead to the hemiparesis of the tongue and associated speech and masticatory impairment. Additionally, facial movements are not spontaneous responses to emotions, but are achieved by voluntary movements of the tongue [8].

Combined techniques can decrease the functional sequelae, like in the case of the hypoglossal-facial side-to-end jump nerve anastomosis that uses a greater auricular nerve graft to gap the distance between the proximal ends of the facial nerve and the hypoglossal nerve, using a side-to-end anastomosis in order to avoid complete impairment of the hypoglossal function [6]. Other regional nerves have been tried for the same type of anastomosis, such as the accessory nerve or parts of the cervical plexus and the descending branch of the hypoglossal nerve, but the results were shown to be less satisfactory and the sequelae at the donor site more debilitating for the patient [9].

In the particular case of extended tumors leading to extensive postoperative defects and the need for free flap reconstruction, it is always an option to perform the reconstruction of the facial nerve by anastomosing the proximal end to the nerve of the flap or use it as a vascularized nerve graft to bridge the existing defect [9]. Especially when there are no sufficient soft tissues left after tumor ablation to cover the facial nerve [10], or in the case of preoperative radiotherapy, revision surgery with existing adherences, or when performing a late reconstruction, a free vascularized nerve graft can offer an optimal solution with good functional recovery [11]. The dorsal nerve of the latissimus dorsi flap can be harvested as part of a neuromusculocutaneous flap aiming to achieve a functional muscular transfer by direct anastomosis to the proximal end of the facial nerve. Depending on the characteristics of the defect, when a more pliable thin flap is desired, a radial flap harvested together with the superficial branch of the radial nerve as a neurofasciocutaneous flap can offer great results by using the nerve as a vascularized graft to connect the proximal and distal ends of the facial nerve [12]. The neuromuscular free flaps can also be used in association with cross-facial nerve suture for dynamic reanimation when the proximal end of the facial nerve has been resected during tumor ablation. Given the proportion between the loss of soft tissue volume or skin coverage, a suitable flap is chosen for the reconstruction, and generally for any choice made, a suitable local nerve at the donor site can be elevated together with the flap and used for facial nerve reconstruction [4]. Modern concepts of facial nerve repair aim at obtaining spontaneous facial movements by combining existing techniques, a goal that can be achieved even in the case of plasty following extended parotidectomy and associating transection and unavailability of the main trunk of the nerve, by performing free muscular flaps neurotized by the contralateral facial nerve [13].

Dynamic repair can also be performed using a temporalis, masseter, or digastric muscle plasty. The temporalis muscle can be especially useful for treating the postoperative lagophthalmos and lifting the oral commissure, as an alternative to the more complex techniques of nerve grafting, in certain cases where fast results are desired by means of a simple procedure [14]. Another simple but static alternative method is the upper lid loading by insertion of a gold plate, and it can be completed by suspension of the cheek region or lower lid surgery to improve palpebral competence. Additional procedures to help improve the appearance are represented by brow lift, lateral canthopexy, tarsorrhaphy, and minor adjustments with the use of botulinum toxin [7]. The various methods used for treating postoperative lagophthalmos make the subject of Chap. 22.

Static reanimation procedures by suspension of the soft tissues are especially important when dealing with extended parotid malignancy, in cases where the extensive removal of soft tissues restricts the possibility of a dynamic reconstruction. They offer a simple solution to improve symmetry and tonus and therefore help perform certain functions. The static techniques are also useful in association with dynamic procedures or in the case of failure of the dynamic reconstruction [5]. The lifting of the tissues will even help eye closure by volume effect, as well as mastication by lifting the corner of the mouth. The overall improvement of the facial appearance, especially when smiling, increases the quality of life of the patients with the advantage of a minimally invasive and short procedure that can be performed under local anesthesia (Fig. 21.2a, b). The same principle can be applied even for the suspension of bulky flaps used for the plasty of the defect, such as the latissimus dorsi. The use of such a heavy flap will initially pull down on

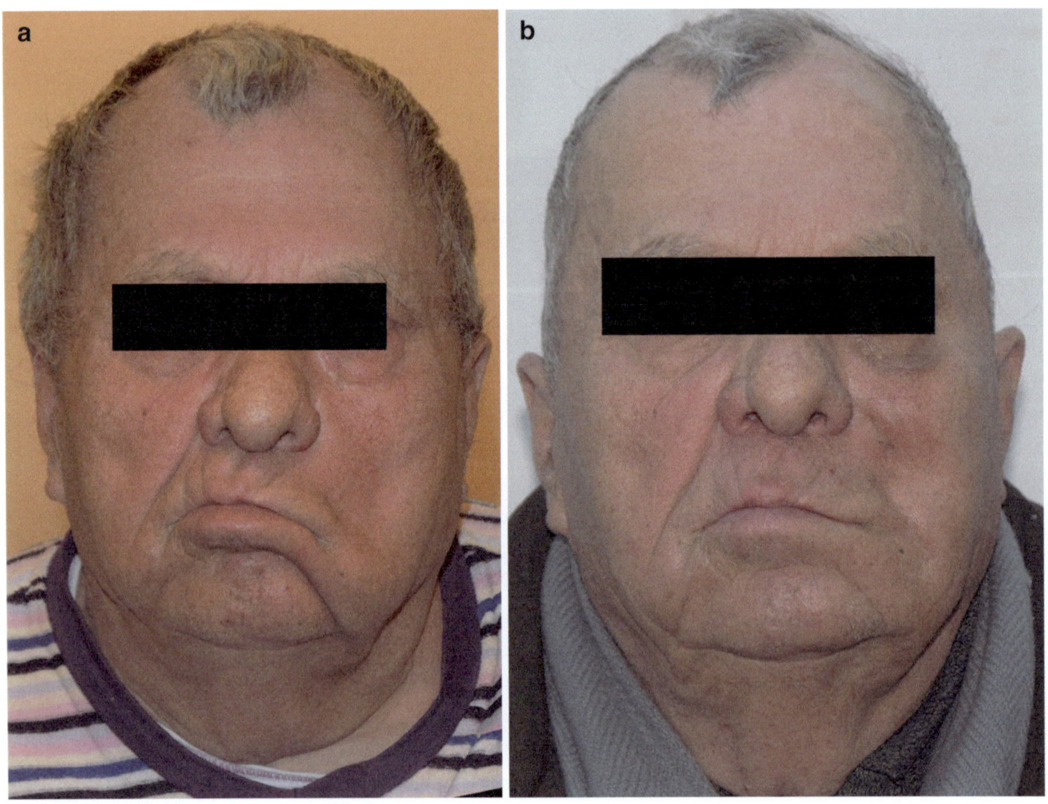

Fig. 21.2 (**a**) Postoperative paralysis of the facial nerve. (**b**) The result of the static facial reanimation by the use of sling sutures suspended in the temporal region is a favorable one, with good aesthetic results by raising of the oral commissure and reinforcement of the cheek musculature that allows the improvement of phonation, mastication, and deglutition, with excellent results regarding the oral competence

the tissues, accentuating the signs of facial paralysis, but this inconvenience can be overcome by the use of sling sutures.

References

1. Preis M, Soudry E, Bachar G, Shufel H, Feinmesser R, Shpitzer T. Predicting facial nerve invasion by parotid gland carcinoma and outcome of facial reanimation. Eur Arch Otorhinolaryngol. 2010;267(1):107–11. doi:10.1007/s00405-009-0968-x.
2. Liebig C, Ayala G, Wilks JA, Berger DH, Albo D. Perineural invasion in cancer: a review of the literature. Cancer. 2009;115(15):3379–91.
3. Gupta S, Mends F, Hagiwara M, Fatterpekar G, Roehm PC. Imaging the facial nerve: a contemporary review. Radiol Res Pract. 2013. doi:10.1155/2013/248039.
4. Iseli TA, Harris G, Dean NR, Iseli CE, Rosenthal EL. Outcomes of static and dynamic facial nerve repair in head and neck cancer. Laryngoscope. 2010;120(3):478–83. doi:10.1002/lary.20789.
5. Renkonen S, Sayed F, Keski-Säntti H, Ylä-Kotola T, Bäck L, Suominen S, Kanerva M, Mäkitie AA. Reconstruction of facial nerve after radical parotidectomy. Acta Otolaryngol. 2015;10:1–5.
6. Volk GF, Pantel M, Guntinas-Lichius O. Modern concepts in facial nerve reconstruction. Head Face Med. 2010;6:25. doi:10.1186/1746-160X-6-25. PMCID: PMC2984557.
7. Tate JR, Tollefson TT. Advances in facial reanimation. Curr Opin Otolaryngol Head Neck Surg. 2006; 14(4):242–8.
8. Myers EN, Ferris RL. Salivary gland disorders. Berlin: Springer; 2007.
9. Terzis JK, Konofaos P. Nerve transfers in facial palsy. Facial Plast Surg. 2008;24:177–93. doi:10.1055/s-2008-1075833.
10. Chuang DC. Free tissue transfer for the treatment of facial paralysis. Facial Plast Surg. 2008;24(2):194–203. doi:10.1055/s-2008-1075834.
11. Kimata Y1, Sakuraba M, Hishinuma S, Ebihara S, Hayashi R, Asakage T. Free vascularized nerve grafting for immediate facial nerve reconstruction. Laryngoscope. 2005;115(2):331–6.
12. Urken ML, Weinberg H, Vickery C, Biller HF. The neurofasciocutaneous radial forearm flap in head and neck reconstruction: a preliminary report. Laryngoscope. 1990;100(2 Pt 1):161–73.
13. Gousheh J, Arasteh E. Treatment of facial paralysis: dynamic reanimation of spontaneous facial expression-apropos of 655 patients. Plast Reconstr Surg. 2011;128(6):693e–703. doi:10.1097/PRS.0b013e318230c58f.
14. Boahene KD. Dynamic muscle transfer in facial reanimation. Facial Plast Surg. 2008;24(2):204–10. doi:10.1055/s-2008-1075835.

The Management of Lagophthalmos in Facial Nerve Paralysis

22

Orlando Guntinas-Lichius

Abstract

Restoring the eyelid and tearing function is challenging for the head and neck surgeon performing facial reanimation surgery. A detailed eye examination is the basis to choose the best options for the individual patient. Treatment normally starts with medical treatment like using eye drops and ointments to protect the eye. In case of permanent facial palsy and especially when nonsurgical treatment fails to solve the problems, surgical treatment is indicated. There are a variety of standardized surgical techniques available to improve the function of the upper eyelid, the lower eyelid, the brow, and the forehead. The most important procedures are presented in this chapter. Treatment of periocular synkinesis is primarily an indication for botulinum toxin injections but surgery might also be an option. Finally, the treatment of the lacrimal system should not be overseen, that is, most often performed in collaboration with an ophthalmologist.

22.1 Introduction

A facial palsy caused by a parotid tumor infiltrating the extratemporal facial nerve or as a consequence of parotid surgery causes primarily two major problems: abnormalities of the upper and lower eyelid position and defective tearing. Incomplete eye closure (i.e., lagophthalmos) leads to a dry eye. The consequence could be acute and chronic inflammation of the eye with ocular irritation, ulceration, or even loss of corneal sensation, corneal perforation, and blindness. Defective tearing is the result of decreased tear production. Furthermore, the paralytic ectropion of the lower eyelid can additionally influence the flow of the tears. Besides the functional deficits, the incomplete eye closure and especially an ectropion in patients with long-term palsy are visible to any counterpart and promote the stigmatization of the patients. In this chapter, a systematic evaluation of the function of the patient's eye with major focus on the lagophthalmos is presented. The medical management of such problems is presented. Surgery to reanimate the eyelid

O. Guntinas-Lichius, MD
Department of Otorhinolaryngology,
University Hospital Jena, Jena, Germany
e-mail: orlando.guntinas@med.uni-jena.de

© Springer International Publishing Switzerland 2016

V.-V. Costan (ed.), *Management of Extended Parotid Tumors*, DOI 10.1007/978-3-319-26545-2_22

function is indicated if medical management fails [1, 2]. Of course, facial nerve reanimation surgery (details in Chap. 21) will produce the best results in patients with permanent facial palsy concerning corneal protection and to correct malposition eyelid. If such surgery is not possible or as adjuvant measures, some smaller surgical procedures might be helpful and will be presented.

22.2 Clinical Examination

The patient history is focused on the reasons, duration, and severity of the eye and tearing problems [3]. It is important to get information on the severity of the facial nerve damage and of the probability of a sufficient regeneration. In case of a permanent facial nerve lesion or of the nerve branches responsible for the muscles involved in eye closure, the management will differ from a patient in whom a restoration of the eye closure can be expected within the next months. Concerning the ocular complaints, symptoms for first complications have to be asked. It is important to know if the patient already developed symptoms like redness, irritation, or dryness. The absence of the reflex rolling up and out of the cornea to close the eye is known as Bell's phenomenon. The so-called BAD syndrome consists of a lack of Bell's phenomenon, anesthetic cornea, and a dry eye. Ocular problems like refractive errors not related to the palsy can aggravate the situation.

The basis of the physical examination is an evaluation of the visual acuity and the visual fields of both eyes. The pupils are controlled. The conjunctivae are inspected for irritation and inflammation. The corneal sensation should be tested. One may need the help from an ophthalmologist. The photodocumentation, which is normally used in any patient with facial palsy, helps to quantify the level of the eyebrow. A brow ptosis is evaluated at rest and with elevation of the forehead and compared to the healthy side. The eyelid approximation is tested with involuntary blink and during voluntary effort. At best, this effort is also photographically documented. The eyelid approximation is primarily a function of the upper eyelid. The lower eyelid may be affected by an ectropion. This leads to a punctual eversion which leads then to epiphora and corneal drying. Schirmer's test helps to quantify the tear production. In case of complication of incomplete eye closure, the patients should be examined every few days during treatment. If nonsurgical treatment occurs to be insufficient, decision making for surgery should not be hesitated.

22.3 Nonsurgical Treatment

Medical treatment accomplices the surgical treatment or may be the primary treatment of choice in patients with favorable diagnosis not needing a surgical therapy [4, 5]. The aim of the medical treatment is to improve the humidification of the affected eye. There are manifold eye drops and ointments on the market to protect the cornea. Often, the patient has to test several products as the tolerance is very variable. Taping is a simple method to keep the eye open, or vice versa, to keep the eye closed to protect the cornea. Taping the brow to the upper lid holds the upper lid in an upward position and therefore simply improves the vision. When taping should be used for eye closure, an ointment is used to protect the cornea. The tape should not rub against the bulbus. During daytime there should be period with an open eye. Taping can also be used to overcome an ectropion of the lower eyelid: The tape is first fixed to the center of the lower lid. Then it is pulled laterally and fixed to the lateral orbital margin with tension upward and laterally. Botulinum toxin A injection into the supratarsal fold to paralyze the levator palpebrae muscle induces a ptosis and is therefore a nonsurgical alternative to close the eye. Of course, reversible restriction of the vision is a disadvantage of such a chemical procedure. This method is helpful if a transient coverage of the cornea is needed in cases of corneal ulceration. Other nonsurgical measures to protect the eye are to use protective soft lenses, special sun glasses, and moisture chambers (Fig. 22.1a). Moisture chambers are cheap and therefore popular. Take care that the patient does not use them day and night because the periorbital skin will suffer from a permanent humidification. A better alternative is to fix an external lid weight on the skin of the upper eyelid (see Fig. 22.1b). These weights are derived from the implantable lid weights (see Sect. 22.5) but of much cheaper material. Finally, conservative management also includes hairstyle, eyeglasses, and makeup to camouflage facial asymmetry in the eye region compared to the healthy side.

22.4 Surgical Treatment

In case of permanent facial palsy, first it should be evaluated if reconstruction of the facial nerve is possible (details in Chap. 21). Surgical reanimation to induce a reinnervation of the facial nerve branches for the eye region will produce the best functional results concerning the eye function. But such reinnervation needs time. For instance, reconstruction of the main trunk of the facial nerve needs at least 12 months to yield a sufficient active eye closure. Therefore, additional surgical measures might be indicated to bridge this period. Furthermore, such adjuvant surgery, presented in the next subsection, applied synchronously or in a later session can support the results of facial nerve surgery.

22.5 Surgery of the Upper Eyelid

The simplest surgery is to use lid sutures but it is a last possibility if other methods fail to reach sufficient eye closure to protect, for instance, an eye with corneal ulceration. Non-resorbable sutures are placed in the center of the upper eyelid skin, pulled downward, are fixed with downward tension to the cheek. Alternatively, the suture is sewn through both upper and lower lids. Nowadays, the implantation of an upper lid

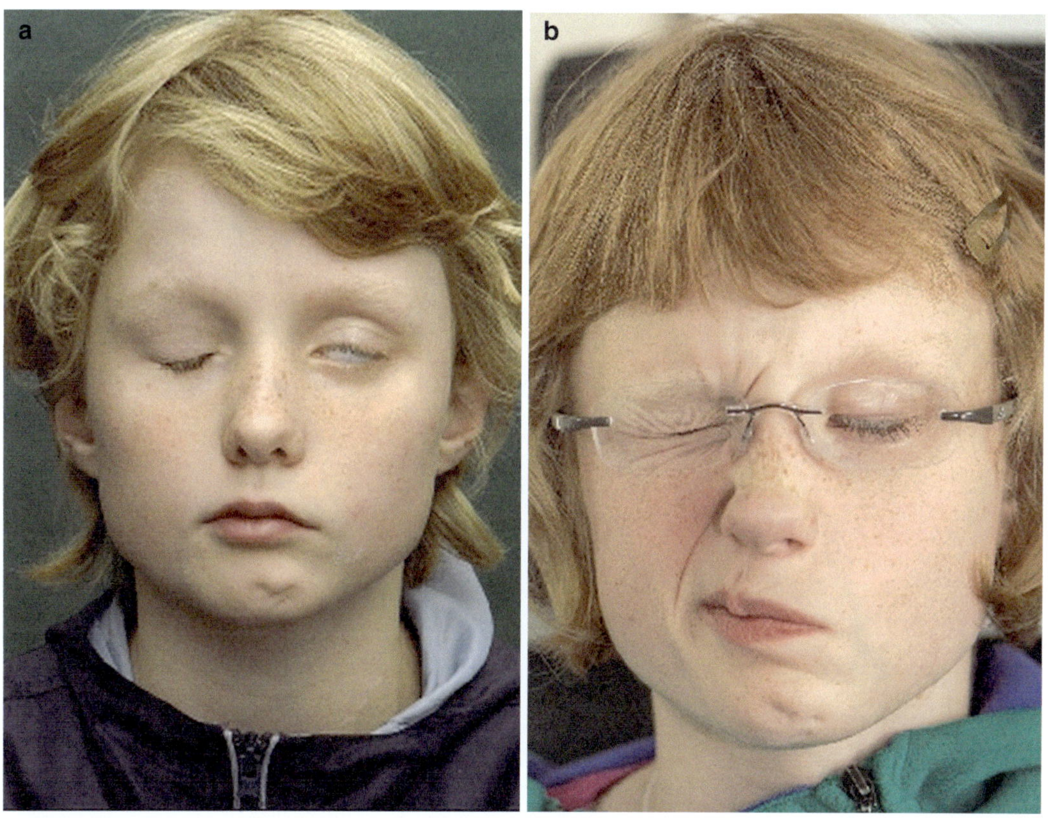

Fig. 22.1 Young patient with facial palsy of the left side. (**a**) Incomplete eye closure. (**b**) Improved situation after implantation of a upper gold lid weight

weight is a good option to improve the closure of the upper lid (Figs. 22.2 and 22.3) [6, 7]. Custom-made gold implants and platinum chains are available. Especially in patients with incomplete paresis instead of complete paresis, the results are often excellent. Negative preoperative factors for good results are complete paresis, upper lid retraction, no Bell's phenomenon, absence of supratarsal fold, and very thin upper lid skin. The optimal weight for the individual patient is selected prior to surgery on the alert patient. Implants of different weight are pasted on the upper eyelid. The optimal weight allows the patient to open and close the eye easily without effort in upright and supine position. The procedure itself can be performed in local or general anesthesia. The incision is made along the supratarsal fold. A pocket is prepared to fix the implant on the tarsal plate. The optimal position is about 3 mm from the lid margin. An alternative to upper lid weight implantation is to use a wire spring implant. As this procedure like lateral and medial canthoplasty are primarily propagandized by ophthalmologists, therefore please see ophthalmological literature for more details.

Although upper lid weights produce much better functional results, tarsorrhaphy still is performed frequently, especially by general ophthalmologists. Tarsorrhaphy cannot completely cover and therefore incompletely protects the cornea and limits the patient's vision. If reversed in case of recovery of the facial palsy, an entropion can remain. Finally, the aesthetic appearance of a tarsorrhaphy is insufficient. Therefore, tarsorrhaphy

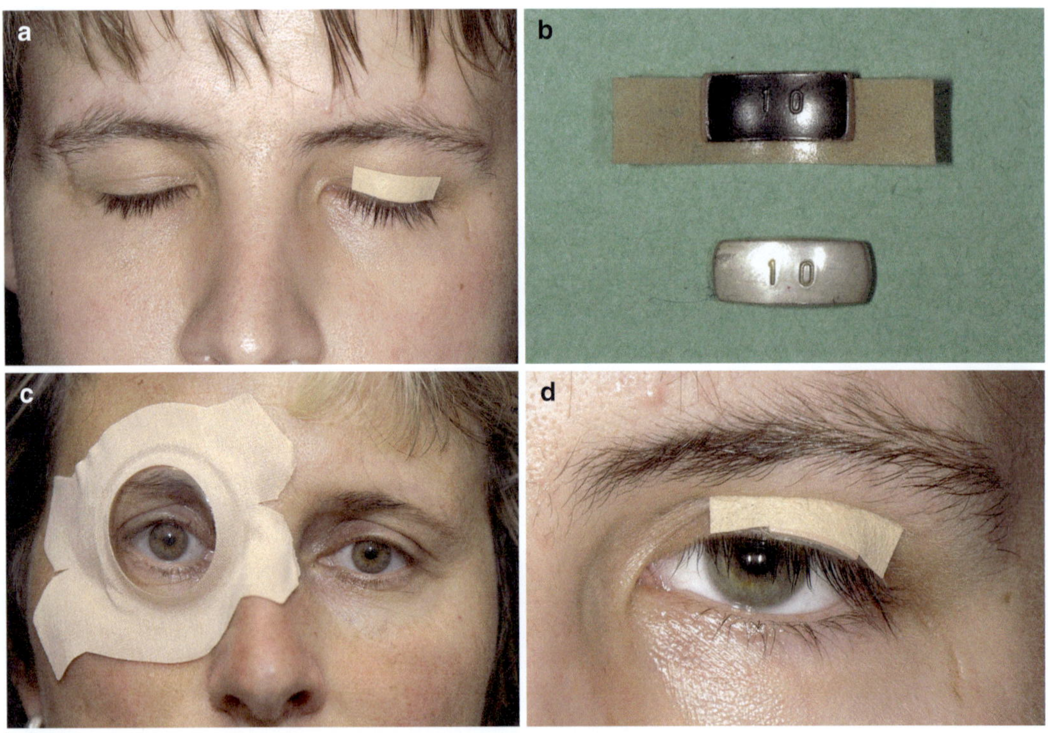

Fig. 22.2 Nonsurgical treatment to improve the closure of the eye for better humidification. (**a**) External upper lid weight with eye closed. (**b**) Material needed for external upper lid weighting. (**c**) Watch glass bandage to improve humidification of the eye. (**d**) External upper lid weight with the eye open

Fig. 22.3 Correction of incomplete closure of the eye and of an ectropion. (**a**) Incision lines for the upper lid weight positioning and lateral lower lid resection. (**b**) Positioning of a gold weight on the tarsal plate of the upper lid. (**c**) Wedge resection of the lower lid. (**d**) Final situs after skin closure

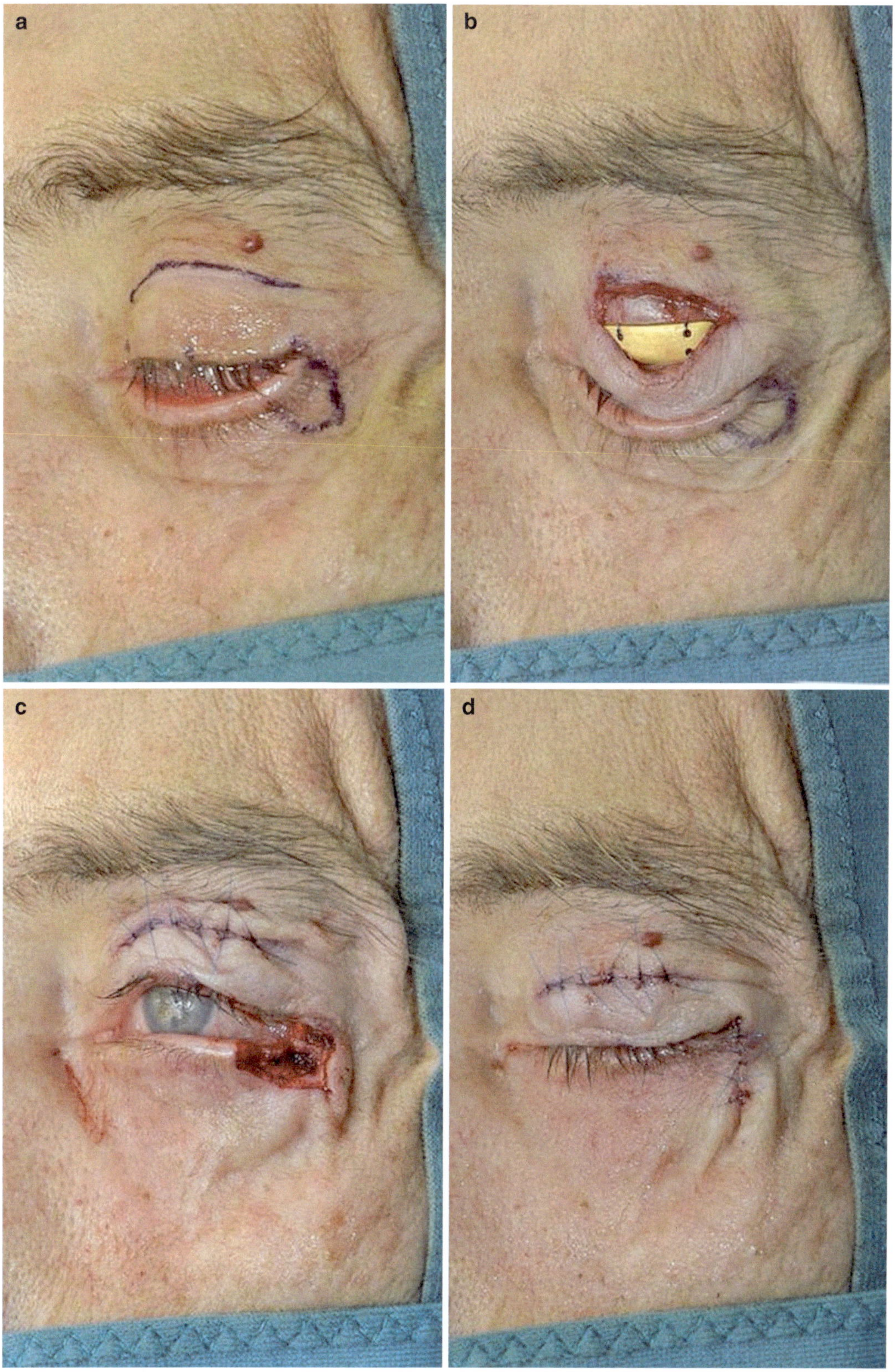
a
b
c
d

cannot be recommended as a good option to improve the eye closure and protection.

22.6 Surgery of the Lower Eyelid

Lower eyelid surgery should improve the margin approximation of the lower lid to the eye globe. While performing lower eyelid surgery, it is very important not to change to position of the lacrimal puncta, if in normal position. Otherwise, drainage of the tears can be disturbed. A medial canthoplasty can correct a medial canthal laxity [8]. Briefly, the canthal tendon is exposed after minimal skin resection in the inner corner of the eye above and below while preserving the lacrimal puncta. Splinting the puncta helps for protection. The upper and lower tendon is then joined in the exposed area with sutures. Finally, the skin is closed. Several modifications of the medial canthoplasty technique have been proposed. Equivalently, a lateral canthoplasty, often combined with lateral cantholysis, corrects lateral canthal laxity (Fig. 22.4) [9]. Up to one-third of the lid margin can be resected. Again, take care not to disturb the lacrimal puncta. Very important is to fix the new lateral margin of the tarsus to the lateral canthal tendon at the end of the procedure. The implantation of a cartilage strut can help to stabilize the lower eyelid [10]. The cartilage is typically harvested from the cavum conchae of the ear. After subciliary incision, the cartilage implant is placed into a pocket prepared under the medial aspect of the tarsus at its inferior border. The results are better than with a temporalis sling as a shortcoming of this procedure is often the mass movement which occurs with mouth movements. Another technique for lower lid

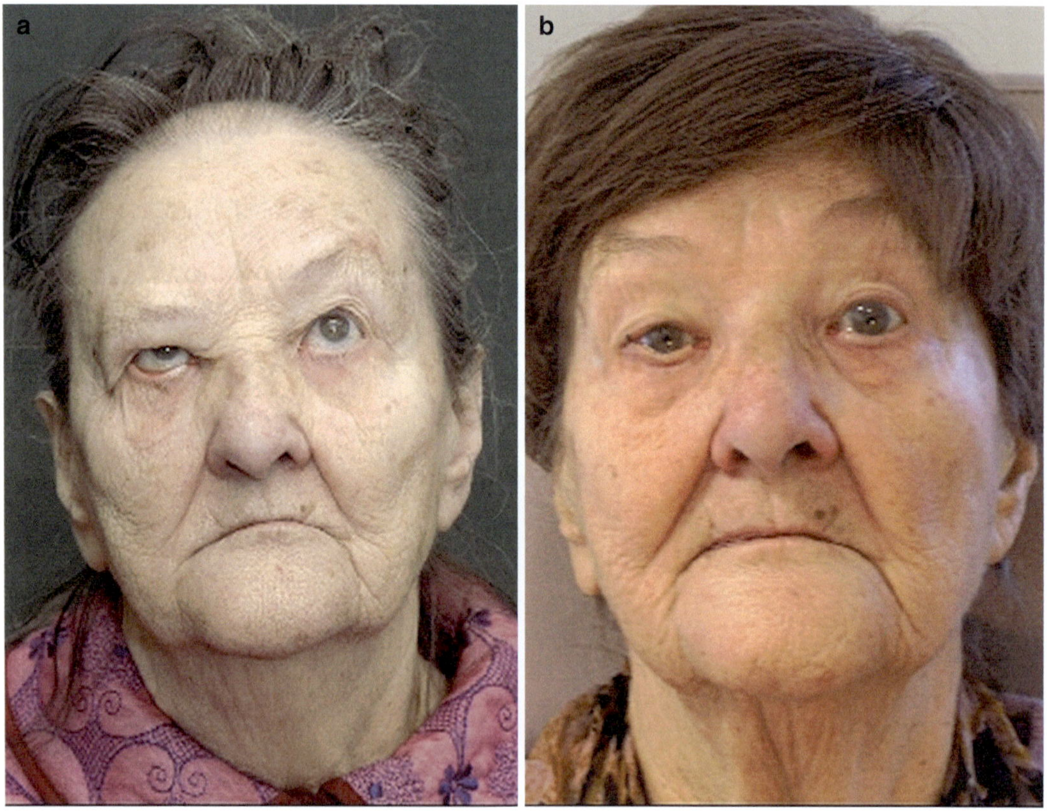

Fig. 22.4 Patient with incomplete facial palsy of the right side with emphasis on the periorbital region. (**a**) Brow ptosis and ectropion of the lower lid are obvious. (**b**) Situation after brow lift and lateral canthoplasty and camouflage of the forehead using side parting of the hair

shortening is lower lid wedge resection (see Fig. 22.3). Here, a full-thickness part of the lid is excised.

22.7 Surgery of Brow Ptosis and of the Forehead

Because the constant comparison of the paralyzed with the healthy side is of importance, the treatment can include surgery of the paralyzed side to improve the resting tone and movements but also by toning down the activity of the forehead of the normal side by resection of the forehead muscle using a forehead lift or the use of botulinum toxin. This subsection will focus on measures for the paralyzed side. A dropped brow may impair the patient's vision. Indirectly, it can also impair the upper eyelid retraction. A brow lift is a good option to correct the eyebrow (see Fig. 22.4) [11, 12]. But be careful if you want to combine the brow lift (producing traction on the upper lid) with other procedures on the upper lid. In such a situation an impaired eyelid closure might be an undesired result that has to be avoided. Therefore, it is very important to plan the extent of resection on the alert patient. The brow is held in its normal position in relation to the healthy side and it is observed if this would impair the eyelid closure. The surgery is performed at best under local anesthesia so that the patient can close the eye during surgery when requested. The incision is marked directly superior to the eyebrow. In most cases, the resection area is larger for the lateral two-thirds. Avoid loss of brow hairs. Skin resection is often but not always necessary. Obligatory is the resection of subcutaneous tissue and of parts of the frontal muscle. The most important step is to fix the lower wound edge to the periosteum superior to the upper incision line. The skin is closed in two layers. Alternatively, it is also possible to perform the brow lift endoscopically [13]. The incision line for an endoscopic brow lift is the temporalis fossa. Typically sutures (eventually together with screws) and fascia are used to produce tension between orbital rim and the temporal region.

22.8 Treatment of Periocular Synkinesis

Periocular synkinesis is a consequence of misdirected reinnervation of the facial nerve after facial nerve injury without or with facial nerve repair. The abnormal movements occur about 3–6 months after injury or facial nerve repair. Characteristically is that the patient cannot raise the eyebrow and the eye is closed without intention slightly or even completely during intentional movements in the mouth region and vice versa. Synkinesis can affect the complete hemiface but this section only will focus on the periocular synkinesis. The clinical examination will illustrate the severity of the synkinesis. Electromyography helps to quantify the status and helps to define the muscle areas mostly involved. Primary treatment of choice is botulinum toxin A injection (Fig. 22.5) [14]. As in cases with blepharospasm, the target muscle for botulinum toxin A injections is the orbicularis oculi muscle. Typical injection sites are lateral and medial upper eyelid (here, injections into the levator palpebrae have to be avoided not to produce a ptosis) and the temporal lower eyelid. Because botulinum toxin A is very effective, surgical myectomy is nowadays the only method of second choice [15]. Upper myectomy can be combined with a brow plasty. Target muscles can be, depending on the localization of the most important sites of synkinesis, the corrugator muscle, the procerus muscle, or parts of the orbicularis oculi muscle. Lower myectomy for removal of lower parts of the orbicularis oculi muscle is often combined with lower eyelid blepharoplasty but without orbital fat resection.

22.9 Treatment of the Lacrimal System

Treatment to improve the tear function or dysfunction might be of additional value [16]. In case of epiphora, the implantation of a lacrimal pump system or lacrimal gland resection should be discussed. In case of a dry eye, punctual occlusion is a good option.

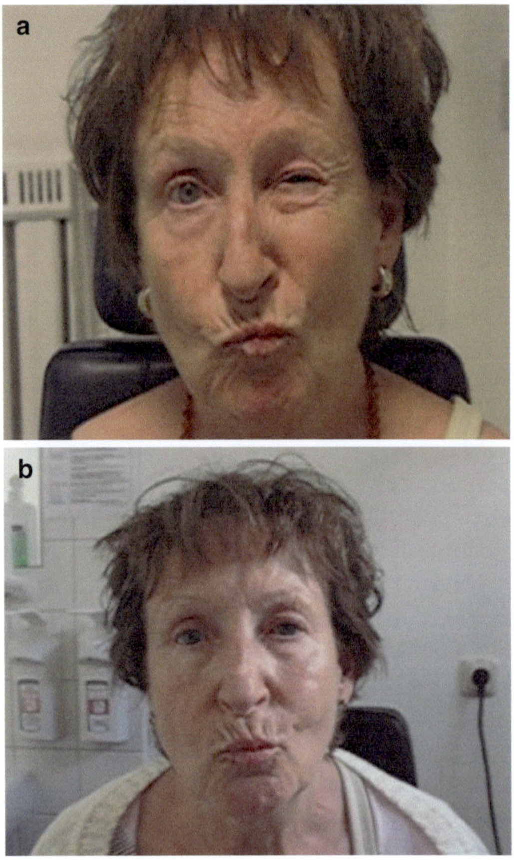

Fig. 22.5 Patient with severe synkinesis after facial nerve trauma on the left side. (**a**) Hyperkinesis of the orbicularis oculi muscle while pursing the lips. (**b**) Situation 3 weeks after botulinum toxin A injection into the orbicularis oculi muscle

References

1. Volk GF, Pantel M, Guntinas-Lichius O. Modern concepts in facial nerve reconstruction. Head Face Med. 2011;6:25. PubMed eng.
2. Bhama P, Gliklich RE, Weinberg JS, Hadlock TA, Lindsay RW. Optimizing total facial nerve patient management for effective clinical outcomes research. JAMA Facial Plast Surg. 2014;16:9–14.
3. McGinnigle S, Naroo SA, Eperjesi F. Evaluation of dry eye. Surv Ophthalmol. 2012;57(4):293–316. PubMed.
4. Nelson JD, Helms H, Fiscella R, Southwell Y, Hirsch JD. A new look at dry eye disease and its treatment. Adv Ther. 2000;17(2):84–93. PubMed.
5. Fiscella RG. Understanding dry eye disease: a managed care perspective. Am J Manag Care. 2011;17 Suppl 16:S432–9. PubMed.
6. Kim DW, Ali MJ. Modified retrograde approach to upper eyelid static loading. Laryngoscope. 2007; 117(12):2110–4. PubMed.
7. Razfar A, Afifi AM, Manders EK, Myers EN, Johnson JT, Ferris RL, et al. Ocular outcomes after gold weight placement and facial nerve resection. Otolaryngol Head Neck Surg. 2009;140(1):82–5. PubMed eng.
8. Sakamoto Y, Nakajima H, Tamada I, Kishi K. New technique for medial canthoplasty that incorporates modified v-w epicanthoplasty. Arch Facial Plast Surg. 2012;14(1):59–61. PubMed.
9. Bartsich S, Swartz KA, Spinelli HM. Lateral canthoplasty using the Mitek anchor system. Aesth Plast Surg. 2012;36(1):3–7. PubMed.
10. Liebau J, Schulz A, Arens A, Tilkorn H, Schwipper V. Management of lower lid ectropion. Dermatol Surg. 2006;32(8):1050–6; discussion 6–7. PubMed.
11. Bastidas N, Zide B. Suspension of the brow in facial paralysis and frontalis loss. Plast Reconstr Surg. 2010;126(2):486–8. PubMed.
12. Henstrom DK, Lindsay RW, Cheney ML, Hadlock TA. Surgical treatment of the periocular complex and improvement of quality of life in patients with facial paralysis. Arch Facial Plast Surg. 2011;13(2):125–8. PubMed Epub 2011/03/23. eng.
13. Jones BM, Grover R. Endoscopic brow lift: a personal review of 538 patients and comparison of fixation

techniques. Plast Reconstr Surg. 2004;113(4):1242–50; discussion 51–2. PubMed.
14. Filipo R, Spahiu I, Covelli E, Nicastri M, Bertoli GA. Botulinum toxin in the treatment of facial synkinesis and hyperkinesis. Laryngoscope. 2012;122(2):266–70. PubMed Epub 2012/01/19. eng.
15. Guerrissi JO. Selective myectomy for postparetic facial synkinesis. Plast Reconstr Surg. 1991;87(3):459–66. PubMed.
16. Bergeron CM, Moe KS. The evaluation and treatment of upper eyelid paralysis. Facial Plast Surg. 2008;24(2):220–30. PubMed.

Autologous Fat Transfer to Reconstruct Facial Defects After Parotidectomy

23

Victor-Vlad Costan, Daniela A. Trandafir, Eugenia I. Popescu, and Cristian Ilie Drochioi

Abstract

Parotidectomy (superficial, total, or extended) is a surgical procedure that may be associated with a number of aesthetic and functional complications. Some of them (like facial asymmetry due to the presence of tissue depression following the removal of invaded structures, and Frey syndrome) particularly requested the attention of researchers aiming to find the optimal correction methods. A widely used technique in aesthetic and reconstructive surgery – autologous fat transfer – may be a great option for compensating the defect caused by extended parotidectomy, demonstrating good and very good results over time, from both aesthetic and functional points of view. Autologous fat grafting is a technique used in reconstructive surgery to reshape the soft parts, as recommended by a lot of advantages: it can be performed under local anesthesia, requires short execution time, has unlimited availability of reconstruction material, no additional scars, no morbidity at the donor site, it can be repeated to achieve the desired effect with minimum discomfort for the patient, and has good aesthetic and functional results stable over time. Additionally, the multipotent mesenchymal cells associated to the fat cells significantly contribute to the improvement in texture and nutrition of the tissues in the area where lipostructure is performed, tissues that are often altered by previous surgery for tumor excision or by additional treatment procedures (radio- and chemotherapy).

V.-V. Costan, MD, DMD, PhD (✉)
Department of Oral and Maxillo-Facial Surgery, Faculty of Dental Medicine, "Grigore T. Popa" University of Medicine and Pharmacy, "St. Spiridon" University Hospital Iasi, Iasi, Romania
e-mail: victorcostan@gmail.com

D.A. Trandafir, MD, PhD • E.I. Popescu, DMD, PhD
Department of Surgery (Dentoalveolar Surgery, Oral and Maxillofacial Surgery), "Grigore T. Popa" University of Medicine and Pharmacy, Faculty of Dental Medicine, Iasi, Romania

C.I. Drochioi, DMD, MD
Department of Oral and Maxillofacial Surgery, "Sfântul Spiridon" Emergency Hospital, Iasi, Romania

© Springer International Publishing Switzerland 2016

V.-V. Costan (ed.), *Management of Extended Parotid Tumors*, DOI 10.1007/978-3-319-26545-2_23

23.1 Introduction

Correction of severe facial contour abnormalities continues to be a challenge for cosmetic surgery. The purpose of plastic surgery is to restore a harmonious and symmetrical facial appearance. Clinical entities with facial deformities requiring surgical correction include Parry-Romberg syndrome, lupus, Melkersson-Rosenthal syndrome, morphea, trauma sequelae, hemifacial microsomia, and, last but not least, postoperative sequelae of mutilating radical interventions for cancer in the oral and maxillofacial territory.

Parotidectomy is a surgical procedure generally followed by a certain degree of facial asymmetry, but the aesthetic damage becomes even more important when a more extensive surgery is performed (such as an extended parotidectomy). To compensate the pretragian and maseterin depression consecutive to extended parotidectomy, one can use autologous fat transfer, a widely used technique in aesthetic and reconstructive surgery, with good results in the long term, measured both cosmetically and physiologically [1].

23.2 Brief History of Fat Graft

The idea of using a fat graft to correct a facial deformity has a long history; Neuber reported in 1893 the results of an autologous fat transfer from the forearm to reconstruct facial defects following bone tuberculosis, emphasizing the loss of the initially obtained results over the course of time due to central graft necrosis determined by the absence of vascularization [2].

Autologous fat grafts have been used in medical practice for over 60 years, although initially regarded with reservation due to the finding that only half of them remain viable over time. As technology progressed, the injections of autologous adipose tissue are now well-defined surgical procedures broadly used in order to restore facial contours.

The technique of fat harvesting and preparation for transfer proposed by Coleman has been used in the last 25 years in aesthetic surgery. Coleman's "lipostructure" is preferred for various complex tissue reconstructions ranging from localized atrophy to large soft tissue defects (following trauma, congenital, or after tumor ablation), due to the achievement of better postoperative results and minimal discomfort [2, 3].

23.3 Current Use of Fat Graft and Its Applicability in the Oro-Maxillo-Facial Territory for Aesthetic Results

Autologous fat graft is an easy technique widely used in cosmetic surgery to correct facial wrinkles (like nasolabial folds) or in reconstructive surgery to reshape the soft tissues, to increase the volume of a segment, or to recover a surface [4, 5]. This technique has several advantages: unlimited availability, no additional scars, absence of donor-site morbidity, requires less time to perform, and good long-term results (from aesthetic and functional point of view). To conserve adipocytes, Coleman emphasizes the importance of practicing the least traumatic technique for harvesting and injecting, insisting that a minimal amount of fat should be transferred into complex nest tunnels, in layers, maximizing the contact with the surrounding tissue and adipocyte neovascularization. Therefore, some modifications were made on the initial procedure of Coleman, regarding harvesting and injection techniques [6].

Fat harvesting is preferred from periumbilical region [2]. Once lidocaine (0.25 %) with adrenaline is injected into the specified levels, the fat is harvested using special cannulas and stored into 5 mL syringes (Fig. 23.1) which are then centrifuged at 3000 RPM for 6 min; in each syringe three layers will be distinguished (Fig. 23.2). After removing the upper layer (oil) as well as the lower layer (serous), the middle layer (fat) is injected into the defect. In one session we can inject the fat ranging from 10 to 45 mL. The injection is performed three dimensionally in very thin layers, in order to allow a good fat graft revascularization and, at the same time, a more accurate recovery of the facial symmetry. Since the thickness of the fatty graft is rather small, in most cases it is necessary to repeat the procedure with an interval of at least 6 months [2]. The interval between two injections of fat can vary from 3 to 12 months, by different authors [7, 8].

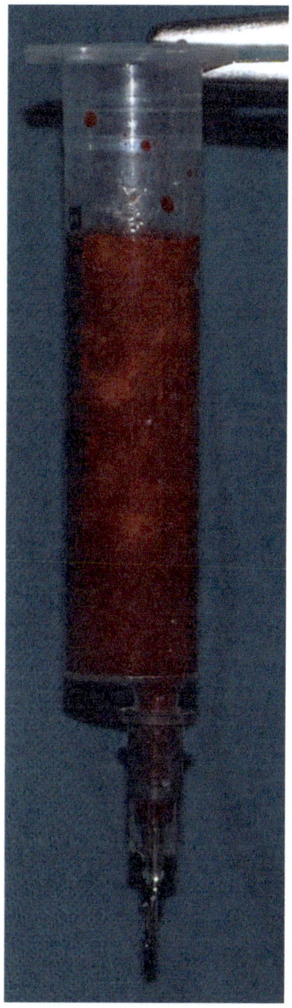

Fig. 23.1 The aspect of the harvested fat

The fat can be currently considered the ideal filler because it is a natural product, stable over time, which does not present the usual complications of the synthetic products: allergic or granulomatous type reactions [5, 9]. It is also an autologous product, inexpensive, and, typically, in a sufficient quantity.

The adipose tissue contains a large amount of fat cells and mesenchymal stem cells, which are able to differentiate into several connective tissue-type cell lines [10]. Therefore, the lipostructure allows not only the volume restoration but it also brings a capital of multipotent mesenchymal cells in the region of the atrophied scar tissue (consecutive to surgery, radiotherapy and/or chemotherapy). Therefore, the texture and nutrition of the skin (and other tissues where lipostructure was performed) will significantly improve [11]. The injected mesenchymal stem cells turn into young fibroblasts and additionally stimulate neovascularization with beneficial effects on the scar tissue, including the increase in its hydration [12].

Another advantage of this technique is the possibility to preserve the graft by freezing the centrifuged fat for up to 20 months; Donofrio [13] found that using the so prepared fat will also lead to an increase in the quality of the reconstruction. In this way, the patient's comfort is also improved, since the graft harvesting is not performed at the time of the lipostructure; only the existing graft will be injected in the receiving region [13].

The complications of this method are represented by the occurrence of minor irregularities in the reconstructed regions or excessive corrections, which can then be shaped [2]. In regions with very thin skin (like the eyelid), we avoid this by using micro-cannulas. The role of the fat injected at this level is very important for the patients in which the facial nerve had to be sacrificed. The injected fat at this level is designed to support the lower lid, so that the decreased tone of the orbicularis muscle will be compensated. This effect contributes to a better eyelid occlusion (see Fig. 23.2e, f). Undercorrection is generally easier to treat than overcorrection. Additional fat may be grafted at a separate time to complete the correction. Removing excess graft is more difficult as the host tissue infiltrates into the graft. Edema is usually evident for 1–2 weeks after the procedure. Bleeding complications usually are limited to transient mild ecchymosis and are associated with the use of sharp needles for fat injection. Superficial ecchymosis tends to resorb rapidly. Small hematomas are more unusual and are associated with the use of sharp needles for graft placement. Damage to underlying structures, particularly around the eye, is possible and generally is prevented using a blunt needle for infiltration. Careful control of the injection to keep the fat in superficial areas as well as the use of a blunt cannula should prevent these complications [6]. Infectious complications may exceptionally occur in the donor or recipient regions. The donor-site scarring is a potential concern. Contour irregularities can result from overly aggressive harvesting in a small area.

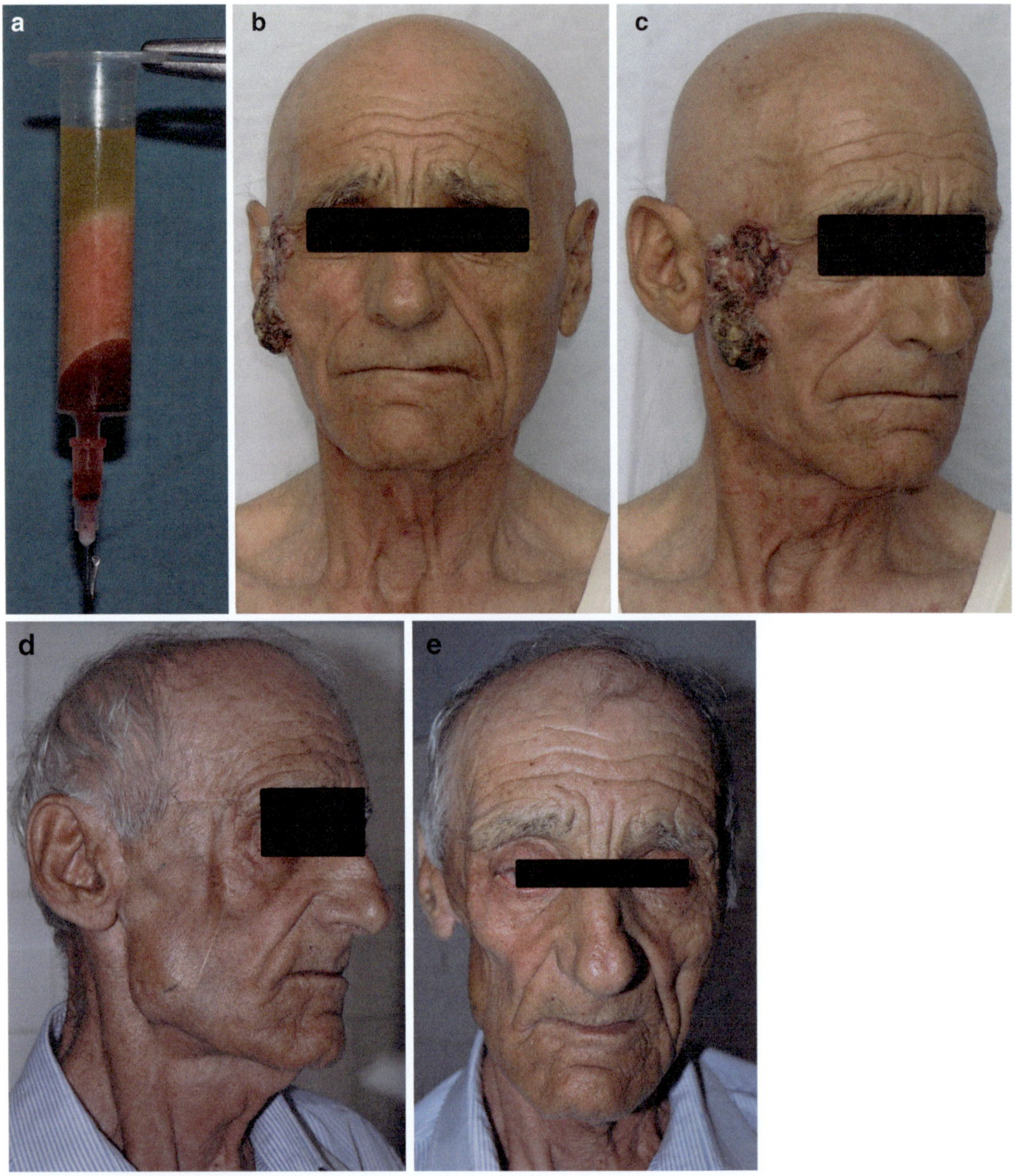

Fig. 23.2 (**a**) The fat appearance after centrifugation at 3000 RPM for 6 min. There are three layers: the upper one, represented by the oil from the destroyed adipocytes; the one in the middle, represented by the purified adipocytes obtained by centrifugation; and the lower one, represented by debris from the blood. (**b**, **c**) A patient with an adenoid cystic carcinoma originating in the skin of the right parotid region, which has later extended in the parotid gland. (**d**, **e**) After the parotidectomy extended to the skin and the right zygomatic bone and the sacrifice of the facial nerve, the defect plasty was performed using a radial free flap transfer with obvious postoperative facial asymmetry. (**f**, **g**) The patient's appearance after two sessions of lipostructure, performed in a period of 6 months. The patient noted the significant improvement of the facial symmetry and, not least, the functioning of the right lower eyelid, supported by the injected fat

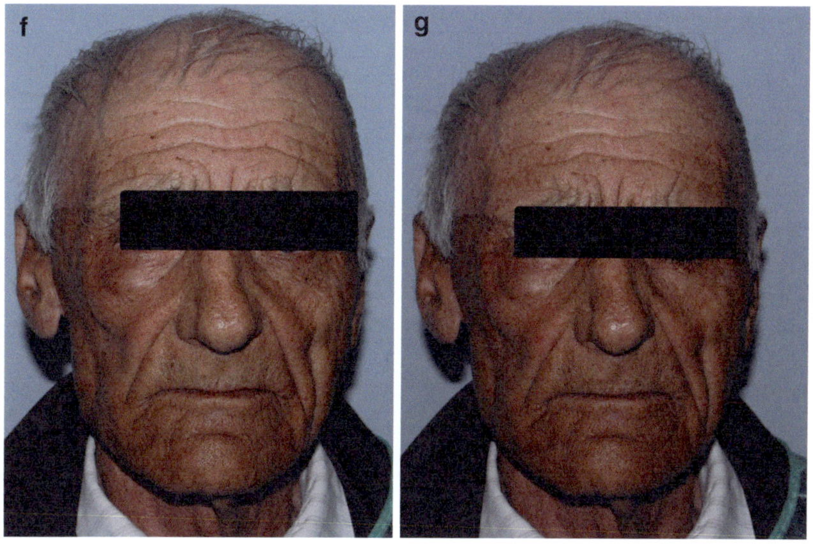

Fig. 23.2 (continued)

23.4 Physiological Outcome of Fat Graft within the Oro-Maxillo-Facial Territory

Besides the good and very good aesthetic results of autologous fat transfer after extensive parotidectomy, the physiological effect is a highly rated one [1]. The Frey syndrome, also called the gustatory sweating or auriculotemporal syndrome, is characterized by sweating and congestion or redness of the cheek during chewing after parotidectomy. It affects between 2.6 and 14.3 % of patients with superficial or total parotidectomy [14], but also extended parotidectomy. It is caused by regeneration of the sectioned secretomotor parasympathetic fibers between the facial nerve and branches of the auriculotemporal or the great auricular which is responsible for aberrant innervation of sweat glands and subcutaneous vessels, explaining the pathophysiology of the syndrome. Several authors believe that autologous fat transfer not only corrects the distortion of the preauricular area post-parotidectomy but also avoids the Frey syndrome [1, 15–17].

Autologous fat injection in the parotid area may be a minimally invasive option as the fat would create a barrier between the skin and the residual parotid gland and may prevent abnormal nerve neo-anastomoses to the sweat glands. In addition to being useful for treating the unpleasant salivary sweating and flushing typical of post-parotidectomy Frey syndrome, autologous fat injection could also have a positive aesthetic impact as it may fill the gap left by the excision of the parotid. It can be performed in a one day hospital stay under local anesthesia and sedation, but it needs to be preceded by careful marking of the entire affected area identified by the help of the Minor's iodine starch test. This consists of applying an iodine solution (iodine 1.5 g, castor oil 10 g, and 95 % ethanol 125 mL) to the parotid skin surface and then sprinkling it with white starch powder; when the patient starts to eat, sweating in the skin areas affected by post-parotidectomy Frey syndrome turns the white solution to dark purple. Minimally invasive autologous fat injection of the parotid area can be considered safe and effective in post-parotidectomy Frey syndrome and also has an aesthetic impact as it can fill the gap left by the parotid gland excision. However, patients should be informed that the procedure may need to be repeated to achieve a definitive result.

23.5 Applicability's Details and Other Effects for Autologous Fat Graft

Guerrerosantos [18], Coleman [5, 11], Ellenbogen [19], and Trepsat [20] are just a few of the authors who enthusiastically supported autologous fat transplantation for reconstruction of facial deformities, reporting high rates of survival for autologous fat graft and fewer complications. Some of the comments offered by those with experience in the use of these tissue grafts relates to (1) the need for injection of small or moderate amounts of fat in each treatment, (2) the best results are seen when fatty grafts are injected subfascially or intramuscularly, (3) fat injections should be made deep in several places in the form of fine droplets or small rolls, and (4) massage the areas injected with fat to ensure the fat penetration.

Autologous fat injections have been shown to be clinically effective in patients with adverse effects of radiation and severe burns. These results are encouraging not only aesthetically but also have a good effect on skin texture. Histologically, the tissue biopsy shows neovascularization, increased collagen, and dermal hyperplasia. It is believed that these effects are influenced by a residual population of stem cells in the stroma vascular fraction of the harvested tissue by liposuction that is able to differentiate into multiple tissue types [10, 12, 21–24].

Conclusion

Autologous fat transfer is a very interesting option to correct sequelae of extended parotidectomy, both to restore the facial contours and to prevent Frey syndrome. The reasons supporting the use of this method of correction are unlimited availability of adipose tissue, the absence of additional scars, absence of donor-site morbidity, and shorter duration for outgoing, good, and excellent results maintained over time, both from the aesthetic and functional point of view.

References

1. Vico PG, Delange A, De Vooght A. Autologous fat transfer: an aesthetic and functional refinement for parotidectomy. Surg Res Pract. 2014;2014, Article ID 873453, 6 pages. doi:10.1155/2014/873453.
2. Costan VV, Vicol C, Drochioi C, Boişteanu O, Popescu E. The value of lipostructure in reconstruction of the maxillo-facial soft tissue defects. J Chir (Iaşi). 2012;8(1):53–6.
3. Mojallal A, Breton P, Delay E, Foyatier JL. Greffe d'adipocytes: applications en chirurgie plastique et esthétique. Encyclopédie Médico-chirurgicale: Techniques chirurgicales. Amsterdam: Elsevier SAS; 2004.
4. Kaufman MR, Miller TA, Huang C, Roostaeian J, Wasson KL, Ashley RK, et al. Autologous fat transfer for facial recontouring: is there science behind the art? Plast Reconstr Surg. 2007;119(7):2287–96.
5. Coleman SR. Structural fat grafts: the ideal filler? Clin Plast Surg. 2001;28(1):111–9.
6. Coleman SR. Structural fat grafting. St. Louis: Quality Medical Publishing; 2004.
7. Faghahati S, Delaporte T, Toussoun G, Gleizal A, Morel F, Delay E. Traitement par transfert graisseux des séquelles postradiques de tumeur faciale maligne de l'enfance. Ann Chir Plast Esthet. 2010;55:169–78.
8. Clauser LC, Tieghi R, Galiè M, Carinci F. Structural fat grafting: facial volumetric restoration in complex reconstructive surgery. J Craniofac Surg. 2011; 22(5):1695–701.
9. Requena C, Izquierdo MJ, Navarro M, Martínez A, Vilata JJ, Botella R, et al. Adverse reactions to injectable aesthetic microimplants. Am J Dermatopathol. 2001;23:197–202.
10. Zuk PA, Zhu M, Ashjian P, De Ugarte DA, Huang JI, Mizuno H, et al. Human adipose tissue is a source of multipotent stem cells. Mol Biol Cell. 2002;13:4279–95.
11. Coleman SR. Structural fat grafting: more than a permanent filler. Plast Reconstr Surg. 2006;118 Suppl 3:108–120S.
12. Rigotti G, Marchi A, Galiè M, Baroni G, Benati D, Krampera M, et al. Clinical treatment of radiotherapy tissue damage by lipoaspirate transplant: a healing process mediated by adipose-derived adult stem cells. Plast Reconstr Surg. 2007;119(5):1409–22; discussion 1423–4.
13. Donofrio LM. Technique in facial fat grafting. Aesthet Surg J. 2008;28:681–7.
14. Ambro BT, Goodstein LA, Morales RE, Taylor RJ. Evaluation of superficial musculoaponeurotic system flap and fat graft outcomes for benign and malignant parotid disease. Otolaryngology. 2013;148(6):949–54.
15. Fasolis M, Zavattero E, Iaquinta C, Berrone S. Dermofat graft after superficial parotidectomy to prevent Frey syndrome and depressed deformity. J Craniofac Surg. 2013;24(4):1260–2.
16. Mazzola RF, Cantarella G, Torretta S, Sbarbati A, Lazzari L, Pignataro L. Autologous fat injection to face and neck: from soft tissue augmentation to regenerative medicine. Acta Otorhinolaryngol Ital. 2011;31:59–69.
17. Bayram Y, Sever C, Karagoz H, Kulahci Y, Genc G. Two-stage surgical approach with dermofat graft and lipofilling for the treatment of established Frey syndrome and facial depression deformity. J Craniofac Surg. 2012;23(4):e311–4.

18. Guerrerosantos J. Long-term outcome of autologous fat transplantation in aesthetic facial recontouring. Sixteen years of experience with 1936 cases. Clin Plast Surg. 2000;27(4):515.
19. Ellenbogen R. Fat transfer. Current use in practice. Clin Plast Surg. 2000;27(4):545.
20. Trepsat F. Volumetric face lifting. Plast Reconstr Surg. 2001;108:1358.
21. Klinger M, Marazzi M, Vigo D, Torre M. Fat injection for cases of severe burn outcomes: a new perspective of scar remodeling and reduction. Aesthetic Plast Surg. 2008;32(3):465–9.
22. Tholpady SS, Llull R, Ogle RC, Rubin JP, Futrell JW, Katz AJ. Adipose tissue: stem cells and beyond. Clin Plast Surg. 2006;33(1):55–62, vi.
23. Viard R, Bouguila J, Voulliaume D, Comparin JP, Dionyssopoulos A, Foyatier JL. Fat grafting in facial burns sequelae. Ann Chir Plast Esthet. 2012; 57(3):217–29.
24. Brzoska M, Geiger H, Gauer S, Baer P. Epithelial differentiation of human adipose tissue-derived adult stem cells. Biochem Biophys Res Commun. 2005; 330(1):142–50.

Radiotherapy in Advanced Parotid Tumors

24

Dragos Iancu, Christian N. Mihaila, and Daniela A. Trandafir

Abstract

Radiotherapy is one of the main methods of locoregional treatment for parotid cancer, as in the cases of malignant tumors from other sites. Primary irradiation (definitive) is a viable alternative in the case of inoperable tumors (because of the associated comorbidities or in the cases of bulky tumors). Most authors argue that a good local tumor control is obtained after surgical removal of the salivary tumor followed by adjuvant radiotherapy versus single surgical treatment, reaching about 60–95 % local control. Postoperative radiotherapy is particularly indicated in the aggressive tumors, especially when complete surgical removal could be achieved. If the parotid tumor is bulky, the local tumor control achieved only by irradiation is still unsatisfactory. Therefore, if there are no contraindications for operability, subtotal tumor resection is preferred before irradiation. Usually, the radiotherapy with high linear energy transfer (neutrons) is recommended in cases of aggressive tumors, knowing that the relative biological effectiveness for this type of tumor is high. But new techniques with intensity-modulated radiotherapy (IMRT) have opened a modern way of treatment for large and/or aggressive tumors both by achieving better compliance of the irradiation plan and by the possibility of increasing the total dose prescribed, protecting the nearby organs.

D. Iancu, MD, PhD (✉)
Department of Radio-oncology, "Grigore T. Popa" Regional Institute of Oncology, University of Medicine and Pharmacy, Iasi, Romania
e-mail: dt_iancu@yahoo.com

C.N. Mihaila, MD
Department of Radio-oncology, Hôpital du Valais, Sion, Valais, Switzerland

D.A. Trandafir, MD, PhD
Department of Surgery (Dentoalveolar Surgery, Oral and Maxillofacial Surgery), Faculty of Dental Medicine, "Grigore T. Popa" University of Medicine and Pharmacy, Iasi, Romania

24.1 Malignant Tumors of the Parotid Gland

Most salivary gland tumors arise in the parotid glands, and the main therapeutic method is surgical intervention followed by radiation in cases of local unfavorable prognosis [1]. Various retrospective studies have been demonstrated that adjuvant postoperative radiation purpose can reduce the risk of locoregional recurrences over

© Springer International Publishing Switzerland 2016

V.-V. Costan (ed.), *Management of Extended Parotid Tumors*, DOI 10.1007/978-3-319-26545-2_24

30 % at 10 %, but failed to improve overall survival [2].

Postoperative radiotherapy is recommended in stages T3–T4, in incomplete resections with positive margins or perineural invasion bone, and in forms with increased aggression or recurrences [3]. In such situations, adjuvant chemotherapy appears to be effective.

In advanced, inoperable, or locoregional recurrences, local irradiation with heavy particles (neutrons or carbon ions) appears to have superior effects in terms of local control compared with standard photon radiation, with no data concerning improvement of overall survival [4].

Adjuvant radiotherapy to the tumor bed is recommended for all forms of aggressive/intermediate salivary tumors – high-grade mucoepidermoid, high-grade adenocarcinoma, and carcinoma arising from pleomorphic adenoma – except stage T1 completely excised with clear margins. Ipsilateral lymphatic levels Ib, II, and III must be irradiated prophylactic because of high risk of occult metastases, except when lymph node dissections were performed selective. Adjuvant radiation therapy is indicated for stage N2/N3 or in the presence of extracapsular spread.

In low-grade tumors – mucoepidermoid carcinoma, low-grade adenocarcinoma, and acinic cell carcinoma – adjuvant irradiation is recommended where excision margins are positive or close (<5 mm) generally after a preliminary discussion with the surgeon and pathologist. Special attention is necessary for deep excision margin close to the facial nerve. In case of occult metastases, N0 risk is lower than in aggressive forms, so prophylactic irradiation is not recommended.

Adenoid cystic carcinomas have a relatively high risk of locoregional recurrence and a propensity of perineural spread; therefore adjuvant radiation therapy is recommended for all forms (except the few stages T1 without perineural invasion).

Pleomorphic adenomas, although benign, are difficult to control only through surgery so radiotherapy is indicated in cases of excision with positive margins or outdated surgical cases (invasive tumors along the facial nerve). Prophylactic radiotherapy should be considered to prevent further recurrences in patients who have had a pleomorphic adenoma excised on more than one occasion previously, particularly if there is a short interval between recurrences relative to the life expectancy of the patient or if further compromise cosmetic or function [5].

24.2 Sequences and Multimodal Treatment Steps

Adjuvant radiation therapy should be initiated ideally 4–6 weeks after surgery. There is still no clear evidence about the role of concomitant chemotherapy.

Clinical examination can reveal invasion of local structures such as skin, facial nerve (palsy), or pterygoid muscles (trismus) or spread to draining lymph nodes. Fine-needle biopsy guided by ultrasound can confirm the presence or malignancy.

Cross-sectional imaging is performed to assess tumoral extension (particularly with deep edges positioned opposite to the parapharyngeal spaces) and to assess local lymph nodes (Figs. 24.1 and 24.2).

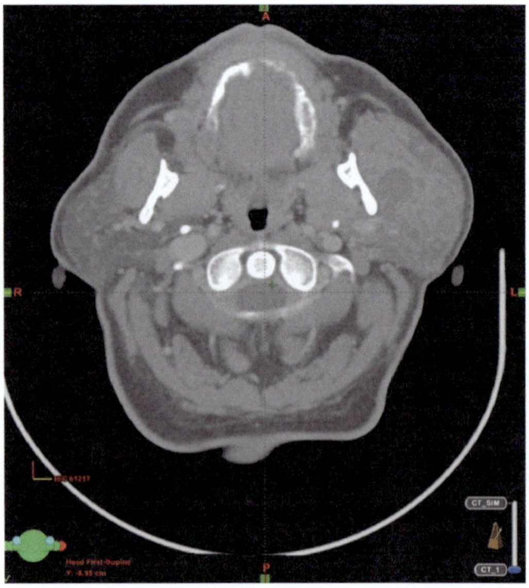

Fig. 24.1 CT scan for a left parotid tumor. Note that the tumoral mass has a deep necrotic area

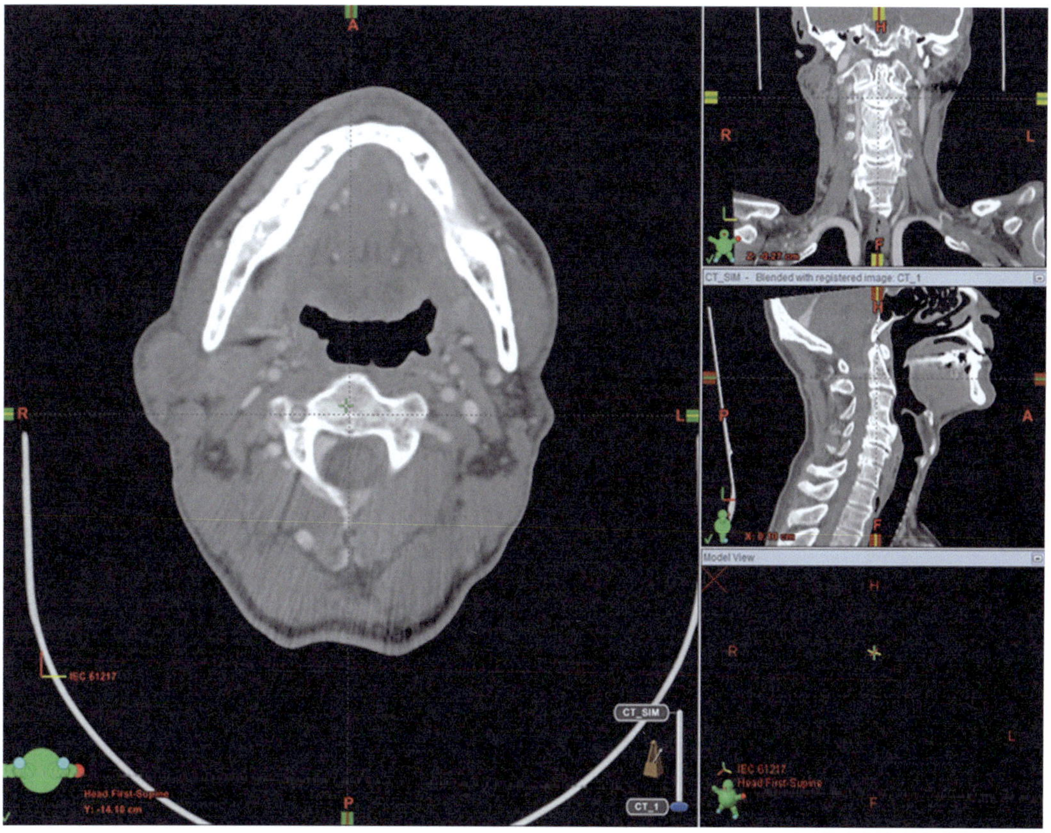

Fig. 24.2 CT scan for a right parotid tumor. This original image is the result of fusion between CT image with contrast and the simulation image (without contrast). The local lymph nodes are well individualized

MRI examination (Fig. 24.3) is preferred to CT because examinations may indicate a greater accuracy of perineural invasion. The scan volume starts from skull base and include all viscerocranium and cervical lymph areas. Preoperative scanning is compulsory and improves prognosis for defining volumes irradiated in postoperative radiotherapy.

Patients should be immobilized in a lying position with the neck in hyperextension and eyes directed posterior superior (to reduce the risk of eye damage). Immobilization is achieved using special systems of contention (Fig. 24.4) – for an ideal grip in thermoplastic masks five points should be used, even if the neck is not covered in the volume of radiation (to minimize errors and to reduce CTV-PTV margins).

After the complete fixe contention the patient is scanned using with a CT simulator, which performs multiple sections of 3 mm (or up to 5 mm) starting from the skull base until the aortic arch.

CT images fused with preoperative MRI are carefully evaluated to detect lymph nodes or macroscopic residual outstanding. The volume of irradiation is determined by pathological features such as perineural invasion of a major nerve and eventually after discussions with the surgeon and pathologist. The delineation of the clinical target volume will be individualized based on the extent of the disease and surgery. Considering that irradiation is adjuvant to surgery, the GTV cannot be limited even in the presence of residual masses.

CTV60 is made based on locoregional extension and on the surgical act. Particular attention is given to the deep excision margin that is likely to be close or involved if the facial nerve has been preserved. Parapharyngeal and infratemporal fossa spaces must be covered adequately. In

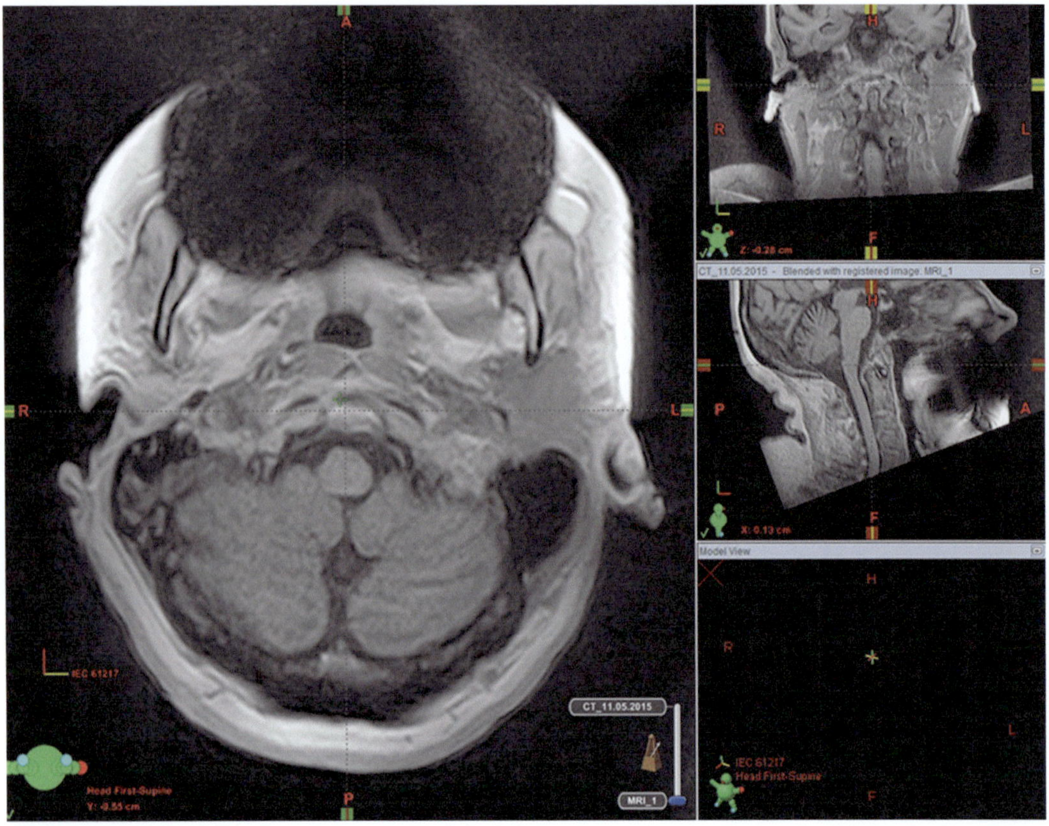

Fig. 24.3 MRI scan of the left parotid tumor before excision. This image was fused with CT simulation image (without contrast)

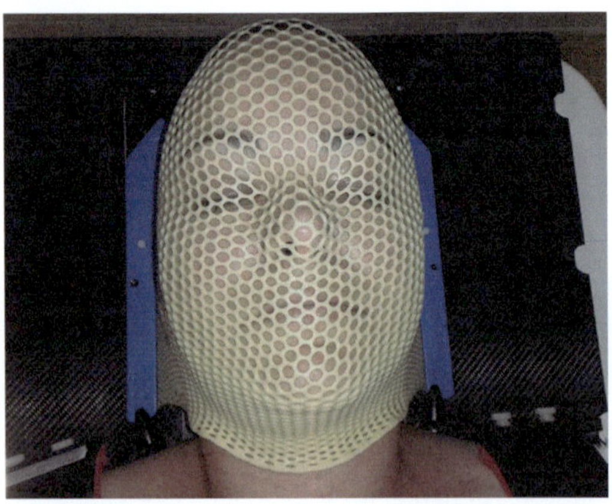

Fig. 24.4 Device for immobilization systems that ensure only the head and neck. There are also more performed devices that can make immobilization for head and neck in six places

general CTV60 medial limit must be tangent to the side of the internal jugular vein, but when the tumor affects the deep lobe of the parotid, irradiation volume should include the parapharyngeal space. CTV60 lateral limit must be just under the skin, without inclusion of postoperative scar. The position of contralateral parotid on the planning CT can be a useful guide to the superior and inferior limit of the CTV60.

In adenoid cystic carcinomas, the CTV60 must include the entire path of the facial nerve starting from stylomastoidian foramen at the skull base. Primary irradiation volume must include ipsilateral infragastric lymph nodes because the inferior pole of the parotid reaches on this region [6].

If there are indications of adjuvant radiation after neck dissection, cervical lymph levels I–V must be included in CTV60 volume. There is still no concrete data about bilateral elective neck irradiation. The recommended dose in such cases of positive lymph nodes is 60 Gy/30 fractions. If prophylactic irradiation areas include nodal irradiation volumes Ib, II, and III, an intermediate CTV44 volume can be defined.

In terms of extracapsular spread or positive resection margins, CTV66 should be defined including all levels without compromise. CTV once defined is extended in all directions with safety margins (set-up margins) of 3–5 mm according to each department of radiotherapy protocols.

As organs at risk (OAR), besides classical (spinal cord, brainstem, lens, optic nerves) should be outlined contralateral parotid, internal ear, and cochlea. The contralateral parotid does not receive a higher dose as 28 Gy (more than xerostomia occurs). The inner ear should be defined as an OAR, as reducing dose to the cochlea may reduce the risk of deafness.

Similar principles can be applied for volume definition for tumors of the submandibular or minor salivary glands. In adenoid cystic carcinomas, the nerve innervating the primary tumor site should be included up to the skull base. In adenoid cystic carcinomas of the submandibular gland, this should include the lingual nerve (a branch of the mandibular nerve, V_3) back to the foramen ovale and the marginal mandibular branch of the facial nerve to the stylomastoid foramen. For tumors arising in or close to the midline (e.g., hard palate), prophylactic lymph node volumes should be outlined bilaterally if lymph nodes are to be included in the CTV.

Parotid gland irradiation depends on the available equipment, staff training, and the possibility of initiating therapy in an optimal range. In principle there are using ^{60}Co machines, linear accelerators, and neutron therapy, and as basic therapy, there are three approaches using conventional, 3D-conformational irradiation (3D-CRT) and intensity-modulated radiation therapy (IMRT) planning.

Conventional therapy uses two to three oblique photons beams and is available on older ^{60}Co machines and linear accelerators (energies of 4 or 6 MV). In principle, this technique can provide the uniformity of the dose distribution on the CTV without increasing dose to the adjacent critical organs. For this purpose are used the unilateral anterior and posterior wedged-pair fields. A slight inferior angulation of the beams avoids an exit dose through the contralateral eye. An additional third lateral photon beam may provide a more homogenous distribution but will increase dose to the contralateral parotid gland and possibly to the spinal cord.

Optional – only for multiple energy LINACS – simpler technique uses homolateral fields with 12 or 16 MeV electrons (which provide up to 80 % of the delivered dose) in combination with fields 4 or 6 MV photons in order to reduce oral mucositis and decrease the skin reaction produced by electrons. Conventional techniques do not allow for tissue heterogeneity (air cavity, dense bones, and tissues) [7].

3D-conformational irradiation (*3D-CRT*) uses conformal geometrically shaped beams of uniform intensity (Fig. 24.5). It provides superior coverage and enhanced protection of organs at risk and more normal tissues may be spared with technique [6]. Hot spots in the mandible of >107 % should be avoided in order to reduce the risk of osteoradionecrosis. Excessive dose in the temporomandibular joint should avoid reducing the risk of long-term temporomandibular joint dysfunction and trismus. The cochlear dose should be kept below 50 Gy if possible to minimize the risk of hearing damage.

IMRT techniques produce convex distributions and step dose gradients. Coplanar conformation solutions 5-7-9 spaced beams provide excellent coverage with sparing the mandible, cochlea, spinal cord, brainstem, and oropharynx, but may increase the dose to the contralateral parotid. An ipsilateral four beam IMRT beam planning solution has been used but may not be better than 3D-CRT beam arrangement [8] (Figs. 24.6 and 24.7).

IMRT is a new technology in radiation oncology that delivers radiation more precisely to the tumor while relatively sparing the surrounding normal tissues. It also introduces new concepts of inverse planning and computer-controlled radiation deposition and normal tissue avoidance in contrast to the conventional trial-and-error approach. IMRT has a wide application in most aspects of radiation oncology because of its ability to create multiple targets and multiple avoidance structures, to treat different targets simultaneously to different doses as well as to weight targets and avoidance structures according to their importance. By delivering radiation with greater precision, IMRT has been shown to minimize acute treatment-related morbidity, making dose escalation feasible that may ultimately improve local tumor control. IMRT has also introduced a new accelerated fractionation

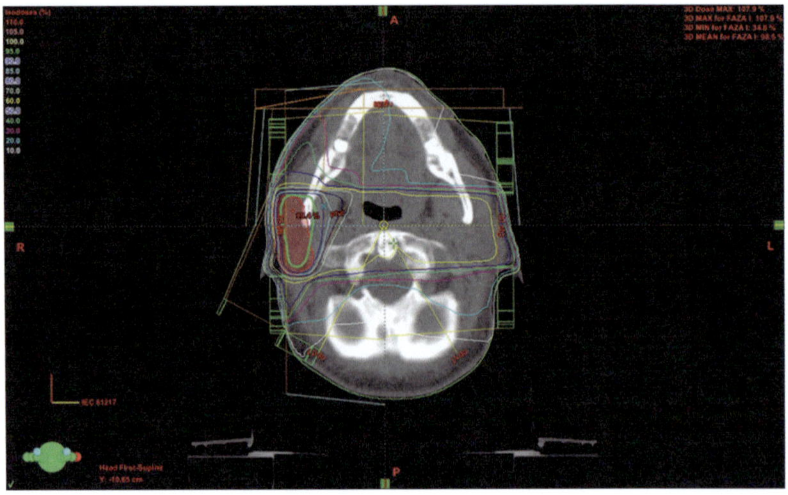

Fig. 24.5 3D-conformational irradiation for a right parotid tumor in the first phase of treatment. Noted that the ideal dose 95 % did not covered all tumoral volume and present a hot spot inside the irradiated volume

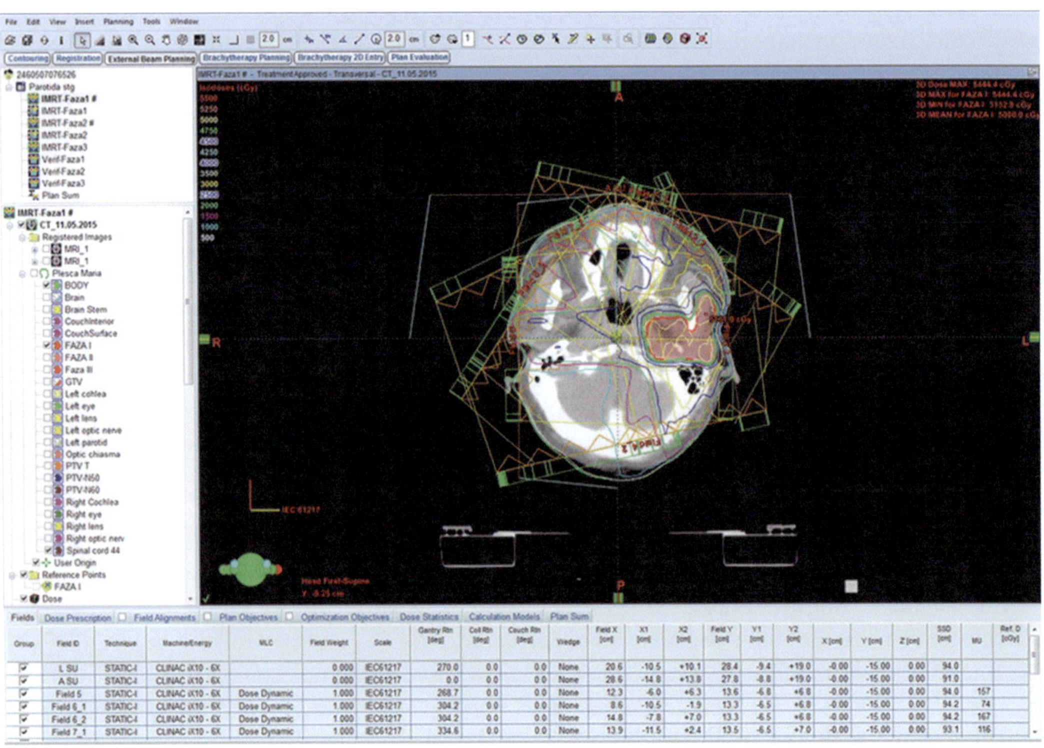

Fig. 24.6 IMRT dose solution for the left parotid tumor with a better coverage of PTV-T. There is an arrangement of seven fields from all sides around creating a perfect coverage of tumoral volume

scheme known as SMART (simultaneous modulated accelerated radiation therapy) boost. By shortening the overall treatment time, SMART boost has the potential of improving tumor control in addition to offering patient convenience and cost savings.

More recently, there has been some interest in arc-based or rotational therapies in an attempt to overcome some of the limitations associated with fixed-field IMRT. The basic concept of arc therapy is the delivery of radiation from a continuous rotation of the radiation source and allows the patient to be treated from a full 360° beam angle. Arc therapies have the ability to achieve highly conformal dose distributions and are essentially an alternative form of IMRT. However, a major advantage over fixed-gantry IMRT is the improvement in treatment delivery efficiency as a result of the reduction in treatment delivery time and the reduction in MU usage with subsequent reduction of integral radiation dose to the rest of the body. In addition to the subsequent advantages from the shorter treatment delivery time, a further potential benefit is the availability of extra time within a set treatment appointment time slot to employ image-guided radiotherapy (IGRT). IGRT involves the incorporation of imaging before and/or during treatment to enable more precise verification of treatment delivery and allow for adaptive strategies to improve the accuracy of treatment. The main drawback of IGRT is the requirement for more time on the treatment couch and an increase in the total amount of radiation to the patient, especially with daily IGRT imaging schedules. These disadvantages are less of an issue with arc therapies, which have shorter treatment delivery times and fewer MU.

Neutron therapy, when they can be accessed, is the first choice for inoperable tumors, residual masses, or major relapses. Various studies have shown a higher local control rate risk however of a higher toxicity [9]. A study from Heidelberg for advanced, inoperable, recurrent, or incompletely resected adenoid cystic carcinoma compared results of treatment with neutrons, photons, or mixed beam. Severe grade 3 and 4 toxicity was

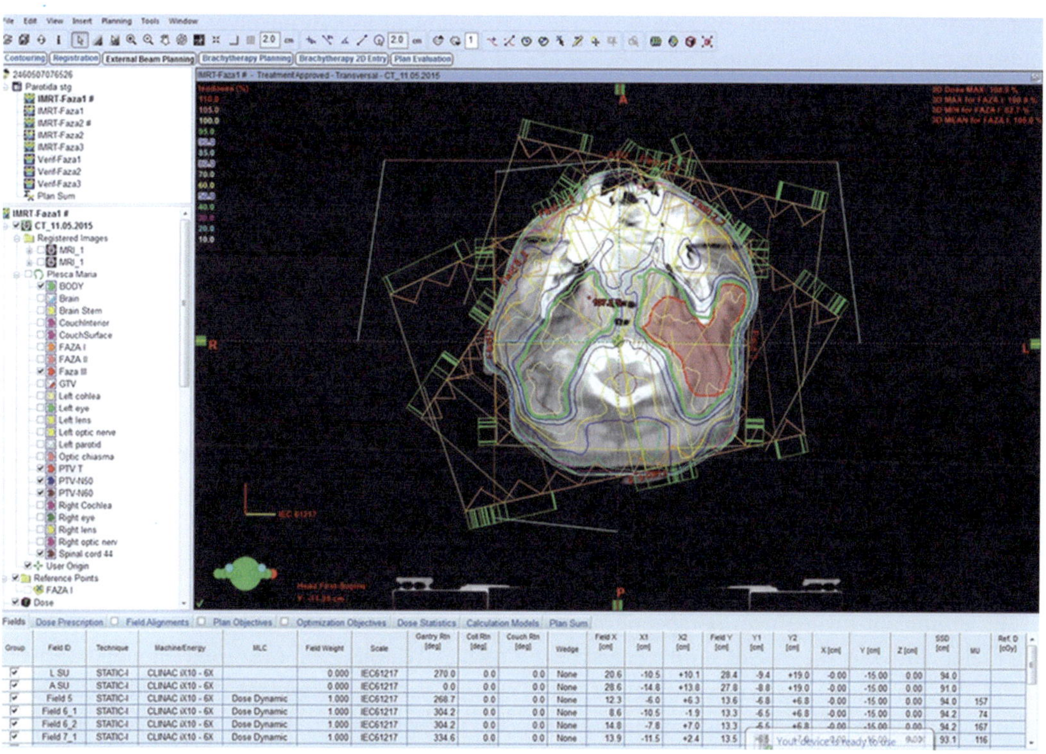

Fig. 24.7 Fields-IMRT uniformity dose solutions for a right parotid tumor

19 % with neutrons, compared to 10 % with mixed beam and 4 % with photon therapy. The 5-year local control was 75 % for neutrons and 32 % for mixed beams and photons survival was identical [10].

Total or partial preservation of facial nerve followed by postoperative radiotherapy is the preferable treatment unless the facial nerve is involved by the tumor. An aggressive surgery does not improve disease-free survival, but a decrease in extended surgery resulting in a decrease of sacrifice of the facial nerve has been shown [11]. Cable facial nerve grafting with the greater auricular or sural nerve decreases the incidence of facial palsy postoperatively, especially if branches and not the main trunk are involved. Adjuvant postoperative radiotherapy has no negative effect on facial nerve function [12].

Postoperative radiotherapy is generally indicated in all case to improve locoregional control. Indications for radiotherapy are compulsory in case of microscopic positive margins after surgical resection and large and deep lesions that may not allow complete surgical excision with adequate margins or require complete sacrificing of the facial nerve or in case of recurrent disease. Radiotherapy may decrease the risk of a second recurrence only, not for uninodular disease.

When a named branch of cranial nerve is involved by a salivary gland carcinoma (especially adenoid cystic), the nerve pathways to the base of skull should be electively treated. When only focal perineural invasion of small unnamed nerves is present, the treatment of the base of skull depends on the site. In this case IMRT may reduce the high-dose volume, compared to the conventional opposed fields, especially when total dose escalade until 70 Gy. Despite combined treatment, there are cases such as salivary duct carcinoma with a very aggressive course and the patients die of the disease.

In an attempt to improve therapeutic results for tumors invading the base of skull, several new techniques have been developed. Mixes of neutron therapy with, after a 4-week split, Gamma Knife stereotactic radiosurgical boost have been used for tumors invading the base of skull. Another option is a combination of photons (54 Gy) and carbon ion (18 Gy) radiotherapy. The results appear to be encouraging, with increased local control, with relatively low side effects, but are encumbered with relatively low access to these techniques [13].

Parotid gland therapy shows generally long-term sequelae. The most notable complication is represented by facial paralysis caused by peripheral surgical procedure, salivary fistulae, and acoustic neuromas of Frey's syndrome.

Primary or adjuvant radiation therapy induces almost permanent dry mouth, temporomandibular joint fibrosis, and loss of hearing when the cochlea receives more than 60 Gy [14]. Some authors have reported late and rarely osteoradionecrosis and some ocular complications (dry eye syndrome, optic atrophy, nasolacrimal duct obstruction, cataract, retinopathy, and even perforated eyeball) [15].

24.3 Treatment of Recurrence

Retreatment usually involves additional surgery, if feasible and postoperative irradiation in previously unirradiated patients. In this case the facial nerve preservation and obtaining local control are more difficult to obtain, but therapy should be performed in an aggressive way if we are to achieve a long-term survivals [16]. Chemotherapy also has been used for recurrent disease. Polychemotherapy for recurrent high-grade disease may result in around 45 % response rate, with a median duration of 7.5 months.

24.4 Treatment Delivery and Patient Care

The amount of oral cavity and oropharynx included in the treatment volume can predict the degree of swallowing problems seen during treatment. Treatment of mucositis should be given within a multidisciplinary team, which reviews the patient weekly. Advice on jaw exercises can reduce the risk of trismus and temporomandibular joint dysfunction.

Conductive hearing loss due to middle ear effusions can occur during radiotherapy and take several months to improve after treatment has finished. If subjective hearing loss persists 2 months after treatment, an audiogram should be performed. If there is evidence of conductive hearing loss, a grommet may be indicated [17].

Conclusion

Radiotherapy is used in the treatment of advanced malignant parotid tumors as adjuvant therapy in combination with enlarged surgical removal, or as monotherapy (primary or definitive irradiation) for inoperable cases, or as palliative treatment.

A good local tumor control is obtained after surgical removal of the salivary tumor followed by adjuvant radiotherapy.

The new radiotherapy modalities (such as intensity-modulated radiotherapy) allow the use of high doses of radiation with favorable radiobiological effects but with increased protection of the healthy tissues.

References

1. Ang KK, Kaanders J, Peters IJ. Radiotherapy for head and neck cancers: indications and techniques. Philadelphia: Lea & Febiger; 1994. p. 109–18.
2. Garden AS, el-Naggar AK, Morrison WH, Callender DL, Ang KK, Peters LJ. Postoperative radiotherapy for malignant tumors of the parotid gland. Int J Radiat Oncol Biol Phys. 1997;37:79–85.
3. Kirkbride P, Liu FF, O'Sullivan B, Payne D, Warde P, Gullane P, et al. Outcome of curative management of malignant parotid gland tumors of the parotid gland. J Otolaryngol. 2001;30:271–9.
4. Douglas JG, Koh W, Austin-Seymour M, Laramore GE. Treatment of salivary gland cancer with fast neutron radiotherapy. Head Neck Surg Arch Otolaryngol. 2003;129:944–8.
5. Chen AM, Garcia J, Lee NY, Bucci MK, Eisele DW. Patterns of nodal relapse after surgery and postoperative radiation therapy for carcinomas of the major salivary glands and minor: what is the role of the elective neck irradiation? Int J Radiat Oncol Biol Phys. 2007;67(4):988–94.
6. Nutting CM, Rowbottom LP, Cosgrove VP, Henk JM, Dearnaley DP, Robinson MH, et al. Optimisation of radiotherapy for carcinoma of the parotid gland: a comparison of conventional 3D conformal, IMRT and techniques. Radiother Oncol. 2001;60:163–72.
7. Yaparpalvi R, Fonteneau DP, Tyerech SK, Boselli LR, Beitler JJ. Parotid gland tumors: a comparison of postoperative radiotherapy techniques using three dimensional (3D) dose distributions and dose-volume histograms (DHVS). Int J Radiat Oncol Biol Phys. 1998;40:43–9.
8. Bragg CM, Conway J, Robinson MH. The intensity-modulated radiotherapy rolls of in the treatment of parotid tumors. Int J Radiat Oncol Biol Phys. 2002; 52:729–38.
9. Douglas JG, Koh W, Austin-Seymour M, Laramore GE. Treatment of salivary gland neoplasms radiotherapy with fast neutrons. Arch Otolaryngol Head Neck Surg. 2003;129:944–8.
10. Huber PE, Debus J, Latz D, Zierhut D, Bischof M, Wannenmacher M, et al. Radiotherapy for advanced adenoid cystic carcinoma: neutrons, photons or mixed beam? Radiother Oncol. 2001;59:161–7.
11. Spiro RH, Armstrong J, Harrison I, Geller NL, Lin SY, Strong EW. Carcinoma of major salivary glands. Arch Otolaryngol Head Neck Surg. 1989;115: 316–21.
12. Brown PD, Eshlemann JS, Foote RL, et al. An analysis of facial nerve function in irradiation of perineural spread or extension of head and neck tumors. Radiographics. 1998;18:737–43.
13. Schulz-Ertner D, Nikoghosyan A, Jäkel O, Haberer T, Kraft G, Scholz M, et al. Feasibility and toxicity of combined photon and carbon ion radiotherapy for locally advanced adenoid cystic carcinomas. Int J Radiat Oncol Biol Phys. 2003;56(2):391–8.
14. Jerenczek-Fossa BA, Zarowski A, Milani F, Orecchia R, et al. Radiotherapy-induced ear toxicity. Cancer Treat Rev. 2003;29:417–30.
15. Jiang GI, Tucker SI, Guttenberger R, Peters LJ, Morrison WH, Garden AS, et al. Radiation induced injury to the visual pathway. Radiother Oncol. 1994; 30:17–25.
16. Simson JR, Thawley SE, Matsubase HM. Adenoid cystic carcinoma of salivary gland: treatment with irradiation and surgery. Radiology. 1984;151:509.
17. Barrett A, Dobbs J, Morris S, Roques T. Practical radiotherapy planning. 4th ed. Boca Raton: CRC Press; 2009. p. 184.

Chemotherapy in Extended Parotidectomy

25

Lucian Miron and Mihai V. Marinca

Abstract

Salivary gland tumors (SGTs) comprise a heterogeneous group of cancers, with high variability in their natural history. Surgery (with adjuvant radiation therapy in high-risk patients) remains the standard curative treatment. Systemic chemotherapy alone has yielded modest results, although its association with radiation therapy is still actively studied. Recent progress in molecular medicine has prompted initiation of many clinical trials of targeted agents. Still, while new specific biological targets have been identified in the main histological subtypes of SGTs, the results of these trials are so far disappointing. Further prospective studies, as well as identification of new molecular pathways, could contribute to therapeutic improvements in this group of diseases.

25.1 Introduction

Salivary gland tumors (SGTs) are a relatively rare and heterogeneous group of neoplasia, representing around 5 % of all head and neck cancers. Annually, approximately three new cases (mostly males over 60) are diagnosed per 100,000 individuals; almost 80 % originate in the parotid gland and the rest in the submandibular, sublingual, and minor salivary glands [1, 2].

The World Health Organization (WHO) classification lists 24 histologic subtypes of epithelial malignant SGTs, of which 5 make up to 80 % of cases: mucoepidermoid carcinoma (MEC), adenoid cystic carcinoma (ACC), acinic cell carcinoma (AcCC), carcinoma ex pleomorphic adenoma (CexPA), and adenocarcinoma not otherwise specified (AC-NOS) [3].

Mucoepidermoid carcinoma is the most frequent neoplasm of the major and minor salivary glands; 50 % of cases occur in the parotid. It is classified as low, intermediate, and high grade (the latter being the most invasive and metastasizing in up to 50 % of cases), but natural history of each subgroup is equally unpredictable. The second most frequent tumor subtype found in the parotid gland (15 %) is AcCC, which is usually a slow-growing cancer, with low mortality. On the other hand, ACC (which makes up to 10 % of parotid gland tumors) is an aggressive, albeit slowly progressing, and usually

L. Miron, MD, PhD • M.V. Marinca, MD, PhD (✉)
Medical Oncology, Faculty of Medicine, "Grigore T. Popa" University of Medicine and Pharmacy, Iasi Regional Oncology Institute, Iasi, Romania
e-mail: mvmarinca@oncol.umfiasi.ro

© Springer International Publishing Switzerland 2016

V.-V. Costan (ed.), *Management of Extended Parotid Tumors*, DOI 10.1007/978-3-319-26545-2_25

lethal cancer (mostly due to the 40 % incidence of lung metastasis). Described in terms of a mixed phenotype, CexPA is defined as a malignant tumor (most frequently a poorly differentiated adenocarcinoma but also of other histologic subtypes) arising from a primary or relapsed benign adenoma of the salivary glands. Adenocarcinomas of the salivary glands behave clinically as they would when located in any other organ.

Pathology findings show great inter- and intra-subtype variability, and many of these tumors have a long natural history, although it does not always translate to a favorable prognosis [4].

Surgery is the primary treatment modality for SGTs. Surgical removal techniques (detailed in Chap. 12) are virtually the same as for benign tumors, the aim in this case being resection within oncological limits, with as low as possible morbidity and side effects. Radical surgery is curative, but SGTs are usually progressing slowly and indolently and are often discovered in advanced, unresectable stages.

Adjuvant radiation therapy further increases local control and possibly survival in certain histologic subtypes such as high-grade carcinomas (those derived from the salivary gland duct), in T3–T4 and/or N+ tumors, or in the case of perineural/lymphovascular invasion.

Definitive irradiation is a valuable alternative for localized disease when surgery is not feasible, although rarely achieves complete responses. Various methods of enhancing radiation therapy effectiveness (such as the use of fast neutrons, carbon ions, protons, altered fractionation, or brachytherapy) are presented in Chap. 24.

Management of relapsed, locally advanced or metastatic SGTs, is difficult, since conventional chemotherapy has low efficacy in this type of tumors [5]. Most systemic therapy choices are drawn from experience gained either in other head and neck tumors (for MEC and undifferentiated carcinomas) or in breast cancer (for ACC), based on resemblance in histology and clinical behavior. With the exception of cisplatin-based chemotherapy, high-level evidence for any of these options (chemotherapy, hormone therapy, or targeted agents) is lacking. Nevertheless, the usually late diagnosis and the high relapse rates (30–50 %) after failure of locoregional therapies substantiate the need for systemic treatment in malignant SGTs.

25.2 Chemotherapy

Chemotherapy is a systemic therapy for cancer, based on drugs (or combinations thereof) which interfere with DNA replication and/or cellular metabolism and determine cell death. Malignant SGTs are generally considered chemotherapy resistant, although up to 50 % of patients may obtain objective responses; virtually none of these responses are, however, complete and/or maintained [6].

Historically, chemotherapy has been used as a primary treatment for incurable patients or in clinical trials, but these have been scarce and of low quality in SGTs due to the low frequency and heterogeneity of these tumors. In the last 20 years, a very limited number of SGT patients (around 500) have been included in clinical trials or otherwise formally evaluated in terms of chemotherapy results. Most of these were retrospective studies, and the few published prospective analyses of activity for different chemotherapeutic agents were based on small series, frequently including mixed histologic SGT subtypes and/or mainly ACCs, which are known for having a lengthy natural history [7]. While the efficacy of several associations of these agents has also been investigated, none of the trials was sufficiently powered to impose a particular combination as standard regimen [8].

Postoperative, definitive, and even neoadjuvant chemotherapy (concomitant or not with radiation therapy) have been evaluated in some of these trials (most of which are, notably, more than two decades old), but results yielded no compelling evidence to support the use of systemic treatment in these settings.

Currently, there is no established place for cytotoxic chemotherapy in the curative intent treatment of SGTs; its role is limited to relapsed, unresectable, and/or metastatic disease and is mainly palliative [9].

25.2.1 Concomitant Chemoradiation

Convincing results from several clinical trials, as well as long-term bedside experience have clearly established concomitant chemotherapy and external beam radiation therapy (CT-EBRT) as a standard alternative to surgery in inoperable or unresectable head and neck cancers, as an efficient preoperative treatment in selected patients or as definitive treatment in locoregional relapses after surgery. The potential benefits of any of these approaches, however, are not supported by compelling evidence in SGTs.

Small sample size, nonrandomized trials have published results on the use of CT-EBRT as neoadjuvant, adjuvant, or definitive treatment. Several chemotherapeutic drugs or regimens (mainly platinum based, but also including pyrimidine analogs, anthracyclines, or others) have been proposed; a few studies also employed molecular targeted agents in conjunction with radiation therapy. A significant activity of combined treatment has been shown in most trials, suggesting a possible benefit in these settings (particularly post-surgery, in high-risk patients), but none of these trials have been sufficiently powered to offer practice-changing data [10–13]. An excellent review of these individual trials has recently been published [14].

In 2010, The Radiation Therapy Oncology Group (RTOG) has initiated a prospective randomized phase II study (RTOG 1008), aiming to compare weekly cisplatin plus radiation therapy with radiation therapy alone as adjuvant treatment. The results of this trial (which will however take several years to mature) are eagerly awaited and if positive will prompt initiation of a phase III trial in the same setting [15].

While concomitant CT-EBRT remains subject to investigation, it might be proposed to good performance status patients at high risk for developing distant metastases after complete resection of SGT (low tumor differentiation; advanced tumor stage/size; positive regional lymph nodes; extracapsular, lymphovascular, and perineural invasion) and in patients with close or positive resection margins [16, 17]. Current guidelines, such as the National Comprehensive Cancer Network (NCCN) Clinical Practice Guidelines in Oncology, do neither oppose nor fully endorse concurrent chemoradiotherapy, and data of a higher level of evidence are an obvious requisite [18].

25.2.2 Single-Agent Chemotherapy

Results of chemotherapy in the setting of a local or distant relapse of SGT are difficult to interpret, due to the low patient numbers and lack of randomized controlled trials (RCTs). Cisplatin [19, 20] and also epirubicin [21], vinorelbine [22, 23], and 5-fluorouracil (5-FU) or other fluoropyrimidines [24] have been considered for the last 30 years as the most active cytotoxics in monotherapy, in spite of the tumor response rates to these drugs being poor (range 10–20 %); moreover, available data come mainly from retrospective studies and preclinical research [25, 26].

The advent of taxanes (inhibitors of the microtubule disassembly during mitosis) and gemcitabine (antimetabolite drug acting as a pyrimidine analogue) in the 1990s entailed new research in SGTs, which stemmed from the relative success of these agents in advanced head and neck cancers. However, the initial enthusiasm was not sustained by further evidence.

Gemcitabine has proven only minor efficacy in several small phase II studies, performed mostly in ACC patients. The best response in these studies has been long-term stable disease, in around 50 % of patients, arguably also pertaining to the protracted, indolent evolution of this tumor subtype [27]. Similarly, studies with paclitaxel in monotherapy have not shown impressive results. In the Eastern Cooperative Oncology Group (ECOG) study E1394, one-third of the patients with MEC or adenocarcinoma (but none of those with ACC) achieved a partial response; overall survival was 12.5 months, and ACC patients reached the highest 3-year survival rate (43 %, as compared to 11 % for MEC and 20 % for adenocarcinomas) [28]. In a series of four patients with recurrent high-grade SGTs not previously treated with systemic therapy, docetaxel (shown in vitro to have Fas-mediated proapoptotic activity) obtained two complete and two partial responses, with a maximum duration of over 2 years [29, 30].

25.2.3 Combination Chemotherapy

Chemotherapy doublets (or triplets) increase the tumor response rates (from 20 % to around 30 %), but without any additional improvement of overall survival and coming at the price of an increased toxicity. Response seems to depend on histologic subtype. Cytotoxics used in squamous cell carcinomas of the head and neck (SCCHN) – such as cisplatin, 5-FU, taxanes, Adriamycin, or methotrexate – also represent a relatively efficient chemotherapy backbone in high-grade MEC and undifferentiated carcinomas, but not in low-grade SGTs. Even in responsive patients in this setting, combination chemotherapy does not appear to increase survival [7].

Platinum-based chemotherapy regimens (especially when including cisplatin, a pseudo-alkylant compound widely used in head and neck cancers) appear to be associated with the best response rates (around 30 % overall, 10–15 % in ACC). Still, these responses seem to be generally short-lived, with a reported median duration of 6–9 months [31–33].

A literature review and meta-analysis on 205 patients with incurable SGTs has found cisplatin-based chemotherapy to be the only independent predictor of survival in multivariate analysis (HR 0.565, 95 % CI 0.36–0.89, $p=0.01$) [34].

The most effective associations proposed have included cisplatin plus 5-FU plus or minus epirubicin/doxorubicin (PF or PEF/PAF regimens) [35–37] or cyclophosphamide, Adriamycin, and cisplatin (CAP regimen) [38–41]; some authors have even proposed quadruple associations (e.g., cyclophosphamide, doxorubicin, cisplatin, and 5-fluorouracil – CAPF regimen) [42]. Up to 60–70 % of patients included in these trials experienced objective responses (including some complete responses), but interpretation of these results should be cautioned by the high number of the limited sample trials from which they were drawn, and the various drug schedules used even within the same protocol.

The combination of cisplatin plus vinorelbine in various histologic subtypes of malignant SGTs has shown higher response rates when compared with vinorelbine alone (44 % vs. 20 %) [23].

As no responses have been identified in ACC patients treated with paclitaxel alone (as opposed to MEC or adenocarcinoma), a combination of carboplatin plus paclitaxel has been advocated in these tumors; however, it only achieved limited success [43, 44].

A National Cancer Institute of Canada (NCIC) phase II trial evaluated gemcitabine in combination with either cisplatin or carboplatin in 33 patients with advanced SGTs (mostly ACCs and adenocarcinomas). The trial was negative, and objective response rates were not even encouraging (20 % in ACC, 26 % in other histologic subtypes) [45].

Other combinations including irinotecan, methotrexate, mitoxantrone, or bleomycin were equally unsuccessful.

When obtained, responses to any of the above regimens did not last over a long period, and chemotherapy triplets or quadruplets did not seem to offer an additional advantage when compared to doublets.

Given the paucity of data and its generally low efficacy in these tumors, current consensus is that chemotherapy should be administered in overtly symptomatic patients with relapsed SGTs, but not in asymptomatic or oligosymptomatic patients (even if metastatic), in whom a "watchful waiting" strategy is advisable.

25.3 Molecular Targeted Therapy

Molecular targeted therapy (MTT) comprises medications or substances that block growth and dissemination of cancer cells, by interfering specific molecules or signaling pathways; these agents usually involve distinctive cellular mechanisms which are vital to the cancer cells (e.g., gene and/or protein expression, growth regulation, cell cycle control, apoptosis, angiogenesis) and as such are less toxic to the normal cells.

Considering the need to improve therapeutic results for both potentially curable and incurable

SGTs, association of radiation therapy with molecular targeted agents such as cetuximab (chimeric monoclonal antibody against the epidermal growth factor receptor, EGFR) has been proposed on the same grounds as for other head and neck cancers. While this approach proved to be feasible in small studies or singular cases, its results (given also the very low patient numbers) could be considered encouraging at best [46, 47].

Some individual molecules have shown promising activity in some studies, but have yet to be confirmed as standard treatment options. Others did not prove effective at all, but our knowledge on cancer biology is building up fast, and new opportunities become available every year. Combining targeted agents between them, or with conventional chemotherapy, did not show any particular complementary or synergistic activity, but did increase toxicity across all SGT subtypes.

Clinical trials are still the "golden standard" in relapsed or metastatic SGTs, and in the last years, many of these trials have focused on MTT. This has been made possible by the current progress in our understanding of tumor genetics and biology, which has led to the identification of genetic alterations ("driver mutations") and of several histologic and molecular profiles of salivary cancers that can be targeted by specific biologic therapies [9].

Also similar to SCCHN, the most extensively studied of these agents are those targeting the EGFR, either alone or combined with other treatment modalities. However, a number of other molecular targets (from which the most promising are detailed below) have been evaluated so far in basic, translational, and clinical research.

25.3.1 Targeted Agents against the EGFR

Effective as they are in other cancers (SCCHN, non-small cell lung cancer, or colorectal tumors), targeting the EGFR pathway (either with monoclonal antibodies or small molecules) seems not the "weapon of choice" in SGTs. However, it might still prove useful in specific situations, in the palliative setting.

Mutations in the EGFR gene are extremely rare in SGTs – particularly in ACC, although the gene itself is activated in more than one-third of this tumor subtype, which is probably the main reason why treatment with EGFR inhibitors has not proved to be particularly effective [48].

However, a translocation t(11;19)(q21-22;p13) resulting in a fusion gene named CRTC1/MAML2 (CREB-regulated transcription coactivator 1/mastermind-like 2) is characteristic for MEC. It encodes for a protein that activates DNA transcription and is involved in upregulating amphiregulin, a ligand for EGFR [49]. While the CRTC1/MAML2 abnormal gene is also present in benign conditions such as Warthin's tumor, it may be regarded as a biomarker that can differentiate "true," more aggressive MECs from other MEC-like tumors [50]. Also the gene's potential to enhance signaling through the AREG-EGFR pathway even in the absence of activating EGFR mutations makes it a potential candidate for targeting with an EGFR inhibitor such as cetuximab, erlotinib, or gefitinib [51].

25.3.2 Targeted Agents against HER2/neu

The epidermal growth factor receptor-2 (ErbB2 or HER2/neu) is a member of the same family of receptors as HER1/ErbB1 (commonly known as EGFR, discussed above). It activates the MAPK (mitogen-activated protein kinase) proliferation pathway, but its unique ability to form dimers with any other HER family member – including itself, but especially HER3, the only one that can activate the PI3K (phosphoinositol-3-phosphate) survival pathway – makes it a major turntable in tumor cell signaling.

Trastuzumab (a humanized monoclonal antibody binding to the extracellular domain of the HER2/neu protein) has shown limited efficacy in various SGT subtypes, since many of those tumors (75 %) do not appear to express the protein [52]. Even in those tumors that do overexpress HER2 in immunohistochemistry, less than 50 % have shown amplification of the gene itself; this discordance has been proposed as explanation for the disappointing clinical results, and the use of more advanced methods for the identification of susceptible mutations is advocated [53]. On the other hand, low-level evidence points to the fact that patients with ductal carcinoma evolved from pleomorphic adenomas (a type of CexPA that frequently shows HER2/neu amplification/overexpression) might benefit significantly from trastuzumab treatment, similarly to their breast cancer counterparts. Also, in a phase II study, trastuzumab treatment prompted a prolonged response in one patient with a HER2-positive MEC [54, 55].

Lapatinib, an oral tyrosine kinase inhibitor of both ErbB1 and ErbB2 receptors, is indicated after trastuzumab failure in HER2/neu overexpressing breast cancer. This warranted investigation also in SGTs, but none of the 36 patients included in the first phase II trial of lapatinib experienced an objective response. Although the disease stabilized in 79 % of patients with ACC and almost half of those with other histologies, in some cases for over 6 months, the study was in fact negative [56].

25.3.3 Targeted Agents against the Kit Receptor

Kit is a surface receptor (encoded by the c-Kit gene) associated with cell migration, differentiation, and proliferation; it is overexpressed in 90 % of ACCs, yet no repeating mutations have been identified in this SGT subtype [57]. Imatinib, a competitive multi-kinase inhibitor (including mutant Kit), has been investigated as a potential treatment for advanced ACC. While a few published case reports have shown imatinib efficacy in patients with high c-Kit expression, no significant tumor response was observed in the two formal studies performed to date (although stable disease has been frequently obtained in treated patients), and toxicity has been moderate [58, 59]. Results may have been hampered by the premature closing of both trials, and – as for HER2/neu or other putative targets – a possible explanation for the lack of efficacy is the low c-Kit mutation rate in these tumors (unlike gastrointestinal stromal tumors (GIST) and chronic myeloid leukemia (CML), where imatinib has shown very impressive results).

25.3.4 Targeted Agents against the PI3K/Akt/mTOR Pathway

Another translocation t(12;15)(p13;q25), first identified in secretory breast cancer and later in up to 90 % of ACCs, results in the ETV6/NTRK3 (ETS transcription factor variant 6/neurotrophic tyrosine kinase receptor, type 3) fusion gene. It constitutively activates the Trk receptor, which will in turn signal downstream through the RAS/RAF/MEK1/ERK/MAPK and especially the PI3K/Akt/mTOR pathway. Data coming from research in breast cancer have hinted to the fact that blockage of IGF-1R (insulin-like growth factor-1 receptor, involved in PI3K signaling) or the Trk kinase itself by novel molecules (such as BMS-536924, NVP-AEW541, or AZD7451, respectively) might suspend cell malignant transformation and delay tumor growth [60–62]. These abnormalities could also translate into potential targets for inhibitors of mTOR (mammalian target of rapamycin) already in clinical use in other cancers (e.g., everolimus, temsirolimus).

Occasionally, silencing of the APC (adenomatous polyposis coli) and PTEN (phosphatase and tensin homolog) tumor suppressor genes leads to activation of the Wnt and mTOR signaling pathways, which promote a more rapid proliferation of AcCC cells. Should these prove to be “driver” mutations, mTOR inhibitors might prove as effective in AcCC as they are in other mTOR-addicted malignant tumors, such as renal or neuroendocrine neoplasia [63].

25.3.5 Targeted Agents against Other Signaling Pathways

Eighty percent of ACC cases feature a specific chromosomal translocation t(6;9)(q22-23; p23-24). This enables the association of the c-MYB (v-myb avian myeloblastosis viral oncogene homolog) and NFIB (nuclear factor I/B) oncogenes (encoding for transcription factors that control cell proliferation, differentiation, and apoptosis through the platelet activation/signaling/aggregation and the Wnt pathways, and through modulation of the RNA polymerase II activity, respectively). In addition, c-MYB is apparently able to cooperate with the fibroblastic growth factor-2 (FGF2) to stimulate bone marrow cell (and possibly tumor cell) proliferation and preclude differentiation to erythrocytes. In vitro research findings suggest that inhibition of either the MYB/NFIB fusion protein or FGF2 may be potential therapeutic targets in ACC.

Several cases of ACC have exhibited BRAF (v-raf murine sarcoma viral oncogene homolog B) and HRAS (Harvey rat sarcoma viral oncogene homolog) mutations [64]. Still, the role of tyrosine kinase inhibitors (TKIs) against the BRAF (e.g., vemurafenib, dabrafenib) or other pathways is unclear.

Chromosomal aberrations specific for, but not limited to, CexPA – including the PLAG1/HMGA2 (pleomorphic adenoma gene 1/high mobility group AT-hook 2) fusion gene, amplification of the MDM2 (mouse double minute 2) or HMGA2 genes, or p53 mutations – have also been identified. These findings suggest that targeting the p53-dependent intracellular pathways by small molecule MDM2 inhibitors (e.g., MI-219, Nutlin-3a analogs) might be able to restore p53 function and induce apoptosis of malignant cells through the NF-κB (nuclear factor kappa-B) pathway [65, 66]. Bortezomib, an inhibitor of the proteasome and of the NF-κB pathway already in clinical use in multiple myeloma, has also been the subject of a phase II trial on 25 advanced ACC patients. Although well tolerated, it only induced a median 4-month stable disease and no objective response, except for one patient (who was also administered doxorubicin) [67].

The use of VEGF inhibitors (e.g., sunitinib, sorafenib) has not yielded any particular benefit, except for a few anecdotal cases, and this research path is not being actively pursued [68, 69].

25.4 Hormone Therapy

Endocrine agents have also been tested in several hormone receptor-positive SGT subtypes. Since estrogen receptors are infrequently expressed and progesterone receptors are always negative, tamoxifen or the aromatase inhibitors most likely have no therapeutic value. Androgen receptors (AR) are also a rare finding (10–15 %), except in "secretory" tumors – salivary duct carcinomas and AC-NOS – where they are revealed in 66 % and 33 % of cases, respectively [70, 71]. Some authors have even proposed – based on their histologic similitude with ductal carcinomas of the breast – a classification of salivary duct tumors in luminal AR-positive, HER2-positive, and basal-like subtypes [72]. There is at least one report on complete remission obtained under antiandrogen therapy in a relapsed, AR-positive parotid adenocarcinoma; in another study, five out of ten patients locally advanced or metastatic SGTs treated with bicalutamide (a nonsteroidal antiandrogen used in prostate cancer) showed tumor regression or maintained stable disease for more than 1 year [73, 74].

25.5 Future Directions

Current therapeutic options for unresectable, extended, recurrent, and/or metastatic parotid cancers are not optimal. Tumors that cannot be treated with curative intent may have a protracted natural history, but their prognosis is uniformly poor. Half of the patients will survive for 5 years, but actually overall survival varies greatly (according to histologic subtype, tumor grading, and a few putative molecular prognostic markers), from around 80 % in low-grade MECs to under 20 % in high-grade MECs and undifferentiated carcinomas.

From all conventional chemotherapeutic drugs, only cisplatin gathered enough positive data to possibly be recommended as a "standard of care" in SGTs. It may be used alone, in association with radiation therapy, or in doublets; in patients with good performance status, combinations including paclitaxel for MEC and adenocarcinomas and 5-FU for ACC seem to have the best risk/benefit ratio.

Irrespective of the molecular or histologic tumor subtypes or the way they were used (alone or in combinations with other agents), targeted therapies so far yielded disappointing results, and none can be recommended for use outside clinical trials.

Further research is ongoing in SGTs, from surgical methods to radiation therapy, from optimal treatment sequencing to novel molecules, or various combinations thereof. A search performed on the US National Institutes of Health website with the string ["salivary gland tumors" OR "salivary gland cancer" OR "parotid tumors" OR "parotid cancer" | Open Studies | Exclude Unknown | Interventional Studies] produced 28 active therapeutic trials [75]. Almost all are phase I or phase II; we manually excluded two phase III trials, which actually investigated symptomatic therapy for patients undergoing radiation therapy for SCCHN. The study population in few of these trials includes only SGTs, but most are performed in head and neck cancers as a whole. It is worth mentioning that 25 (90 %) of these studies were initiated in the USA and Canada. Interventions include surgical procedures (quadrant parotidectomy vs. superficial parotidectomy), irradiation methods (proton radiation therapy, intensity-modulated radiation therapy (IMRT), image-guided adaptive radiation therapy (IGART), brachytherapy), and a number of cytotoxics or targeted agents (some of them still in development). Examples include (but are not limited to) platinum compounds, doxorubicin, paclitaxel, bicalutamide, triptorelin, sorafenib, cetuximab, lapatinib, eribulin mesylate (an inhibitor of microtubule dynamics), afatinib (a HER2/neu and EGFR TKI), dovitinib (a FGFR, VEGFR, and PDGFR TKI), BKM120 (a PI3K inhibitor), and VTX-2337 (an agonist of the toll-like receptor 8 – TLR8, involved in activation of innate immunity).

While SGTs are obviously not incident or lethal enough to constitute a public health issue, the magnitude of lung or breast cancer and the current relative lack of treatment options clearly justify continuation of efforts to find new therapeutic targets or make better use of those already known.

References

1. American Cancer Society. Salivary gland cancer detailed guide. Learn about cancer. Atlanta: American Cancer Society [Internet]; 2014. [updated 2014/01/13; cited 2014 Mar 09]. Available from: http://www.cancer.org/cancer/salivaryglandcancer/detailedguide/salivary-gland-cancer-what-is-key-statistics.
2. Speight PM, Barrett AW. Salivary gland tumours. Oral Dis. 2002;8(5):229–40.
3. Eveson JW, Auclair P, Gnepp DR, El-Naggar AK, Ellis G, Simpson RHW, et al. Tumours of the salivary glands. In: Barnes L, Eveson JW, Reichart P, Sidransky D, editors. Pathology and genetics. Head and neck tumours. WHO/IARC classification of tumours, vol. 9. 3rd ed. Geneva: WHO Press; 2005. p. 210–81.
4. Regezi JA. Salivary gland diseases. In: Regezi JA, Sciubba JJ, Jordan RCK, editors. Oral pathology: clinical pathologic correlations. 4th ed. St. Louis: Saunders; 2003. p. 179–216.
5. Mendenhall WM, Werning JW, Pfister DG. Treatment of head and neck cancer. In: DeVita VT, Lawrence TS, Rosenberg SA, editors. DeVita, Hellman, and Rosenberg's cancer: principles & practice of oncology. 9th ed. Philadelphia: Wolters Kluwer Health/Lippincott Williams & Wilkins; 2011. p. 729–80.
6. Scianna JM, Petruzzelli GJ. Contemporary management of tumors of the salivary glands. Curr Oncol Rep. 2007;9(2):134–8.
7. Day TA, Deveikis J, Gillespie MB, Joe JK, Ogretmen B, Osguthorpe JD, et al. Salivary gland neoplasms. Curr Treat Options Oncol. 2004;5(1):11–26.
8. Laurie SA, Licitra L. Systemic therapy in the palliative management of advanced salivary gland cancers. J Clin Oncol. 2006;24(17):2673–8.
9. Carlson J, Licitra L, Locati L, Raben D, Persson F, Stenman G. Salivary gland cancer: an update on present and emerging therapies. Am Soc Clin Oncol Educ Book. 2013; 49th Annual Meeting (2013): 257–63.
10. Tanvetyanon T, Qin D, Padhya T, McCaffrey J, Zhu W, Boulware D, et al. Outcomes of postoperative concurrent chemoradiotherapy for locally advanced major salivary gland carcinoma. Arch Otolaryngol Head Neck Surg. 2009;135(7):687–92.
11. Pederson AW, Salama JK, Haraf DJ, Witt ME, Stenson KM, Portugal L, et al. Adjuvant chemoradiotherapy for locoregionally advanced and high-risk salivary gland malignancies. Head Neck Oncol. 2011;3:31.
12. Rosenberg L, Weissler M, Hayes DN, Shockley W, Zanation A, Rosenman J, et al. Concurrent chemoradiotherapy for locoregionally advanced salivary gland malignancies. Head Neck. 2012;34(6):872–6.
13. Schoenfeld JD, Sher DJ, Norris Jr CM, Haddad RI, Posner MR, Balboni TA, et al. Salivary gland tumors treated with adjuvant intensity-modulated radiotherapy with or without concurrent chemotherapy. Int J Radiat Oncol Biol Phys. 2012;82(1):308–14.

14. Cerda T, Sun XS, Stéphane V, Marcy P-Y, Baujat B, Baglin A-C, et al. A rationale for chemoradiation (vs radiotherapy) in salivary gland cancers? On behalf of the REFCOR (French rare head and neck cancer network). Crit Rev Oncol Hematol. 2014; in press. http://dx.doi.org/10.1016/j.critrevonc.2014.1002.1002.
15. Radiation Therapy Oncology Group. Radiation therapy with or without chemotherapy in treating patients with high-risk malignant salivary gland tumors that have been removed by surgery. Bethesda: National Library of Medicine (US); 2010. ClinicalTrials.gov [Internet]; 2010- [updated 2014/03/20; cited 2014 Mar 23]. Available from: http://clinicaltrials.gov/show/NCT01220583.
16. Terhaard CHJ, Lubsen H, Rasch CRN, Levendag PC, Kaanders HHAM, Tjho-Heslinga RE, et al. The role of radiotherapy in the treatment of malignant salivary gland tumors. Int J Radiat Oncol Biol Phys. 2005; 61(1):103–11.
17. Adelstein DJ, Koyfman SA, El-Naggar AK, Hanna EY. Biology and management of salivary gland cancers. Semin Radiat Oncol. 2012;22(3):245–53.
18. National Comprehensive Cancer Network. Clinical practice guidelines in oncology: head and neck cancers (version 2.2013). Fort Washington: NCCN [Internet]; 2013. [updated 2013/05/29; cited 2014 Mar 23]. Available from: http://www.nccn.org/professionals/physician_gls/pdf/head-and-neck.pdf.
19. Schramm Jr VL, Srodes C, Myers EN. Cisplatin therapy for adenoid cystic carcinoma. Arch Otolaryngol (Chicago, IL: 1960). 1981;107(12):739–41.
20. Licitra L, Marchini S, Spinazze S, Rossi A, Rocca A, Grandi C, et al. Cisplatin in advanced salivary gland carcinoma. A phase II study of 25 patients. Cancer. 1991;68(9):1874–7.
21. Vermorken JB, Verweij J, de Mulder PH, Cognetti F, Clavel M, Rodenhuis S, et al. Epirubicin in patients with advanced or recurrent adenoid cystic carcinoma of the head and neck: a phase II study of the EORTC Head and Neck Cancer Cooperative Group. Ann Oncol. 1993;4(9):785–8.
22. Airoldi M, Bumma C, Bertetto O, Gabriele P, Succo G, Pedani F. Vinorelbine treatment of recurrent salivary gland carcinomas. Bull Cancer. 1998; 85(10):892–4.
23. Airoldi M, Pedani F, Succo G, Gabriele AM, Ragona R, Marchionatti S, et al. Phase II randomized trial comparing vinorelbine versus vinorelbine plus cisplatin in patients with recurrent salivary gland malignancies. Cancer. 2001;91(3):541–7.
24. Kaplan MJ, Johns ME, Cantrell RW. Chemotherapy for salivary gland cancer. Otolaryngol Head Neck Surg. 1986;95(2):165–70.
25. Ma B, Liang LZ, Liao GQ, Liang YJ, Liu HC, Zheng GS, et al. Inhibition of autophagy enhances cisplatin cytotoxicity in human adenoid cystic carcinoma cells of salivary glands. J Oral Pathol Med. 2013; 42(10):774–80.
26. Harada K, Kawaguchi SI, Supriatno, Onoue T, Yoshida H, Sato M. Enhancement of apoptosis in salivary gland cancer cells by the combination of oral fluoropyrimidine anticancer agent (S-1) and radiation. Int J Oncol. 2004;25(4):905–11.
27. van Herpen CML, Locati LD, Buter J, Thomas J, Bogaerts J, Lacombe D, et al. Phase II study on gemcitabine in recurrent and/or metastatic adenoid cystic carcinoma of the head and neck (EORTC 24982). Eur J Cancer. 2008;44(17):2542–5.
28. Gilbert J, Li Y, Pinto HA, Jennings T, Kies MS, Silverman P, et al. Phase II trial of taxol in salivary gland malignancies (E1394): a trial of the Eastern Cooperative Oncology Group. Head Neck. 2006;28(3):197–204.
29. Piechocki MP, Lonardo F, Ensley JF, Nguyen T, Kim H, Yoo GH. Anticancer activity of docetaxel in murine salivary gland carcinoma. Clin Cancer Res. 2002; 8(3):870–7.
30. Raguse JD, Gath HJ, Bier J, Riess H, Oettle H. Docetaxel (Taxotere) in recurrent high grade mucoepidermoid carcinoma of the major salivary glands. Oral Oncol Extra. 2004;40(1):5–7.
31. Agulnik M, Siu LL. An update on the systemic therapy of malignant salivary gland cancers: role of chemotherapy and molecular targeted agents. Curr Med Chem Anticancer Agents. 2004;4(6):543–51.
32. Surakanti SG, Agulnik M. Salivary gland malignancies: the role for chemotherapy and molecular targeted agents. Semin Oncol. 2008;35(3):309–19.
33. Vattemi E, Graiff C, Sava T, Pedersini R, Caldara A, Mandara M. Systemic therapies for recurrent and/or metastatic salivary gland cancers. Expert Rev Anticancer Ther. 2008;8(3):393–402.
34. Rizk S, Robert A, Vandenhooft A, Airoldi M, Kornek G, Machiels J-P. Activity of chemotherapy in the palliative treatment of salivary gland tumors: review of the literature. Eur Arch Otorhinolaryngol. 2007; 264(6):587–94.
35. Hill ME, Constenla DO, A'Hern RP, Henk JM, Rhys-Evans P, Breach N, et al. Cisplatin and 5-fluorouracil for symptom control in advanced salivary adenoid cystic carcinoma. Oral Oncol. 1997;33(4):275–8.
36. Venook AP, Tseng Jr A, Meyers FJ, Silverberg I, Boles R, Fu KK, et al. Cisplatin, doxorubicin, and 5-fluorouracil chemotherapy for salivary gland malignancies: a pilot study of the Northern California Oncology Group. J Clin Oncol. 1987;5(6):951–5.
37. Ross PJ, Teoh EM, A'Hern RP, Rhys-Evans PH, Harrington KJ, Nutting CM, et al. Epirubicin, cisplatin and protracted venous infusion 5-Fluorouracil chemotherapy for advanced salivary adenoid cystic carcinoma. Clin Oncol (R Coll Radiol). 2009;21(4):311–4.
38. Creagan ET, Woods JE, Rubin J, Schaid DJ. Cisplatin-based chemotherapy for neoplasms arising from salivary glands and contiguous structures in the head and neck. Cancer. 1988;62(11):2313–9.
39. Alberts DS, Manning MR, Coulthard SW, Koopmann Jr CF, Herman TS. Adriamycin/cis-platinum/cyclophosphamide combination chemotherapy for advanced carcinoma of the parotid gland. Cancer. 1981;47(4):645–8.

40. Belani CP, Eisenberger MA, Gray WC. Preliminary experience with chemotherapy in advanced salivary gland neoplasms. Med Pediatr Oncol. 1988;16(3): 197–202.
41. Licitra L, Cavina R, Grandi C, Palma SD, Guzzo M, Demicheli R, et al. Cisplatin, doxorubicin and cyclophosphamide in advanced salivary gland carcinoma. A phase II trial of 22 patients. Ann Oncol. 1996;7(6):640–2.
42. Dimery IW, Legha SS, Shirinian M, Hong WK. Fluorouracil, doxorubicin, cyclophosphamide, and cisplatin combination chemotherapy in advanced or recurrent salivary gland carcinoma. J Clin Oncol. 1990;8(6):1056–62.
43. Airoldi M, Fornari G, Pedani F, Marchionatti S, Gabriele P, Succo G, et al. Paclitaxel and carboplatin for recurrent salivary gland malignancies. Anticancer Res. 2000;20(5c):3781–3.
44. Jennings T, Li Y, Pinto HA, Kies MS, Mansour E, Forastiere AA. Phase II trial of paclitaxel in advanced or metastatic salivary gland malignancies: an Eastern Cooperative Oncology Group study. Proc Am Soc Clin Oncol. 2001;20:236a. abstr 942.
45. Laurie SA, Siu LL, Winquist E, Maksymiuk A, Harnett EL, Walsh W, et al. A phase 2 study of platinum and gemcitabine in patients with advanced salivary gland cancer: a trial of the NCIC Clinical Trials Group. Cancer. 2010;116(2):362–8.
46. Balermpas P, Hambek M, Seitz O, Rodel C, Weiss C. Combined cetuximab and reirradiation for locoregional recurrent and inoperable squamous cell carcinoma of the head and neck. Strahlenther Onkol. 2009;185(12):775–81.
47. Milanovic D, Jeremic B, Kayser G, Rischke HC, Pfeiffer J, Henke A. Relapsing high grade mucoepidermoid carcinoma. Long-lasting complete response following reirradiation and EGFR blockade. Strahlenther Onkol. 2012;188(6):518–22.
48. Locati LD, Bossi P, Perrone F, Potepan P, Crippa F, Mariani L, et al. Cetuximab in recurrent and/or metastatic salivary gland carcinomas: a phase II study. Oral Oncol. 2009;45(7):574–8.
49. Coxon A, Rozenblum E, Park Y-S, Joshi N, Tsurutani J, Dennis PA, et al. Mectl-Maml2 fusion oncogene linked to the aberrant activation of cyclic AMP/CREB regulated genes. Cancer Res. 2005;65(16):7137–44.
50. Schwarz S, Stiegler C, Muller M, Ettl T, Brockhoff G, Zenk J, et al. Salivary gland mucoepidermoid carcinoma is a clinically, morphologically and genetically heterogeneous entity: a clinicopathological study of 40 cases with emphasis on grading, histological variants and presence of the t(11;19) translocation. Histopathology. 2011;58(4):557–70.
51. O'Neill ID. Gefitinib as targeted therapy for mucoepidermoid carcinoma of the lung: possible significance of CRTC1-MAML2 oncogene. Lung Cancer. 2009;64(1):129–30.
52. Glisson B, Colevas AD, Haddad R, Krane J, El-Naggar A, Kies M, et al. HER2 expression in salivary gland carcinomas: dependence on histological subtype. Clin Cancer Res. 2004;10(3):944–6.
53. Williams MD, Roberts DB, Kies MS, Mao L, Weber RS, El-Naggar AK. Genetic and expression analysis of HER-2 and EGFR genes in salivary duct carcinoma: empirical and therapeutic significance. Clin Cancer Res. 2010;16(8):2266–74.
54. Sharon E, Kelly RJ, Szabo E. Sustained response of carcinoma ex pleomorphic adenoma treated with trastuzumab and capecitabine. Head Neck Oncol. 2010;2:12.
55. Haddad R, Colevas AD, Krane JF, Cooper D, Glisson B, Amrein PC, et al. Herceptin in patients with advanced or metastatic salivary gland carcinomas. A phase II study. Oral Oncol. 2003;39(7):724–7.
56. Agulnik M, Cohen EWE, Cohen RB, Chen EX, Vokes EE, Hotte SJ, et al. Phase II study of lapatinib in recurrent or metastatic epidermal growth factor receptor and/or erbB2 expressing adenoid cystic carcinoma and non adenoid cystic carcinoma malignant tumors of the salivary glands. J Clin Oncol. 2007; 25(25):3978–84.
57. Wetterskog D, Wilkerson PM, Rodrigues DN, Lambros MB, Fritchie K, Andersson MK, et al. Mutation profiling of adenoid cystic carcinomas from multiple anatomical sites identifies mutations in the RAS pathway, but no KIT mutations. Histopathology. 2013;62(4):543–50.
58. Hotte SJ, Winquist EW, Lamont E, MacKenzie M, Vokes E, Chen EX, et al. Imatinib mesylate in patients with adenoid cystic cancers of the salivary glands expressing c-kit: a Princess Margaret Hospital phase II consortium study. J Clin Oncol. 2005;23(3):585–90.
59. Pfeffer MR, Talmi Y, Catane R, Symon Z, Yosepovitch A, Levitt M. A phase II study of Imatinib for advanced adenoid cystic carcinoma of head and neck salivary glands. Oral Oncol. 2007;43(1):33–6.
60. Ivanov SV, Panaccione A, Brown B, Guo Y, Moskaluk CA, Wick MJ, et al. TrkC signaling is activated in adenoid cystic carcinoma and requires NT-3 to stimulate invasive behavior. Oncogene. 2013;32(32): 3698–710.
61. Tognon CE, Somasiri AM, Evdokimova VE, Trigo G, Uy EE, Melnyk N, et al. ETV6-NTRK3-mediated breast epithelial cell transformation is blocked by targeting the IGF1R signaling pathway. Cancer Res. 2011;71(3):1060–70.
62. Browne BC, Eustace AJ, Kennedy S, O'Brien NA, Pedersen K, McDermott MSJ, et al. Evaluation of IGF1R and phosphorylated IGF1R as targets in HER2-positive breast cancer cell lines and tumours. Breast Cancer Res Treat. 2012;136(3):717–27.
63. Ettl T, Schwarz-Furlan S, Haubner F, Muller S, Zenk J, Gosau M, et al. The PI3K/AKT/mTOR signalling pathway is active in salivary gland cancer and implies different functions and prognoses depending on cell localisation. Oral Oncol. 2012;48(9):822–30.
64. Tetsu O, Phuchareon J, Chou A, Cox DP, Eisele DW, Jordan RCK. Mutations in the c-Kit gene disrupt mitogen-activated protein kinase signaling during tumor development in adenoid cystic carcinoma of the salivary glands. Neoplasia. 2010;12(9):708–17.

65. Persson F, Andren Y, Winnes M, Wedell B, Nordkvist A, Gudnadottir G, et al. High-resolution genomic profiling of adenomas and carcinomas of the salivary glands reveals amplification, rearrangement, and fusion of HMGA2. Genes Chromosomes Cancer. 2009;48(1):69–82.
66. Shangary S, Wang S. Small-molecule inhibitors of the MDM2-p53 protein-protein interaction to reactivate p53 function: a novel approach for cancer therapy. Annu Rev Pharmacol Toxicol. 2009;49:223–41.
67. Argiris A, Ghebremichael M, Burtness B, Axelrod RS, Deconti RC, Forastiere AA. A phase 2 trial of bortezomib followed by the addition of doxorubicin at progression in patients with recurrent or metastatic adenoid cystic carcinoma of the head and neck: a trial of the Eastern Cooperative Oncology Group (E1303). Cancer. 2011;117(15):3374–82.
68. Chau NG, Hotte SJ, Chen EX, Chin SF, Turner S, Wang L, et al. A phase II study of sunitinib in recurrent and/or metastatic adenoid cystic carcinoma (ACC) of the salivary glands: current progress and challenges in evaluating molecularly targeted agents in ACC. Ann Oncol. 2012;23(6):1562–70.
69. Thomson DJ, Silva P, Denton K, Bonington S, Mak SK, Swindell R, et al. Phase II trial of sorafenib in advanced salivary adenoid cystic carcinoma of the head and neck. Head Neck. 2013. doi:10.1002/hed.23577.
70. Locati LD, Perrone F, Losa M, Mela M, Casieri P, Orsenigo M, et al. Treatment relevant target immunophenotyping of 139 salivary gland carcinomas (SGCs). Oral Oncol. 2009;45(11):986–90.
71. Nasser SM, Faquin WC, Dayal Y. Expression of androgen, estrogen, and progesterone receptors in salivary gland tumors. Frequent expression of androgen receptor in a subset of malignant salivary gland tumors. Am J Clin Pathol. 2003;119(6):801–6.
72. Di Palma S, Simpson RHW, Marchio C, Skalova A, Ungari M, Sandison A, et al. Salivary duct carcinomas can be classified into luminal androgen receptor-positive, HER2 and basal-like phenotypes*. Histopathology. 2012;61(4):629–43.
73. Jaspers HCJ, Verbist BM, Schoffelen R, Mattijssen V, Slootweg PJ, van der Graaf WTA, et al. Androgen receptor-positive salivary duct carcinoma: a disease entity with promising new treatment options. J Clin Oncol. 2011;29(16):e473–6.
74. Locati LD, Quattrone P, Bossi P, Marchiano AV, Cantu G, Licitra L. A complete remission with androgen-deprivation therapy in a recurrent androgen receptor-expressing adenocarcinoma of the parotid gland. Ann Oncol. 2003;14(8):1327–8.
75. U.S. National Institutes of Health. ClinicalTrials.gov: search for studies. Bethesda: National Library of Medicine (US); 2014. ClinicalTrials.gov [Internet]; 2014 [updated 2014/03/20; cited 2014 Mar 23]. Available from: http://www.clinicaltrials.gov/ct2/results?term=%22salivary+gland+tumors%22+OR+%22salivary+gland+cancer%22+OR+%22parotid+tumors%22+OR+%22parotid+cancer%22&recr=Open&no_unk=Y&type=Intr.

Index

© Springer International Publishing Switzerland 2016
V.-V. Costan (ed.), *Management of Extended Parotid Tumors*, DOI 10.1007/978-3-319-26545-2

MIX
Papier aus verantwortungsvollen Quellen
Paper from responsible sources
FSC® C105338

If you have any concerns about our products,
you can contact us on
ProductSafety@springernature.com

In case Publisher is established outside the EU,
the EU authorized representative is:
Springer Nature Customer Service Center GmbH
Europaplatz 3, 69115 Heidelberg, Germany

Printed by Libri Plureos GmbH
in Hamburg, Germany